Immunology
and Aging

Comprehensive Immunology

Series Editors: ROBERT A. GOOD and STACEY B. DAY

Sloan-Kettering Institute for Cancer Research
New York, New York

Immunology and Aging

Edited by

TAKASHI MAKINODAN

Baltimore City Hospitals
Baltimore, Maryland
and
Veterans Administration Wadsworth Hospital Center
and University of California at Los Angeles

and

EDMOND YUNIS

Sidney Farber Cancer Institute
Harvard Medical School
Boston, Massachusetts

PLENUM MEDICAL BOOK COMPANY
New York and London

Library of Congress Cataloging in Publication Data

Main entry under title:

Immunology and aging.

  (Comprehensive immunology; v. 1)
  Includes bibliographies and index.
  1. Immunity—Addresses, essays, lectures. 2. Aging—Addresses, essays, lectures. I. Makinodan, T. II. Yunis, Edmond J. III. Series. [DNLM: 1. Aging. 2. Immunity—In old age W1 CO4523 v. 1/WT104 I331]
QR186.A33 1976   612.6'7   76-53755
ISBN 0-306-33101-2

©1977 Plenum Publishing Corporation
227 West 17th Street, New York, N. Y. 10011

Plenum Medical Book Company is an imprint of
Plenum Publishing Corporation

Printed in the United States of America

Contributors

Robert E. Anderson   Department of Pathology, University of New Mexico School of Medicine, Albuquerque, New Mexico, and the Albuquerque V.A. Hospital

Kay E. Cheney   Department of Pathology, University of California School of Medicine, Los Angeles, California

William E. Doughty   Department of Pathology, University of New Mexico School of Medicine, Albuquerque, New Mexico, and the Albuquerque V.A. Hospital

Nicola Fabris   Experimental Gerontology Center, INRCA, Ancona, Italy

Gabriel Fernandes   Department of Laboratory Medicine and Pathology, University of Minnesota, Minneapolis, Minnesota

Richard K. Gershon   Department of Pathology, Yale University School of Medicine, New Haven, Connecticut

Robert A. Good   Sloan-Kettering Institute for Cancer Research, New York, New York

Leonard J. Greenberg   Department of Laboratory Medicine and Pathology, University of Minnesota, Minneapolis, Minnesota

W. Hijmans   Institute for Experimental Gerontology of the Organization for Health Research TNO, Rijswijk, The Netherlands

Katsuiku Hirokawa   Department of Pathology, Medical Research Institute, Tokyo Medical and Dental University, Tokyo, Japan

C. F. Hollander   Institute for Experimental Gerontology of the Organization for Health Research TNO, Rijswijk, The Netherlands

John W. Jutila   Department of Microbiology, Montana State University, Bozeman, Montana

Marguerite M. B. Kay   Laboratory of Cellular and Comparative Physiology, Gerontology Research Center, National Institute on Aging, National Institutes of Health, PHS, U.S. Department of Health, Education and Welfare, Bethesda, and Baltimore City Hospitals, Baltimore, Maryland

Ian R. Mackay   Clinical Research Unit of the Walter and Eliza Hall Institute of Medical Research, and The Royal Melbourne Hospital, Victoria, Australia

Takashi Makinodan   Baltimore City Hospitals, Baltimore, Maryland, and Veterans Administration Wadsworth Hospital Center and University of California at Los Angeles.

John D. Mathews   Clinical Research Unit of the Walter and Eliza Hall Institute of Medical Research, and The Royal Melbourne Hospital, Victoria, Australia viii

CONTRIBUTORS

Charles M. Metzler Department of Pathology, Yale University School of Medicine, New Haven, Connecticut

Patricia J. Meredith Department of Pathology, University of California School of Medicine, Los Angeles, California

Gary M. Troup Department of Pathology, University of New Mexico School of Medicine, Albuquerque, New Mexico, and the Albuquerque V.A. Hospital

Roy L. Walford Department of Pathology, University of California School of Medicine, Los Angeles, California

Senga F. Whittingham Clinical Research Unit of the Walter and Eliza Hall Institute of Medical Research, and The Royal Melbourne Hospital, Victoria, Australia

Edmond J. Yunis Department of Laboratory Medicine and Pathology, University of Minnesota, Minneapolis, Minnesota; Present address: Sidney Farber Cancer Institute, Harvard Medical School, Boston, Massachusetts

Jorge J. Yunis Department of Laboratory Medicine and Pathology, University of Minnesota, Minneapolis, Minnesota

Preface

In the classic sense, immunity is the ability of an organism to resist disease. On the one hand, we must distinguish between age and disease; on the other hand, the interaction between them is of considerable theoretical and practical interest. To the gerontologic research community, therefore, immunity also becomes the ability of an organism to resist age. Were the immune and other protective systems of the body able to maintain themselves over the course of time, and if there were no degradation related to age, the everyday loss of energy and vitality that occurs in the lives of older people as a consequence of viruses, arthritis, and other debilitating circumstances would be greatly lessened. The objective of gerontologists is not just to extend the life span but rather to improve the vigor, health, and quality of life.

To date, we have not developed a single index to measure immunity that is of use clinically in the evaluation of older people and of their immunologic competence. It may not be surprising that just such a clinical index may be available in the not-too-distant future. We can also look forward to the assembling of a greater body of information explaining how and why the immune system fails with age while, paradoxically, the incidence of autoimmune diseases increases with age. It is this latter phenomenon that may play a part in a wide range of chronic diseases from rheumatoid arthritis to senile dementia. In addition, we may see the development of a system of "adoptive immunity" in which an immune state is produced by transferring immunologically active lymphocytes or sera from an immunized donor to a nonimmunized recipient. Conceivably, children might then donate their "youthful" immunity directly to their parents. The future of many disciplines will depend on the further development of the field of immunology:

- To the medical historian, the steps in the elucidation of immunity have reflected the opening of an entire era of medical discovery in bacteriology.
- To the epidemiologist, the understanding of immunity has meant immunizations and vaccinations that have contributed significantly to the increased life expectancy of the twentieth century.
- To the public health policy maker, techniques for the further enhancing of the immune capacities of the body could extend the productive, healthy, and vigorous middle years and reduce what is a personally distressing and socially expensive period of dependency in old age.
- To the psychiatrist, breakthroughs in the elimination of autoimmune disorders might mean the prevention of senile dementia, or primary neuronal

degeneration, the condition (or conditions) so destructive to personality and memory.

- To the clinician, the development of a means to bolster the immune system with age could lead to the amelioration of many of the daily discomforts and illnesses of older patients.
- To the scientist, further knowledge about immunity and age would represent important steps in the enhancement of our understanding of the molecular and cellular biology of aging.

This volume, edited by Dr. Takashi Makinodan and Dr. Edmond Yunis, contains many outstanding contributions by the world's leading immunologists. We are grateful to have their attention focused on the relatively new but highly promising field of gerontology.

Robert N. Butler, M.D.
Director
National Institute on Aging

Contents

1

Biology of Aging: Retrospect and Prospect

TAKASHI MAKINODAN

1. Introduction

Aging can be defined as a time-dependent process whereby one's body can no longer cope with environmental stress and change as easily as it once could. Hence loss of physiological adaptability is one of the hallmarks of aging. Suffice it to say, aging is rapidly becoming the most critical issue socioeconomically and biomedically on this planet. It is not surprising, therefore, that in recent years increasing attention is being given to biomedical gerontology, as attested by the creation in 1974 of the National Institute on Aging in the United States.

The goals of most biomedical gerontologists are to extend the productive years of one's life at the expense of the unproductive years of life and to enable one to age graciously with a minimum of mental and physical disabilities. One may ask: What are the productive years of life? Obviously this will vary in part with one's profession. According to Lehman (1953), writers, for example, reach their peak in their second and third decades of life, while heads of religious organizations reach their peak in their seventh and eighth decades. However, when we refer to the productive years of one's life, we are generally thinking in terms of the second to the fifth decades. In any event, to achieve our goals, we need to understand (a) the processes that cause the human body to deteriorate with time, (b) whether the deterioration can be interfered with, and, if so, (c) how and when.

In this introductory chapter, an attempt will be made to present (a) a brief overview of biology of aging, (b) molecular theories of aging, and (c) reasons why the immune system is an excellent model for studies of cellular and molecular etiology of aging, pathogenesis of aging, and approaches to improve the quality of the terminal phases of life.

TAKASHI MAKINODAN • Baltimore City Hospitals, Baltimore, Maryland, and Veterans Administration Wadsworth Hospital Center and University of California at Los Angeles.

TAKASHI
MAKINODAN

2. Past Research Activities

2.1. Life Span Analysis

Early research was centered primarily about population analysis with focus on the life span of different species. This research revealed that each species has a finite and unique life span; e.g., a mayfly has a life span of about a day, a mouse about 3 years, a dog about 20 years, a horse about 40 years, and a human about 110 years. Moreover, the average life span is generally significantly shorter than the maximum life span, and variation between individuals within a species is large. These findings indicate that the life span is genetically regulated and the difference between the maximum and average life span in a species reflects the influence of environment to a great extent.

Support for the genetic basis comes from studies of monozygotic and dizygotic progenies of parents with long and short life spans (Kallman, 1961). These studies revealed that (a) the intrapair life span difference is smaller in monozygotic than dizygotic twins, (b) the life expectancy of progenies of parents with a longer life span is longer than that of progenies of parents with a short life span, and (c) the cause of death is about twice as similar in monozygotic as in dizygotic pairs.

Since the turn of the century, the survival curve is becoming more rectangular or "boxlike" in shape (Figure 1); i.e., the average life span is increasing significantly but the maximum life span is not. This is due to control of deleterious environmental factors through effective dietary, hygienic, and vaccination programs and, in addition, through the use of antibiotics since the late 1940s. If the boxlike trend continues, it is possible that in the near future most of us will live to about the same age, e.g., 90 ± 5 years.

Actuarial analysis of human life spans reveals that different diseases kill off the aging population at increasing but at relatively similar rates (Kohn, 1971). This means that as the maximum life span is approached, individuals will die but the disease they will die of is fortuitous, suggesting that the maximum life span cannot be extended significantly by controlling the environmental factors. This suspicion is borne out by a recent U.S. Bureau of Census report (Siegel and O'Leary, 1973). According to this report, if the cause of death through malignant neoplasma is eliminated today, a child born tomorrow will have an increase in life expectancy of only 2.3 years and an adult 65 years old tomorrow will have an increase of only 1.2 years! Moreover, if all four major causes of death of the aged (i.e., cardiovascular–renal diseases, heart diseases, vascular diseases affecting the central nervous system, and malignant neoplasms) can be eliminated today, there will be only a 20-year gain in life expectancy of babies born tomorrow.

Based on these considerations, it should be apparent that the long-held fear that "breakthroughs" in aging research will enable people to live longer and contribute significantly to the existing problem of population explosion is not justified. The estimates above show that even by increasing the mean life expectancy to its *maximum* the population will increase by no more than 15–20%, and this increase will be only for a brief period of time. In short, population explosion is a socioeconomic problem, for countries with high standards of living seem to contribute relatively little to this problem (Figure 2).

2.2. Organisms and Organs

Physiological functions generally decline with age in a linear fashion. One of the fundamental issues that has confronted biomedical gerontologists over the years is whether the decline in various functions is initiated by the decline in function of only a few cell types or tissues or whether each tissue senesces independently of other tissues. Many investigators, on the basis of actuarial data, feel that aging of individuals is caused by a senescence time clock built into only a few cell types.

2.3. Tissues and Cells

In an attempt to resolve this issue, Krohn (1962) transplanted the skin of old mice into young, healthy mice in a serial manner. He found that the skin has a life span longer than the mouse from which it originated. This means that skin ages *in situ* because of factors extrinsic to it. Comparable results have been reported subsequently with several other tissues including bone and prostate tissues (Franks, 1970). Of course, there have been reports that certain tissues possess a limited *in*

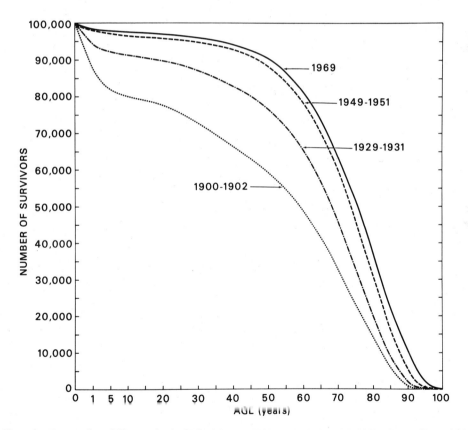

Figure 1. Expectation of life span in the United States, 1900–1969 (Golenpaul, 1973). Curves beyond 80 years of age were kindly extrapolated by Dr. Phillip I. Good and Dr. Noel R. Mohberg of the Upjohn Company, Kalamazoo, Michigan, through the use of extreme value theory for minima.

vivo transfer life (Siminovitch *et al.,* 1964; Cudkowicz *et al.,* 1964; Daniels *et al.,* 1975), suggesting that some tissues age because of changes intrinsic to them. However, the recent study of Harrison (1975) on *in vivo* transfer life span of hematopoietic stem cells of young and old mice indicates that the *in vivo* transfer life span of a tissue is due to the number of traumatic experiences a tissue undergoes during its transfer handling rather than to the *in situ* age of the tissue.

Perhaps a better approach in resolving this issue is to assess senescence of a homogeneous cell population in a defined *in vitro* culture condition. To this end,

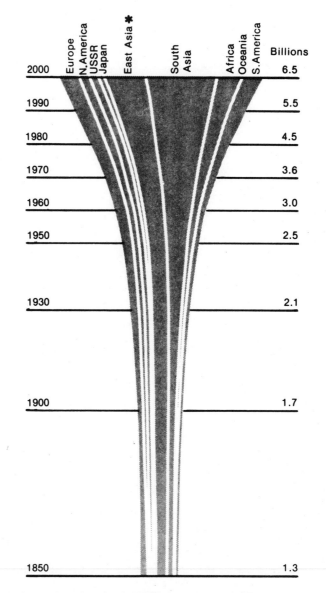

Figure 2. Estimated growth and regional distribution of the world's population, 1850–2000 (with permission from the Federation of American Scientists). *Excluding Japan.

there has been a burst of activities over the past decade centered on the fibroblast, the cell of choice over other cycling cells, resting cells (liver and kidney cells), and postmitotic cells (neurons and heart muscle cells). Hayflick (1965), who addressed himself to the issue of *in vitro* life span of human fibroblasts, found that the cultures undergo about 50 doubling passages before they die (i.e., on the average, one fibroblast can generate 10^{15} fibroblasts or 1 metric ton of fibroblasts). In an attempt to demonstrate that death of passaged fibroblasts is due to a time clock built into them, he mixed fibroblasts that had previously undergone x number of passages with marker fibroblasts that had previously undergone y number of passages and determined the number of passages each type is still capable of undergoing. He found that the former went $(50-x)$ more passages and the latter, $(50-y)$ more passages. These results strongly suggest that the *in vitro* proliferative life span of human fibroblasts is governed by a time clock built into them. The current issues are whether the time clock is in the nucleus or the cytoplasm and whether activation of the clock is genetic or stochastic?

3. Theories on Mechanisms of Aging

In looking back it would appear that the multitude of theories that emerged following studies at the organismic and organ levels stymied rather than enhanced the field of gerontology. Thus, rather than deliberate on the individual theories, it would be more fruitful to focus our attention at the genetic information and processing levels, since aging must emanate at the molecular level.

The various theories can be divided into two broad types. One is that it is an orderly, genetically programmed event which is the consequence of differentiation, growth, and maturation (e.g., Kanungo, 1976). The other is that it is a stochastic event resulting from accumulation of random errors (e.g., Orgel, 1963). Most gerontologists today seem to favor the former, although definitive evidence for or against either type of theory is still lacking. Aging can initiate at the transcriptional level, where it can be manifested as a mutation, DNA deletion, macromolecular crosslinking of DNA, etc. It can also initiate at the translational level where it can be manifested by altered RNA polymerase, tRNA, and tRNA synthetase, etc. It can also initiate at the posttranslational level, where it can be manifested by stochastic alteration of certain vital, slowly-turning-over macromolecules. These could include enzymes that are essential for protein synthesis and DNA repair.

4. Present Research Activities

Since much phenomenological study has been completed, especially at the organismic, organ, and tissue levels, present studies seem to be centered on the mechanism(s) of aging at the cellular and molecular levels. There are several areas of research that appear very promising. They include: (a) age effects on the regulatory role of the neuroendocrine system, (b) *in vitro* cellular aging with emphasis on the role of regulatory factors and site of initiation of the aging process, (c) drug sensitivity with emphasis on receptors, (d) age effects on resting cells with emphasis on their impaired adaptive enzyme systems, and (e) age effects on the immune system, which will be discussed in the subsequent section.

Relative to studies on the mechanism of aging, studies on pathogenesis of aging and on approaches in minimizing the deteriorative processes of aging are very limited for want of better understanding of the etiology of aging.

5. The Immune System, a Cellular and Molecular Aging Model par Excellence

Biomedical gerontologists are now investigating many physiologic systems. Many of those who are biologically oriented are hopeful that there may be at most only a few mechanisms responsible for the various manifestations of aging of individuals and diseases associated with it. Those who are clinically oriented are hopeful that there will be ways in delaying the onset of, lessening the severity of, or preventing the diseases of the aged. Of all the systems being examined systematically, the immune system is perhaps the most attractive from both biologic and clinical points of view. The reasons are compelling:

1. The immune system, which is intimately involved in adaptation of the body to environmental stress and change, declines in its efficiency in performing certain functions.
2. Associated with the decline is the rise in susceptibility to viral and fungal infections, cancer, and autoimmune and immune complex diseases, which can interfere with many physiological functions of the body.
3. We probably know more about differentiation, ontogenetic, and phylogenetic processes of the immune system at the cellular, genetic, and molecular levels than any other system.
4. The immune system is amenable to precise cellular and molecular analysis and therefore offers great promise for successful manipulation.
5. There is a reasonable chance that a delay, reversal, or decrease in the rate of decline in normal immune functions may delay the onset and lessen the severity of diseases of aging, and there are several approaches available.

6. Conclusion

An attempt has been made to present a brief overview of the field of biomedical gerontology, retrospectively and prospectively. It should be apparent that it is a relatively new field in molecular biomedicine and that the aged are becoming the most critical socioeconomic issue of the world. Therefore, it is anticipated that many more investigators will become involved, and hopefully their participation will accelerate the progress of research on aging.

Currently, much research activity is centered on the mechanism(s) of aging at the cellular and molecular levels, since many phenomenological studies at the organismic, organ, and tissue levels have been completed. As our knowledge of aging increases, it is anticipated that research on molecular pathogenesis and approaches in minimizing the deteriorative processes of aging will increase.

Of the various systems being investigated, the immune system is one of the most promising, for it is a well-defined system in which to study cellular and molecular mechanisms of aging. It is also intimately involved with many of the diseases of the aged and offers several approaches to minimizing the deteriorative processes of aging.

References

Cudkowicz, G., Upton, A. C., Shearer, M., and Hughes, W. L., 1964, Lymphocyte content and proliferative capacity of serially transplanted mouse bone marrow, *Nature* **201**:165–167.

Daniels, C. W., Aidells, B. D., Medina, D., and Faulkin, L. J., 1975, Unlimited division potential of precancerous mouse mammary cells after spontaneous or carcinogen-induced transformation, *Fed. Proc.* **34**:64–67.

Franks, L. M., 1970, Cellular aspects of ageing, *Exp. Geront.* **5**:281–289.

Golenpaul, D., 1973, *Information Please Almanac, Atlas and Yearbook,* Dan Golenpaul Associates, New York.

Harrison, D. E., 1975, Normal function of transplanted marrow cell lines from aged mice. *J. Gerontol.* **30**:279–285.

Hayflick, L., 1965, The limited *in vitro* lifetime of human diploid cell strains, *Exp. Cell. Res.* **37**:614–636.

Kallman, F. J., 1961, Genetic factors in aging: comparative and longitudinal observations on a senescent twin population, in: *Psychopathology of Aging* (P. H. Hoch and J. Zubin, eds.), Chapter 13, pp. 227–247, Grune and Stratton, New York.

Kanungo, M. S., 1976, A model for aging, *J. Theor. Biol.* **53**:253–261.

Kohn, R. K., 1971, *Principles of Mammalian Aging,* Prentice-Hall, Englewood Cliffs and New York.

Krohn, P. L., 1962, Review lectures in senescence. II. Heterochromic transplantation in the study of aging, *Proc. Roy. Soc.,* Ser. B, **157**:128–147.

Lehman, H. C., 1953, *Age and Achievement,* Princeton University Press, Princeton, New Jersey.

Orgel, L. E., 1963, The maintenance of the accuracy of protein synthesis and its relevance to aging, *Proc. Nat. Acad. Sci. U.S.* **49**:517–521.

Siegel, J. S., and O'Leary, W. E., 1973, Some demographic aspects of aging in the United States, in: *Current Population Reports,* U.S. Bureau of the Census, Series P-23, No. 43, pp. 1–30, U.S. Government Printing Office, Washington, D.C.

Siminovitch, L., Till, J. E., and McCulloch, E. A., 1964, Decline in colony-forming ability of marrow cells subjected to serial transplantation into irradiated mice, *J. Cell. Comp. Physiol.* **64**:23–32.

2

Cellular Basis of Immunosenescence

TAKASHI MAKINODAN, ROBERT A. GOOD,
and MARGUERITE M. B. KAY

1. Introduction

Certain normal immune functions decline with age in humans, guinea pigs, hamsters, rats, and mice (Walford, 1969; Sigel and Good, 1972) (Figure 1). The onset, magnitude, and rate of decline, however, vary with the type of immune function and the species. It is clinically important that with a decrease in immunologic vigor, the incidence of infections, autoimmune and immune complex diseases, and cancer increases (Walford, 1969; Mackay, 1972; Good and Yunis, 1974) (Figure 2), as is the case in immunodeficient newborns and immunosuppressed adults (Fudenberg *et al.*, 1971; Penn and Starzl, 1972; Good, 1975). What is not clear is whether the diseases compromise normal immune functions, or whether a decline in normal immune functions to threshold levels predisposes individuals to diseases. We favor the latter explanation because of the following observations: (a) the onset of decline in thymus-derived T-cell-dependent immune functions can occur as early as sexual maturity when the thymus begins to involute (Makinodan and Peterson, 1962), which is long before immunodeficiency diseases of the elderly are manifested; (b) immunodeficiency, wasting disease, amyloidosis, and autoimmunity in neonatally thymectomized mice and in genetically susceptible mice can be prevented, or at times even reversed, by reconstituting them with young but not old, syngeneic thymus or spleen grafts (Yunis *et al.*, 1964; Fabris *et al.*, 1972); (c) adult humans subjected to immunosuppressive drug therapy are many times more vulnerable to cancer than are normal adults (Cerilli and Hatten, 1974); (d) patients with primary

TAKASHI MAKINODAN • Baltimore City Hospitals, Baltimore, Maryland, and Veterans Administration Wadsworth Hospital Center and University of California at Los Angeles.   MARGUERITE M. B. KAY • Laboratory of Cellular and Comparative Physiology, Gerontology Research Center, National Institute on Aging, National Institutes of Health, PHS, U.S. Department of Health, Education and Welfare, Bethesda and Baltimore City Hospitals, Baltimore, Maryland.   ROBERT A. GOOD • Sloan-Kettering Institute for Cancer Research, New York.

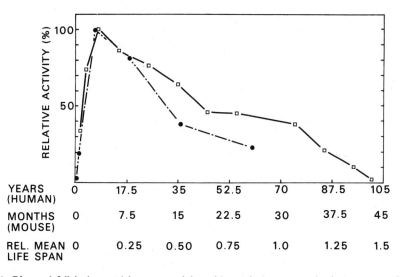

Figure 1. Rise and fall in humoral immune activity with age in humans and mice. □, natural serum Anti-A isoagglutinin titers in the human (Thomsen and Kettel, 1929); ●, peak serum antibody response to sheep red blood cell stimulation by long-lived mice (Makinodan and Peterson, 1964).

immunodeficiencies in which the immunity systems fail to develop normal vigor are vulnerable to autoimmunity, amyloidosis, and certain forms of cancer (Good and Yunis, 1974); and (e) cessation of immunosuppressive therapy following inadvertent transplantation of cancer along with renal transplant leads to the prompt rejection of the tumor and even of widely disseminated cancer (Zukoski *et al.,* 1970).

In any event, the intriguing possibility exists that a delay, reversal, or prevention of the decline in normal immune functions could delay the onset and/or minimize the severity of certain diseases of the elderly (for detail, see chapters by Fernandes *et al.,* and by Walford *et al.,* this volume). However, before any attempt

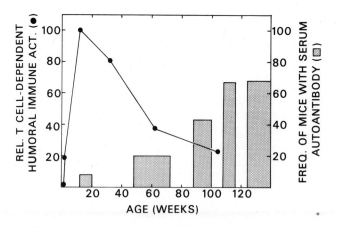

Figure 2. Inverse relationship between age-related T-cell-dependent humoral immune activity and frequency of individual mice with antibodies (Makinodan and Peterson, 1964; Peterson and Makinodan, 1972).

is made to intervene with the disease processes, it would seem that an understanding of the basic mechanism(s) responsible for the loss of immunologic vigor is both desirable and essential. It is not surprising, therefore, that much of the research on immunosenescence has currently been centered on this basic mechanism.

In this chapter, we will present an overview of this rapidly developing area of research by focusing our attention on the changes in the environment in which cells must function and the cellular changes responsible for the decline in immune functions with age.

2. Cellular Environmental Changes

The decline in normal immune functions with age may be due to changes in the cellular environment or milieu, changes in the cells of the immune system, or both. To differentiate between the influences of cells and their environment, we employed the cell transfer method, which assesses immunocompetent cells from young and old mice in immunologically inert old and young syngeneic recipients, respectively (Albright and Makinodan, 1966; Price and Makinodan, 1972a,b). The results revealed that changes both intrinsic and extrinsic to the cells affect the immune response; only about 10% of the normal age-related decline can be attributed to changes in the cellular environment, while 90% of the decline can be attributed to changes intrinsic to the old cells (Price and Makinodan, 1972a,b).

The responsible factor(s) in the cellular environment was shown to be systemic and noncellular (Price and Makinodan, 1972b). Spleen cells from young mice were cultured with the test antigen either in the young (or old) recipient's spleen by the cell transfer method or in the recipient's peritoneal cavity by the diffusion chamber method (Goodman *et al.,* 1972). A twofold difference in response at both sites was observed between young and old recipients, indicating that the factor(s) is systemic. The fact that the effect was observed in cells grown in cell-impermeable diffusion chambers further indicates that a noncellular factor is involved. A comparable twofold difference was also observed when bone marrow stem cells were assessed in the spleens of young and old syngeneic recipients (Chen, 1971), indicating that the systemic, noncellular factor(s) influences both lympho- and hematopoietic processes.

The factor(s) could be a deleterious substance of molecular or viral nature, or it could be an essential substance that is deficient in old mice. We suspect that factors of both types change with age and, further, that several factors of each type may exist.

This area of research will certainly progress more rapidly when a sensitive *in vitro* assay to analyze mouse sera has been perfected. At present, for example, it remains unclear why normal adult mouse serum is toxic for mouse immunocompetent cells grown *in vitro*.

3. Cellular Changes

One of the characteristics of immunosenescence is the increase in variability of immune indices (Makinodan *et al.,* 1971). If more than one factor is responsible for the increase in variability, it is not surprising to find that the decline in humoral immune capacity of aging mice results from deficiencies of both the immune cells and of the milieu in which they must function (Albright and Makinodan, 1966; Price and Makinodan, 1972a,b).

Three types of cellular changes could cause a decline in normal immune functions: (a) an absolute decrease in cell number through death caused possibly by autoimmune cells, (b) a relative decrease in cell number as a result of an increase in the number of "suppressor" cells, and (c) a decrease in functional efficiency possibly caused by somatic mutation. One approach in resolving this problem is first to estimate the frequency with which old mice exhibit various cellular changes. This can be done by assessing the activity of reference immune cells from adult individuals in the presence of immune cells from old individuals. A response of young–old cell mixtures that was less than the sum of the responses given by pure young and pure old cells would indicate that the decreased response of old individuals was due to an increase in suppressor cells. If the response of the mixture was comparable, it would indicate that the decreased response of old individuals was caused either by a decrease in their functional efficiency or by a general loss of immune cells. If the response of the mixture was higher, it would indicate that the decreased response of old individuals was caused by a selective loss of one type of immune cell that exists in excess in young individuals. The results of our ongoing studies indicate that, indeed, all three types of interactions can occur (Peter, 1971; Makinodan *et al.,* 1976). The results of these investigations support our contention that, although there may be a dormant underlying mechanism responsible for the loss of immunologic vigor with age, it is expressed differently between aging individuals, and this fact contributes to the increase in variability of immunologic performance with age.

3.1. Stem Cells

In mouse bone marrow, which contains 90% of all stem cells, the total stem-cell number remains constant with age (Coggle and Proukakis, 1970; Chen, 1971). This indicates that stem cells can replicate *in situ* throughout the natural life span of the mouse, unlike stem cells passaged *in vivo* whose ability to replicate can be exhausted (Siminovitch *et al.,* 1964; Lajtha and Schofield, 1971; Harrison, 1975). Further, stem cells do not lose their lympho-hematopoietic ability with age (Harrison and Doubleday, 1975). On the other hand, subtle changes have been detected with age. Thus the rate of B (bone-marrow-derived) cell formation seems to decline with age (Farrar *et al.,* 1974), as does the ability to repair X-ray-induced DNA damage (Chen, 1974). In addition, alteration in certain kinetic parameters in spleen colony formation has been detected with age (Deitchman and Makinodan, 1975). Interestingly, when attempts were made to reverse these age-related kinetic parameters by enabling "old" stem cells to self-replicate in syngeneic young recipients for an extended period, it was found that kinetically they still behaved as old stem cells. However, when "young" stem cells were allowed to self-replicate in syngeneic old recipients, they behaved as old stem cells kinetically. These results indicate that the milieu of stem cells induced subtle changes which affect their responsiveness to differentiation-homeostatic factors.

3.2. Macrophages

Many of the earlier studies on the mechanism of loss in immunological vigor with age were focused on the macrophages (e.g., see the review by Teller, 1972). It was thought that because macrophages confront antigens before the T (thymus-derived) and B cells, any defect in them could decrease immune functions without appreciable changes in the antigen-specific T and B cells. Studies of this question showed that macrophages are not adversely affected by aging in their handling of antigens during both the induction of immune responses and phagocytosis, i.e., (a) the *in vitro* phagocytic activity of old mice was equal to or better than that of young mice (Perkins and Makinodan, 1971), (b) the activity of at least three lysosomal enzymes in macrophages increased rather than decreased with age (Heidrick, 1972), (c) the ability of antigen-laden macrophages of old mice to initiate primary and secondary antibody responses *in vitro* was comparable to that of young mice (Perkins and Makinodan, 1971), and (d) the capacity of splenic macrophages and other adherent cells to cooperate with T cells and B cells in the initiation of antibody responses *in vitro* was unaffected by age (Heidrick and Makinodan, 1973). Further-more, when their antigen-processing ability was indirectly assessed by injecting young and old mice with varying doses of sheep red blood cells, it was found that both the slope of the regression line of the antigen dose–response curve and the minimum dose of antigen needed to generate a maximum response were signifi-cantly lower in old mice (Price and Makinodan, 1972a). Such results could be explained by assuming that the antigen-processing macrophages prevented antigen-sensitive T cells and B cells from responding maximally to limiting doses of the antigen (Lloyd and Triger, 1975), perhaps because their number or phagocytic efficiency increased with age (Heidrick, 1972). Associated with reduced antigen-processing is the failure of antigens to localize in the follicles of lymphoid tissues of antigen-stimulated old mice (Metcalf *et al.,* 1966; Legge and Austin, 1968). One clinical implication of these results is that the ability of individuals to detect low doses of antigens, especially "weak" antigens, such as syngeneic tumor antigens, can decline with age, contributing to the age-related poor immune surveillance noted against low doses of certain syngeneic tumor cells in mice (Prehn, 1971). It also could explain why the resistance to allogeneic tumor-cell challenge can decline more than a hundredfold with age in mice manifesting only a fourfold decline in T-cell-mediated cytolytic activity against the same tumor cells (Goodman and Maki-nodan, 1975).

3.3. B Cells

The number of B cells in the spleen and lymph nodes does not seem to change appreciably with age in long-lived mice (Makinodan and Adler, 1975) (Figure 3), whereas the number of plasma cells seems to increase in autoimmune-prone, relatively short-lived mice (Good and Yunis, 1974). In humans, studies have been limited primarily to circulating B cells, and they indicate that the number of B cells also remains relatively constant (Diaz-Jouanen *et al.,* 1975). Unfortunately, we do not know as yet whether the number of circulating B cells corresponds to that in the spleen and lymph nodes. In contrast to the constancy with age in the total B cell population, subpopulations of B cells may fluctuate. Support of this view comes from the observations that the number of B cells responsive to a T-cell-independent antigen decreases slightly with age in long-lived mice (Price and Makinodan, 1972a) and that the level of serum IgG and IgA tends to increase with age, while that of serum IgM tends to decrease (Haferkamp *et al.,* 1966; Lyngbye and Kroll, 1971; Buckley *et al.,* 1974).

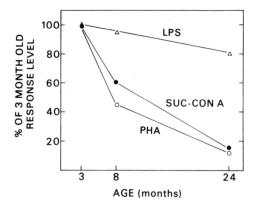

Figure 3. Effect of age on the mitogenic responsiveness of T cells and B cells in mice. LPS. lipopoly-saccharide; Suc-Con A, succinylconcanavalin A; PHA, phytohemagglutinin (Makinodan and Adler, 1975).

Although the number of B cells remains relatively stable with age, their responsiveness to stimulation with certain T-cell-dependent antigens decreases strikingly (Makinodan and Peterson, 1962; Makinodan *et al.*, 1971). When the responses of young and old mice were systematically evaluated by limiting dilution and dose-response methods, they revealed that the decline is caused by (a) a decrease with age in the number of antigen-sensitive immunocompetent (IU) precursor units, which are made up of two or more cell types in various ratios (T_1M_1, T_2M_1, . . ., B_1M_1, B_2M_1, . . ., $T_1M_1B_1$, $T_2M_1B_3$, . . ., etc.) (Groves *et al.*, 1970) and (b) a decrease in the average number of antibody-forming functional cells generated by each IU or the immunologic burst size (IBS) (Price and Makinodan, 1972a,b) (Figure 4). We do not know the cause(s) for the reduction with age in both the relative number of IU and IBS. It could be due to an increase in the number of regulatory T cells, which can inhibit the precursor cells, making up the IU from interacting with each other, as well as inhibit the proliferation of B cells. The reason for this suspicion is that the number of Ig-bearing B cells remains constant with age (Diaz-Jouanen *et al.*, 1975) and the proliferative capacity of mitogen-sensitive B cells also remains unaltered with age (Hung *et al.*, 1975a, b; Makinodan and Adler, 1975). It could also result from an alteration in the ability of certain B cells to interact with other precursor cells making up the IU and in their ability to respond to homeostatic factors during differentiation.

3.4. T Cells

Present evidence suggests that the decline in immune functions which accompanies aging is due primarily to changes in the T cell component of the immune system. The thymic lymphatic mass decreases with age, primarily as a result of cortical atrophy (Figure 5) in both humans and laboratory animals beginning at the time of sexual maturity (Boyd, 1932; Santisteban, 1960; Good and Gabrielsen, 1964; Good *et al.*, 1964). Although the size of lymph nodes and spleen remains the same or decreases slightly with age after adulthood in individuals without lymphatic neoplasia, the cellular composition of the tissue shifts so that there are diminished numbers of germinal centers and increasing numbers of plasma cells and macrophages, as well as an increase in the amount of connective tissue (Chino *et al.*, 1971;

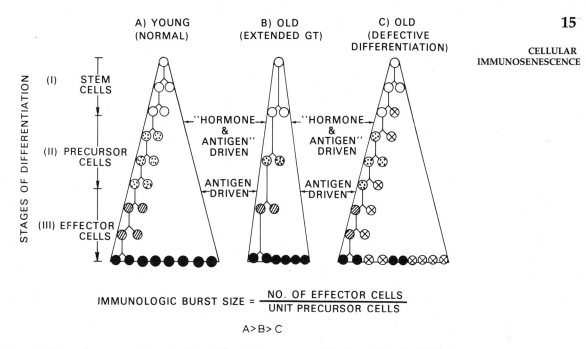

Figure 4. Schematic representation of cellular differentiation process of T cells and B cells (Makinodan and Adler, 1975).

Peter, 1973; Good and Yunis, 1974). The number of circulating lymphocytes decreases progressively during or after middle age in humans to a level that is about 70% of that of a young adult by the sixth decade (Diaz-Jouanen *et al.*, 1975; Augener *et al.*, 1974; Alexopoulos and Babitis, 1976). A proportional decrease in the number of T cells is observed while the number of B cells shows little change.

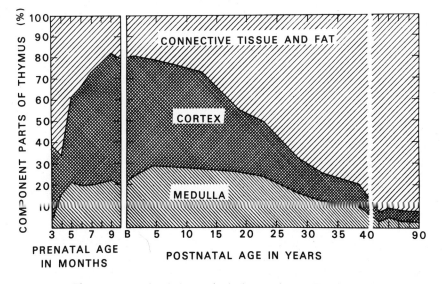

Figure 5. Age-related changes in the human thymus (Boyd, 1932).

However, changes in the number or proportion of T cells in both humans and mice are not sufficient to account for the observed decrease in immunologic functions. Further, as will be discussed later, a decrease in the number of cells bearing surface T cell markers does not mean that the total number of T cells has necessarily decreased; it could mean that the number of T cells in a particular differentiation stage has decreased.

Functional studies have shown an age-related decrease in delayed hypersensitivity to skin test antigens to which an individual has not been sensitized previously (such as dinitrochlorobenzene) (Mackay, 1972). *In vivo* studies in mice indicate that T cell functions decline with age. Cells from old mice have a decreased ability to mount a graft-versus-host (GVH) reaction, even when enriched T cell populations are utilized to compensate for the possibility that old animals may have fewer T cells (Stutman *et al.,* 1968; Teague *et al.,* 1970; Goodman and Makinodan, 1975).

The *in vitro* findings show that the proliferative capacity of T cells of humans and rodents in response to plant mitogens [phytohemagglutinin (PHA) and concanavalin A (Con A)] and allogeneic target cells declines with age (Pisciotta *et al.,* 1967; Adler *et al.,* 1971; Heine, 1971; Hallgren *et al.,* 1973; Hori *et al.,* 1973; Konen *et al.,* 1973; Mathies *et al.,* 1973; Roberts-Thomson *et al.,* 1974) and the decline is most striking in mice, regardless of their life span. In contrast, the decline in the cytotoxic index of T cells of long-lived mice is generally moderate against allogeneic tumor cells (Goodman and Makinodan, 1975) and not readily apparent against certain syngeneic tumor cells (Stutman, 1974). By contrast, in short-lived strains of mice, capacity to mount a cytotoxic killer-cell immunologic response declines sharply during the second half of the first year of life (Fernandes *et al.,* 1976).

There are conflicting reports in the literature on the effect of age on the mixed lymphocyte culture (MLC) reactions. Some investigators reported a marked decrease in the response of cells with age (Adler *et al.,* 1971; Hori *et al.,* 1973). Others reported that cells from old mice are as efficient or more so than cells from young mice both as responding and as stimulating cells in the MLC reaction, but the same cells showed a decreased GVH index (Walters and Claman, 1975).

The helper function of T cells declines with age. This has been demonstrated in intact animals and in *in vivo* assays (Price and Makinodan, 1972a, b; Heidrick and Makinodan, 1973; Hardin *et al.,* 1973). Adult thymectomy accelerates the decline of immune responsiveness, as evidenced by a decrease in the hemagglutinin response in sheep RBC, particularly in the early response (19S) phase (Metcalf, 1965), a marked decrease in the GVH reaction, poor general condition of the mice, and reduced antibody response to BSA (Taylor, 1965). The effect on the latter response was less pronounced than that on the GVH. Recently, Hirokawa and Makinodan (1975) transplanted thymus lobes from mice aged 1 day to 33 months into young adult, T-cell-deprived recipients and assessed kinetically the emergence of T cells. They found that the ability of the thymus tissue to influence the differentiation or maturation of cells into functional T cells decreases with increasing age, and that different T cell indices exhibit differential susceptibility to thymus involution (for detail, see chapter 5, this volume).

These results indicate that thymic involution precedes and is responsible for the age-dependent decline in the ability of the immune system to generate functional T cells. What is the mechanism by which thymic involution leads to a decrease in peripheral effector cells? It appears that the primary effect of involution of the thymus is on a T-cell-differentiation pathway. Evidence suggests that a subset of T cells does not respond to stimulation, due possibly to insufficiency of hormones in the milieu and/or alterations intrinsic to the cells. The following observations support this view:

1. The proportion of lymphocytes bearing the theta antigen decreases with age, as does the amount of theta antigen on cell surfaces; yet, there is no compensatory increase in B lymphocytes, nor does the lymphocyte number change significantly. This suggests an increase in T cells that do not carry detectable theta receptors on their surface (Brennan and Jaroslow, 1975). Alternatively, null cells or third population of lymphocytes may increase in number in a compensatory manner.

2. Although PHA-induced blastogenesis of cells from old mice is significantly reduced (see Figure 3), the same cells bind ^{125}I-labeled PHA equally well as cells from young mice (Hung *et al.,* 1975b). Since there seems to be no significant decrease in binding affinities or receptor sites for PHA on cells of old mice, the defect cannot be in their membrane receptors.

3. The cyclic nucleotide 3′,5′-guanosine monophosphate, which has been shown to increase when T cells are stimulated by mitogens, is found in relatively low concentrations in mitogen-stimulated T cells of old mice, and it is known that the levels of cyclic nucleotides are hormone dependent (Heidrick, 1973). This suggests that the defect in T cells is intracellular and may be hormone-dependent.

4. The life span of hypopituitary dwarf mice, which are T cell deficient, can be extended from 4 months to 12 months by a single intraperitoneal injection of 150×10^6 lymph node cells, but one injection of an equal number of thymocytes or 50×10^6 bone marrow cells is ineffective (Fabris *et al.,* 1972). (Lymph nodes are rich in *mature* T cells, whereas thymus and bone marrow are deficient in *mature* T cells.)

5. Transfer of 5×10^7 to 5×10^8 thymus cells from immunologically mature congenic donors into athymic mice reconstitutes the recipient's capacity to reject allogeneic skin graft, whereas transfer of an equal number of thymus cells from newborn mice will not (Pierpaoli, 1975). Presumably, the ability of thymus cell suspension from adult mice to reconstitute graft rejections depends on the number of "competent" lymphocytes resident in the thymic medulla, or from the recirculating pool, which are trapped in the thymus cell suspension.

6. Studies of *synergy* between subpopulations of lymphocytes in the MLC reaction (Meredith *et al.,* 1975; Gerbase-Delima *et al.,* 1975) suggest that lymph node "T_2" cells (amplifier cells) display a greater functional decline with age than do spleen and thymus "T_1" lymphocytes (the precursors of T_2 cells). This suggests that the mature T cells, which are required for the recruitment of precursor T cells and for the MLC reaction, decline with age.

7. Treatment of thymus cell suspensions with anti-TL serum and complement (which spares the more mature, TL−, thymocytes that have undergone differentiation within the thymus and are about to migrate to the periphery while killing the less mature, TL+, thymocytes) does not reduce the GVH

reactivity of thymocyte suspensions (Tigelaar, 1975). However, the capacity of thymocytes to give superadditive GVH reactions when combined with peripheral blood leukocytes was decreased by treatment with anti-TL. These results indicate that synergy among subpopulations of T cells in GVH reactions involves the participation of "immature" T cells under the influence of mature T cells.

8. Density distribution analysis using BSA and Ficoll discontinuous gradients shows that the frequency of less dense cells (ρ, 1.06–1.08) increases at the expense of the more dense cells (ρ, 1.10–1.12) (Makinodan and Adler, 1975). This density shift within the lymphocyte population can also be seen in young mice shortly after they are immunized with foreign red cells or allogeneic lymphocytes and in tumor-bearing mice. In these cases, however, the spleen cell number increases, whereas in unimmunized old mice it does not. This suggests that there is a relative increase with age in immature T_1 cells at the expense of mature T_2 cells.

9. Shortly after the thymus begins to involute and atrophy, the level of serum thymic hormone(s) decreases with age (Bach *et al.,* 1973). It would seem reasonable to assume that this hormone(s) is necessary for terminal differentiation of T cells. This could lead to a decrease in effector cells for certain immune functions and, thus, to a deficit in T cell responsiveness.

10. The *in vitro* PHA response of T cells from old mice can be significantly increased by addition of certain chemicals (e.g., mercaptoethanol and polynucleotides) to the cultures, as can the antibody response to sheep RBC (Braun *et al.,* 1970; Makinodan *et al.,* 1975). This supports the view that old mice are deficient in a hormone(s) that is essential for the differentiation of T cells to become responsive to a mitogen and, further, suggests that simple chemicals can substitute for this hormone.

Studies on the nature of age-related changes in T cells involved in the regulation of B cell immune responses have been minimal, due in part to our lack of understanding of how these cells function, and due to the inadequacy of prior analysis of the T cell subsets. We do not know for certain whether or not there exist two distinct subpopulations of regulator T cells with the potential to promote or suppress a B cell immune response. However, recent studies by Kisielow *et al.* (1975), Shiku *et al.* (1975, 1976), and Cantor and Boyse (1975a, b) seem to indicate that helper and promoter lymphocytes have a different expression of differentiation alloantigens on their surface from killer or suppressor T lymphocytes (Hirst *et al.,* 1975). In any event, the relative number of T cells participating in a B cell immune response decreases with age in short-lived, autoimmune-prone mice (Hardin *et al.,* 1973). This could account for the emergence of auto-antibodies in the older, short-lived mice. Conversely, the relative number can increase slightly in long-lived mice (Price and Makinodan, 1972a). Because excessive numbers of regulator T cells tend to interfere with the B cell response to antigenic stimulation, this could account for the decline in the number of antibody-responsive IU and IBS. The notion that the number of regulator cells with inhibitory activities increases with age was tested by assessing the antisheep RBC response of spleen cells from young mice in the presence or absence of spleen cells from old mice, as discussed earlier (Peter, 1971;

Gerbase-Delima *et al.*, 1975). These results indicate that spleens of old mice contain regulator cells that can interfere with the immunologic activities of spleen cells from young mice.

19

CELLULAR
IMMUNOSENESCENCE

4. Concluding Remarks

A brief overview of cellular immunosenescence, a rapidly developing area of research, has been presented. The results of ongoing studies show that although there may be a single underlying mechanism responsible for the loss of immunologic vigor with age, it is manifested differently between individuals. This diversity could account for the increase with age in variability in immunologic performances between old individuals.

Foremost among the cellular changes are those in the stem cells, as reflected in their growth properties, and in the T cells, where a shift in subpopulations may be occurring with age. The process(es) regulating involution and atrophy of the thymus could be the key to immunosenescence. Focus in future studies therefore is expected to be on regulation of neuroendocrine–thymus axis.

Advancement in this area of research should contribute not only to the etiology and pathogenesis of aging, but also to developmental biology, for aging is a natural consequence of development, growth, and maturation, as well as a natural perturbation of homeostasis.

References

Adler, W., Takiguchi, T., and Smith, R. T., 1971, Effect of age upon primary alloantigen recognition by mouse spleen cells, *J. Immunol.* **107**:1357–1362.

Albright, J. F., and Makinodan, T., 1966, Growth and senescence of antibody-forming cells, *J. Cell. Physiol.* **67**(Suppl. 1):185.

Alexopoulos, C., and Babitis, P., 1976, Age dependence of T lymphocytes, *Lancet* **1**:426.

Augener, W., Cohnen, G., Reuter, A., and Brittinger, G., 1974, Decrease of T lymphocytes during aging, *Lancet* **1**:1164.

Bach, J. F., Dardenne, M., and Salomon, J. C., 1973, Studies on thymus products. IV. Absence of serum "thymic activity" in adult NZB and (NZB × NZW)F$_1$ mice, *Clin. Exp. Immunol.* **14**:247–256.

Boyd, E., 1932, The weight of the thymus gland in health and in disease, *Am. J. Dis. Child.* **43**:1162–1214.

Braun, W., Yahima, Y., and Ishizuka, M., 1970, Synthetic polynucleotides as restorers of normal antibody forming capacities in aged mice, *J. Reticuloendothel. Soc.* **7**:418–424.

Brennan, P. C., and Jaroslow, B. N., 1975, Age-associated decline in theta antigen on spleen thymus-derived lymphocytes of B6CF$_1$ mice, *Cell. Immunol.* **15**:51–56.

Buckley, C. G., Buckley, E. G., and Dorsey, F. C., 1974, Longitudinal changes in serum immunoglobulin levels in older humans, *Fed. Proc.* **33**:2036–2039.

Cantor, H., and Boyse, E. A., 1975a, Functional subclasses of T-lymphocytes bearing different Ly antigens: I. The generation of functionally distinct T-cell subclasses is a differentiative process independent of antigen, *J. Exp. Med.* **141**:1376–1389.

Cantor, H., and Boyse, E. A., 1975b, Functional subclasses of T lymphocytes bearing different Ly antigens: II. Cooperation between subclasses of Ly$^+$ cells in the generation of killer activity, *J. Exp. Med.* **141**:1390–1399.

Cerilli, J., and Hatten, D., 1974, Immunosuppression and oncogenesis, *Am. J. Clin. Pathol.* **62**:218–223.

Chen, M. G., 1971, Age-related changes in hematopoietic stem cell populations of a long-lived hybrid mouse, *J. Cell. Physiol.* **78**:225–232.

Chen, M. G., 1974, Impaired Elkind recovery in hematopoietic colony-forming cells of aged mice, *Proc. Soc. Exp. Biol. Med.* **145**:1181–1186.

Chino, F., Makinodan, T., Lever, W. H., and Peterson, W. J., 1971, The immune system of mice reared in clean and dirty conventional laboratory farms. I. Life expectancy and pathology of mice with long life spans, *J. Gerontol.* **26**:497–507.

Coggle, J. E., and Proukakis, C., 1970, The effect of age on the bone marrow cellularity of the mouse, *Gerontologia* **16**:24–29.

Deitchman, J. W., and Makinodan, T., 1975, Effect of age on the rate of proliferation of lymphohemato-poietic stem cells, *Proc. 10th Internat. Congr. Gerontol.* **2**:12.

Diaz-Jouanen, E., Williams, R. C., Jr., and Strickland, R. G., 1975, Age-related changes in T and B cells, *Lancet* **1**:688–689.

Fabris, N., Pierpaoli, W., and Sorkin, E., 1972, Lymphocytes, hormones and ageing, *Nature* (London) **240**:557–559.

Farrar, J. J., Loughman, B. E., and Nordin, A. A., 1974, Lymphopoietic potential of bone marrow cells from aged mice: comparison of the cellular constituents of bone marrow from young and aged mice, *J. Immunol.* **112**:1244–1249.

Fernandes, G., Yunis, E. J., and Good, R. A., 1976, Influence of protein restriction on immune functions in NZB mice, *J. Immunol.* **116**:782–790.

Fudenberg, H. H., Good, R. A., Goodman, H. C., Hitzig, W., Kunkel, H. G., Roitt, I. M., Rosen, F. S., Rowe, D. S., Seligmann, M., and Soothill, J. R., 1971, Primary immunodeficiencies, *Bull. WHO* **45**:125–142.

Gerbase-Delima, M., Meredith, P., and Walford, R., 1975, Age-related changes, including synergy and suppression, in the mixed lymphocyte reaction in long-lived mice, *Fed. Proc.* **34**:159–161.

Good, R. A., 1975, The primary immunodeficiency diseases, in: *Textbook of Medicine* (P. B. Beeson and W. McDermott, eds.), pp. 104–109, W. B. Saunders, Philadelphia.

Good, R. A., and Gabrielsen, A. E., editors, 1964, *The Thymus in Immunobiology,* Hoeber-Harper, New York.

Good, R. A., Martinez, C., and Gabrielsen, A. E., 1964, Clinical considerations of the thymus in immunobiology, in: *The Thymus in Immunobiology* (R. A. Good and A. E. Gabrielsen, eds.), pp. 3–48, Hoeber-Harper, New York.

Good, R. A., and Yunis, E. J., 1974, Association of autoimmunity, immunodeficiency and aging in man, rabbits, and mice, *Fed. Proc.* **33**:2040–2050.

Goodman, S. A., and Makinodan, T., 1975, Effect of age on cell-mediated immunity in long-lived mice, *Clin. Exp. Immunol.* **19**:533–542.

Goodman, S. A., Chen, M. G., and Makinodan, T., 1972, An improved primary response from mouse spleen cells cultured *in vivo* in diffusion chambers, *J. Immunol.* **108**:1387–1399.

Groves, D. L., Lever, W. E., and Makinodan, T., 1970, A model for the interaction of cell types in the generation of hemolytic plaque-forming cells, *J. Immunol.* **104**:148–165.

Haferkamp, O., Schlettwein-Gsell, D., Schwick, H. G., and Storiko, K., 1966, Serum protein in an aging population with particular reference to evaluation of immune globulins and antibodies, *Gerontologia* **12**:30–38.

Hallgren, H. M., Buckley, E. C., III, Gilbertson, V. A., and Yunis, E. J., 1973, Lymphocyte phytohem-agglutinin responsiveness, immunoglobulins and auto-antibodies in aging humans, *J. Immunol.* **111**:1101–1107.

Hardin, J. A., Chuseo, T. M., and Steinberg, A. D., 1973, Suppressor cells in the graft vs. host reaction, *J. Immunol.* **111**:650–651.

Harrison, D. E., 1975, Normal function of transplanted marrow cell lines from aged mice, *J. Gerontol.* **30**:279–285.

Harrison, D. E., and Doubleday, J. W., 1975, Normal function of immunologic cells from aged mice, *J. Immunol.* **114**:1314–1317.

Heidrick, M. L., 1972, Age-related changes in hydrolase activity of peritoneal macrophages, *Gerontologist* **12**:28.

Heidrick, M. L., 1973, Imbalanced cyclic-AMP and cyclic-GMP levels in concanavalin-A stimulated spleen cells from aged mice. *J. Cell Biol.* **57**:139a.

Heidrick, M. L., and Makinodan, T., 1973, Presence of impairment of humoral immunity in nonadherent spleen cells of old mice, *J. Immunol.* **111**:1502–1506.

Heine, K. R., 1971, Die Reaktionsfähigkeit der Lymphozyten im Alter, *Folia Haematol.* **96**:29–33.

Hirokawa, K., and Makinodan, T., 1975, Thymic involution: effect on T cell differentiation, *J. Immunol.* **114**:1659–1664.

Hirst, J. A., Beverley, P. C. L., Kisielow, P., Hoffmann, M. K., and Oettgen, H. F., 1975, Ly antigens: markers of T cell function on mouse spleen cells, *J. Immunol.* **115**:1555–1557.

Hori, Y., Perkins, E. H., and Halsall, M. K., 1973, Decline in phytohemagglutinin responsiveness of spleen cells from aging mice, *Proc. Soc. Exp. Biol. Med.* **114**:48–53.

Hung, C-Y., Perkins, E. H., and Yang, W-K., 1975a, Age-related refractoriness of PHA-induced lymphocyte transformation. I. Comparable sensitivity of spleen cells from young and old mice to culture conditions, *Mech. Ageing Develop.* **4**:29–39.

Hung, C-Y., Perkins, E. H., and Yang, W-K., 1975b, Age-related refractoriness of PHA-induced lymphocyte transformation. II. ^{125}I-PHA binding to spleen cells from young and old mice, *Mech. Ageing Develop.* **4**:103–112.

Kisielow, P., Hirst, J. A., Shiku, H., Beverley, P. C. L., Hoffman, M. K., Boyse, E. A., and Oettgen, H. F., 1975, Ly antigens as markers for functionally distinct subpopulations of thymus-derived lymphocytes of the mouse, *Nature* **253**:219–220.

Konen, T. G., Smith, G. S., and Walford, R. L., 1973, Decline in mixed lymphocyte reactivity of spleen cells from aged mice of a long-lived strain, *J. Immunol.* **110**:1216–1221.

Lajtha, L. J., and Schofield, R., 1971, Regulation of stem cell renewal and differentiation: possible significance in aging, *Adv. Gerontol. Res.* **3**:131–146.

Legge, J. S., and Austin, C. M., 1968, Antigen localization and the immune response as a function of age, *Aust. J. Exp. Biol. Med. Sci.* **46**:361–365.

Lloyd, R. S., and Triger, D. R., 1975, Studies on hepatic uptake of antigen. III. Studies of liver macrophage function in normal rats and following carbon tetrachloride administration, *Immunology* **29**:253–263.

Lyngbye, J., and Kroll, J., 1971, Quantitative immunoelectrophoresis of proteins in serum from normal population: season-, age-, and sex-related variations, *Clin. Chem.* **17**:495–500.

Mackay, I. R., 1972, Ageing and immunological function in man, *Gerontologia* **18**:285–304.

Makinodan, T., and Adler, W., 1975, The effects of aging on the differentiation and proliferation potentials of cells of the immune system, *Fed. Proc.* **34**:153–158.

Makinodan, T., and Peterson, W. J., 1962, Relative antibody-forming capacity of spleen cells as a function of age, *Proc. Nat. Acad. Sci. U.S.* **48**:234–238.

Makinodan, T., and Peterson, W. J., 1964, Growth and senescence of the primary antibody-forming potential of the spleen, *J. Immunol.* **93**:886–896.

Makinodan, T., Chino, F., Lever, W. E., and Brewen, B. S., 1971, The immune systems of mice reared in clean and dirty conventional laboratory farms. II. Primary antibody-forming activity of young and old mice with long life spans, *J. Gerontol.* **26**:508–514.

Makinodan, T., Deitchman, J. W., Stoltzner, G. H., Kay, M. M., and Hirokawa, K., 1975, Restoration of the declining normal immune functions of aging mice, *Proc. 10th Internat. Congr. Gerontol.* **2**:23.

Makinodan, T., Albright, J. W., Good, P. I., Peter, C. P., and Heidrick, M. L., Reduced humoral immune activity in long-lived old mice: an approach to elucidating its mechanisms, *Immunology,* 1976.

Mathies, M., Lipps, L., Smith, G. S., and Walford, R. L., 1973, Age related decline in response to phytohemagglutinin and pokeweed mitogen by spleen cells from hamsters and a long-lived mouse strain, *J. Gerontol.* **28**:425–430.

Meredith, P., Tittor, W., Gerbase-Delima, M., and Walford, R., 1975, Age-related changes in the cellular immune response of lymph node and thymus cells in long-lived mice. *Cell. Immunol.* **18**:324–330.

Metcalf, D., 1965, Delayed effect of thymectomy in adult life on immunological competence, *Nature* (London) **208**:1336.

Metcalf, D., Moulds, R., and Pike, B., 1966, Influence of the spleen and thymus on immune responses in ageing mice, *Clin. Exp. Immunol.* **2**:109–120.

Penn, I., and Starzl, T. E., 1972, Malignant tumors arising *de novo* in immunosuppressed organ transplant recipients, *Transplantation* **14**:407–417.

Perkins, E. H., and Makinodan, T., 1971, Nature of humoral immunologic deficiencies of the aged, in: *Proc. 1st Rocky Mt. Symp. on Aging,* pp. 80–103, Colorado State University, Fort Collins, Colorado.

Peter, C. P., 1971, Synergism between spleen cells of immunologically active young and inactive aged mice, *Fed. Proc.* **30**:526.

Peter, C. P., 1973, Possible immune origin of age-related pathological changes in long-lived mice, *J. Gerontol.* **28**:265–275.

Peterson, W., and Makinodan, T., 1972, Autoimmunity in aged mice. Occurrence of autoagglutinating factors in the blood of aged mice with medium and long life-spans, *Clin. Exp. Immunol.* **12**:273–290.

Pierpaoli, W., 1975, Inability of thymus cells from newborn donors to restore transplantation immunity in athymic mice, *Immunology* **29**:465–468.

Pisciotta, A. V., Westring, D. W., Deprey, C., and Walsh, B., 1967, Mitogenic effect of phytohemagglutinin at different ages, *Nature* (London) **215**:193–194.

Prehn, R. T., 1971, Evaluation of the evidence for immune surveillance, in: *Immune Surveillance* (R. T. Smith and M. Landy, eds.), pp. 451–462, Academic Press, New York.

Price, G. B., and Makinodan, T., 1972a, Immunologic deficiencies in senescence. I. Characterization of intrinsic deficiencies, *J. Immunol.* **108**:403–412.

Price, G. B., and Makinodan, T., 1972b, Immunologic deficiencies in senescence. II. Characterization of extrinsic deficiencies, *J. Immunol.* **108**:413–417.

Roberts-Thomson, I., Whittingham, S., Youngchaiyud, U., and Mackay, I. R., 1974, Ageing, immune response, and mortality, *Lancet* **2**:368–370.

Santisteban, G. A., 1960, The growth and involution of lymphatic tissue and its interrelationships to aging and to the growth of the adrenal glands and sex organs in CBA mice, *Anat. Rec.* **136**:117–126.

Shiku, H., Kisielow, P., Bean, M. A., Takahashi, T., Boyse, E. A., Oettgen, H. F., and Old, L. J., 1975, Expression of T-cell differentiation antigens on effector cells in cell-mediated cytotoxicity in vitro, *J. Exp. Med.* **141**:227–241.

Shiku, H., Kisielow, P., Boyse, E. A., and Oettgen, H. F., 1976, Immunogenetic identification of functional T-cell subsets, *Transplant. Proc.,* 1976.

Sigel, M., and Good, R. A., editors, 1972, *Tolerance, Autoimmunity and Aging,* Charles C. Thomas, Springfield, Illinois.

Siminovitch, L., Till, J. E., and McCulloch, E. A., 1964, Decline in colony-forming ability of marrow cells subjected to serial transplantation into irradiated mice, *J. Cell. Physiol.* **64**:23–31.

Stutman, O., 1974, Cell mediated immunity and aging, *Fed. Proc.* **33**:2028–2032.

Stutman, O., Yunis, E. J., and Good, R. A., 1968, Deficient immunologic functions of NZB mice, *Proc. Soc. Exp. Biol. Med.* **127**:1204–1207.

Taylor, R. B., 1965, Decay of immunological responsiveness after thymectomy in adult life, *Nature* (London) **208**:1334–1335.

Teague, P. O., Yunis, E. J., Rodey, G., Fish, A. J., Stutman, O., and Good, R. A., 1970, Autoimmune phenomena and renal disease in mice. Role of thymectomy, aging, and involution of immunologic capacity, *Lab. Invest.* **22**:121–130.

Teller, M. N., 1972, Age changes and immune resistance to cancer, *Adv. Gerontol. Res.* **4**:25–43.

Thomsen, O., and Kettel, K., 1929, Die Stärke der menschlichen Isoagglutinine und entsprechende Blutkörperchenrezeptoren in verschiedenen Lebensaltern, *Z. Immunitätsforsch.* **63**:67–93.

Tigelaar, R. E., Gershon, R. K., and Asofsky, R., 1975, Graft-versus-host reactivity of mouse thymocytes: effect of *in vitro* treatment with anti-TL serum, *Cell. Immunol.* **19**:58–64.

Walford, R. L., 1969, *The Immunologic Theory of Aging,* Munksgaard, Copenhagen.

Walters, C. S., and Claman, H. N., 1975, Age related changed in cell mediated immunity in Balb/C mouse, *J. Immunol.* **115**:1438–1443.

Yunis, E. J., Hilgard, H., Sjodin, K., Martinez, C., and Good, R. A., 1964, Immunological reconstitution of thymectomized mice by injections of isolated thymocytes, *Nature* (London) **201**:784–786.

Zukoski, C. I., Killen, D. A., Ginn, E., Matler, B., Lucas, D. O., and Seigler, H. F., 1970, Transplant carcinoma in an immunosuppressed patient, *Transplantation* **9**:71–74.

3

The Pathogenic Role of Age-Related Immune Dysfunctions

W. HIJMANS and C. F. HOLLANDER

In this review of the pathogenic role of age-related immune dysfunctions, an outline of the main characteristics of the immune system will be given first because any discussion on aging and immunity should be based on the prevailing immunological theories and models. The age-related immune dysfunctions will then be surveyed and the need for in depth analysis will be emphasized. Finally, an outline of age-related pathology, which could be a consequence of the age-related dysfunctions, will be discussed. These dysfunctions could themselves be the results of minor defects and, therefore, difficult to detect. Genetic factors may play a major role in their development.

1. The Normal Immune System

It is customary that the situation in young adults be considered the normal one; hence the data obtained in this period serve as the reference standards. Normality is thus associated with a specified age group; however, one can also choose the period in which a maximum response is found. An example is given by Hori, Perkins, and Halsall (1973) who found a peak response to phytohemagglutinin in BALB/c mice aged four months; in BC_3F_1 animals, this occurred at the age of six to eight months. It is, therefore, not to be assumed that the age of three months is always the optimal reference period in mice. Ideally, information should be collected during the full life cycle of the individual, and the normal period should then be determined from data obtained in this longitudinal study. In practice, it is often sufficient to obtain a number of points in a number of individuals of different ages. These individuals

W. HIJMANS and C. F. HOLLANDER • Institute for Experimental Gerontology of the Organization for Health Research TNO, 151 Lange Kleiweg, Rijswijk (ZH), The Netherlands.

should be checked for signs of disease, with special attention being paid to the lymphoreticular system and the circulating immunoglobulins. The reasons for this will be detailed later.

1.1. Humoral and Cellular Immunity

The humoral is traditionally distinguished from the cellular immunity. The former is responsible for the synthesis of immunoglobulins and it is called the B system because in birds, its source of origin is the bursa of Fabricius. Its analog in mammalians is unknown, but the use of the term B system in these species is justified by the fact that the bone marrow is a major site of antibody production (Benner *et al.*, 1974). The thymus is essential for the full development of cellular immunity. This system has accordingly been termed the T system. It plays a major role in the delayed type of hypersensitivity, including the graft-versus-host and transplantation reactions. It can also modify the activity of the B cell system in a helper or a suppressor function. The T cell system also has a separate influence on the degree of affinity of antibodies (Katz and Steward, 1975).

The morphological substrate of both cell lines is the lymphocyte. The most remarkable aspect of this statement is that it was only two decades ago that the role of this cell in immunology was recognized. The lymphocyte is derived from the hematopoietic stem cell. The end cell of the B system is the plasma cell and the end cell of the T system is the specifically sensitized small lymphocyte. B lymphocytes can easily be distinguished from T lymphocytes on the basis of differences in membrane structures, which can be detected by serological means. The most widely used are anti-immunoglobulin reagents for B cells and antisera against structural components of cell membranes for T cells. A unique characteristic of human T cells is their capacity to form spontaneous rosettes with heterologous red blood cells.

Another lymphocyte subpopulation is comprised of the K, or killer, cells, which are responsible for antibody-dependent cytotoxicity. These cells are still difficult to distinguish from the other lymphocytes and their interaction with them is far from being fully understood. They are mentioned here as a reminder that the immune system includes more than just the B and T cells. A review that aims at completeness should also not omit the macrophages.

1.2. Diversity of Antibodies

The second major characteristic of the immune system is its diversity at the molecular level. This feature has been particularly well analyzed with respect to the immunoglobulins. The structural differences in the common part of the immuno-globulin molecules in man allow a separation into five classes, six subclasses, and two types. Differences in the variable part of heavy and light chains lead to at least eight subgroups. Genetic polymorphism expresses itself in a large number of allotypes. Finally, each antibody molecule, of course, has its specific idiotypic structure, which appears to be intimately associated with the antibody-combining site. This is the basis for the immense number of antibody and idiotype specificities of the immunoglobulin molecules. All possible combinations among the constant and the variable parts finally result in an extremely large antibody repertoire within an individual species and an even larger one within a given species. This number more or less reflects the number of lymphocyte clones, because a basic rule in the production of immunoglobulins is that one plasma cell synthesizes only one kind of antibody with a single specificity. The study of the chemical structure responsible for the specificity of T cell products, which can be designated as IgT, is a very recent undertaking.

1.3.   The Network Model

Jerne (1973, 1976) has recently added a new dimension to the model of the immune system. He developed the concept that the immune system is a network of antibody molecules and lymphocytes that recognize and are recognized by other antibody molecules and lymphocytes. The author emphasizes that this network is not just a formal curiosity, but that it is a functional network and that the properties of this network represent the essential regulatory mechanisms of the immune system. It is a complex system, composed of multiple, mutually interdependent subsystems with possibilities of positive and negative signals and feedback mechanisms. This revised model implies essential additions to and differences from the linear B–T system described.

2.   Age-Dependent Immune Dysfunctions

The increased occurrence of immune dysfunctions in relation to aging has been amply documented. These dysfunctions have been defined as qualitative or quantitative, functional or descriptive, or simply as deviations from the normal situation. They can be classified into three groups: immune deficiency, autoimmunity, and idiopathic paraproteinemia. They are not, however, invariably found. Even in some very old individuals none of these dysfunctions may be detectable, whereas combinations occur in others.

2.1.   Immune Deficiency

Many publications contain convincing data on the decline in function of the immune system during aging. Makinodan and co-workers have recently reviewed this subject (1975). The decline in deficiency involves both the B and T systems. In man, the titers of the natural or isoantibodies, such as the blood group antibodies, decrease slowly during aging. The average level in the seventh decade is about a quarter of the figure in the first decade. In studying the primary response of mice to sheep red blood cells, a thymus-dependent antigen, Makinodan et al. (1971) found values in old animals of only 10% of those seen in young animals. This decrease is largely due to changes associated with the immunocompetent cells; only about 10% may be attributed to age-related changes in the cellular environment, the so-called extrinsic factors. This decrease in old mice is found in the primary as well as the secondary response. The T-cell-independent reactivity to *Escherichia coli* lipopolysaccharide also diminishes slowly upon aging (Gerbase-DeLima *et al.*, 1974). Finally, there is conclusive evidence that the cellular immunity can also be deficient in the terminal period of life, as demonstrated in studies on the response to mitogens, in the rejection of transplantable tumors, in the mixed lymphocyte

W. HIJMANS AND
C. F. HOLLANDER

reaction, and in cell-mediated cytotoxicity (see Goodman and Makinodan, 1975). Recent investigations, however, have shown that the situation is more complicated and, indeed, is often confusing (see Yunis, 1974). It is possible, for instance, to obtain values in old animals that are comparable to those found in young adult animals if the total dose of antigen is given in multiple injections (Jaroslow *et al.*, 1974). Blankwater *et al.* (1975) have even described an increased immune response in aging mice of the BALB/c strain to the thymus-independent *E. coli* lipopolysaccharide. Haaijman (unpublished observations) has determined the number of immunoglobulin containing cells (the majority of which were plasma cells) with the fluorescent antibody technique in CBA mice. There was no decrease in the number of positive cells in the bone marrow of the male subjects on aging and a clear increase was observed in the females. Another observation comes from a study by Rádl *et al.* (1975) on the immunoglobulin levels in the serum of individuals over 95 years of age without overt disease, in which studies by others were confirmed and extended. The IgG and IgA levels were higher than those in the younger age groups, whereas the average IgM levels remained constant after childhood. There was, however, a striking increase with age in the variation in the levels of IgM and of the three major IgG subclasses. Within the IgG class, the increased level was due to increases in the subclasses IgG_1 and IgG_3. The age-related changes were, therefore, selective.

In this connection, a predominant role of genetic factors should receive serious consideration, since it has been shown in several animal species—but so far not in man—that the capability to mount a humoral immune response is controlled by the so-called I region of the major histocompatibility complex. The same region is responsible for the Ia (immune-region associated) antigens. These are located on the cell surface of mainly the B lymphocytes, and they have a function in the interaction of these cells with the T lymphocytes (for review, see Schreffler and Davis, 1975).

The situation with regard to cellular immunity is not clear-cut either. As mentioned above, impressive evidence has been presented by a number of authors to support the fact that cellular immunity is impaired in aged animals. Konen *et al.* (1973) noted a decline in reactivity in the mixed lymphocyte reaction in aged C57BL mice and Goodman and Makinodan (1975) reported on decreased cytolytic activity in old $(C57BL \times C3H)F_1$ hybrids. Depressed delayed-type hypersensitivity reactions have also been observed in aged men (Roberts-Thomson *et al.*, 1974). Recently, however, Stutman (1974) found an intact system for cellular immunity in studying the graft-versus-host reaction, allograft skin reactions, and lymphocyte-dependent cytotoxicity in old mice of the long-lived, nonautoimmune C57BL and CBA strains. This causes him to warn against generalizations: many findings can be strain-specific and the results can depend on the experimental situation.

In man, the evidence of the effect of aging is also conflicting. Grossman *et al.* (1975) concluded from an extensive study that there is no impairment in the ability of healthy elderly individuals to manifest a positive delayed hypersensitivity response when tested with a battery of skin-test antigens. The decreased skin-test reactivity in elderly patients could be a manifestation of serious illness and not an age-related phenomenon. Roberts-Thomson *et al.* (1974) found not only a decreased immune response in a group of very old people, but also an increased mortality rate in the hyporesponsive subjects. This age group was composed of persons over 80 years of age, but in contrast to the younger subjects in this study they were not considered healthy.

2.2. Autoimmunity

A major characteristic of the relationship between immunity and aging is the increased occurrence of autoantibodies. Walford (1969) has devoted a monograph to this subject. It is known from clinical observation that autoantibodies can be found in no less than 50% of aged individuals without overt disease, although titers are usually low. These reduced titers are more frequent in females than in males. Weakly positive tests for rheumatoid factor, low-level antinuclear antibodies, or antithyroglobulin antibodies may, therefore, have little medical significance in aged women, but they can be considered to indicate a disturbance in the homeostatic mechanism. The situation in mice is analogous. Autoantibodies were originally described in mice with autoimmune disease, but in later studies autoantibodies (especially antinuclear antibodies) were also detected in aged mice of long-lived strains (Friou and Teague, 1964). The cause of this phenomenon has not yet been clarified, but the progressive development of these autoantibodies is clearly related to age and strain. One can speculate on a gradual decrease in activity of the T cell and especially of its suppressor function (Teague, 1974). The physiological suppression of the synthesis of autoantibodies would then fail to function adequately.

2.3. Restricted Heterogeneity of the Immunoglobulins

The heterogeneity of the immunoglobulins is the hallmark of humoral immunity. A restricted heterogeneity is observed in certain situations. The extreme case is multiple myeloma. This is a malignant proliferation of plasma cells that can result in a greatly increased level of circulating monoclonal immunoglobulins—the M-component or paraprotein—with a concomitant decrease in the other immunoglobulins. The so-called idiopathic or benign paraproteinemia is a far more frequent finding. In general, it differs from myeloma in that it is not progressive, the level of the paraprotein is lower, and the decrease in the residual immunoglobulins is not as pronounced. From the gerontological point of view, idiopathic paraproteinaemia is of considerable interest because of its increase in frequency on aging. The data of Englisova *et al.* (1968) indicate its importance: they found these changes at a frequency of one out of five in very old individuals. The same was found by Rádl *et al.* (1975) in a group of volunteers over 95 years of age, without overt disease. Less pronounced changes of the same nature, indicating a restriction in heterogeneity, were even more frequent. An animal model has recently been described by Rádl and Hollander (1974). They found homogeneous immunoglobulin components in about 50% of aged mice of the C57BL strain, which were free of lymphoreticular malignancies on histological examination. This allows us to design experiments to study the question of whether the dysfunction is situated at the B cell level, the T cell level, or both, and to evaluate the hypothesis of a restricted repertoire in the aging individual.

3. Age-Related Pathology Due to Immune Dysfunctions

The pathological conditions that will be mentioned here are infection, autoimmune diseases, malignancy, and amyloidosis. This list should not be regarded as exhaustive or definitive. Indeed, a major task for immunogerontology will be to delineate immunopathology due to aging and to analyze these conditions in detail.

W. HIJMANS AND
C. F. HOLLANDER

3.1. Infection

It is generally assumed that aged individuals are more prone to develop infections than are young adults, and clinicians and pathologists agree that these infections are still a major cause of death in spite of the great improvements in antibiotic therapy. The respiratory tract is often involved; pneumonia can still be regarded as "old man's best friend," and the aged are at a high risk for influenza. Infections of the urogenital tract are often incapacitating and involvement of the kidney, as seen in pyelonephritis, may shorten the life expectancy. It is surprising to note that no specific information is available on the impaired immune response to infections in aged persons and experimental studies are lacking. At present it is, therefore, not justified to state that immunological resistance against microorganisms decreases during aging unless the immune system itself is involved as a feature of another disease. Lymphoreticular malignancies are the prime example. Myerowitz and co-workers (1971) report an increased frequency of blood cultures positive for Gram negative bacteria in aged patients. The positive cultures, however, were often obtained in patients with diseases such as leukemia, which itself can unfavorably alter the immune system. There is an obvious need for experimental studies. Observations on the occurrence of infections in aged inbred WAG/Rij rats of our own colony showed that the chance of developing severe infectious diseases increased with age and that this increase was not associated with an increase of lymphoreticular malignancies, which attack the immune system directly (Boorman *et al.,* to be published). The role of bacteria in general on life expectancy will be discussed by Anderson (1976) in his contribution on germfree animals in this volume.

3.2. Autoimmune Diseases

The increased incidence of a number of autoimmune diseases, such as rheumatoid arthritis and autoimmune thyroiditis, with aging is beyond doubt. Other autoimmune disorders, however, are more evenly distributed throughout life and, if one considers juvenile diabetes mellitus as an autoimmune disorder, it obviously represents a different category. The frequency of occurrence of these diseases is often difficult to establish, as they can go unnoticed if no specific studies are performed. The figures are also highly dependent on the classifying criteria that are adopted and on the depth of analysis, as shown in population studies on the incidence of rheumatoid arthritis, where threefold differences were observed (Lawrence and Wood, 1966). Signs of a focal thyroiditis can be found in about 25% of postmortem examinations in females over fifty years of age (Williams and Doniach, 1962), and this figure could well reflect the true incidence of autoimmune thyroiditis, since no qualitative differences have been found between this situation and the fully developed clinical picture. The etiology of this group of diseases is unknown. Viruses have been implicated, especially since it was found that C-type particles can be demonstrated with ease in the NZB mouse and the B/W hybrid with their lupuslike syndromes (Mellors and Huang, 1966). It has also been suggested that the failure to distinguish "self" from "nonself," which leads to the production of autoantibodies, is due to mutations, either in the immune system itself or in the target organ. Another theory is based on the supposition that the absence of autoantibodies results from inhibition of their synthesis. In an impaired immune system, the inhibitory function could fail. Combinations of these mechanisms can be easily visualized and the possibility that different causes operate in different autoimmune diseases should also be entertained.

Concepts concerning pathogenesis center around antigen–antibody complexes, which activate the complement system. This activation can lead to cellular infiltrations and tissue damage (see Cochrane and Koffler, 1973). The next obvious question is: In which situations can these complexes develop? There is evidence that there are two major requirements for their formation. The first is a critical ratio of antigen to antibody and the second is a low affinity of the antibodies. The latter could interfere with efficient elimination of the antigen. Antibodies with a reduced binding capacity have been demonstrated in NZB mice, which develop spontaneous autoimmune diseases (Elkerbout and Hijmans, 1974). In NZB/WF$_1$ mice, the time of onset, time course, and severity of the lupus syndrome are associated with the presence of increasing levels of low avidity anti-DNA antibody in the serum (Steward, Katz, and West, 1975). These results can be interpreted as indicating the presence of a selective defect in the suppressor function of the thymus. This may not, however, be the only defect, because a decreased reaction upon aging to *E. coli* lipopolysaccharide, a T-cell-independent antigen, has also been reported in these animals (Blankwater *et al.,* 1975).

3.3. Malignancy

As early as the beginning of this century, Ehrlich (1906) suggested that immune reactions hold a key position in the defense against cancer. He even emphasized the importance of cellular mechanisms relative to humoral immunity (Ehrlich, 1909). More than half a century later, Thomas (1959) again drew attention to this possibility; but it was only after Burnet (1970) had introduced the term *immune surveillance* that this concept found almost universal acceptance. It was soon realized that the evidence was largely circumstantial, and doubts have recently been voiced about its general validity. There are too many exceptions to the rules that this surveillance mechanism requires. Reports on an increased tumor incidence after neonatal thymectomy or immunosuppressive treatment are conflicting, as recently redis- cussed by Prehn (1974). The data obtained by Boorman *et al.* in this instance (to be published), on the spontaneously occurring tumors in neonatally thymectomized WAG/Rij rats, are not impressive and indicate that the situation is more complex than originally envisaged. In the naturally occurring immune deficiency diseases in man, a tumor incidence, which is several hundred times higher than that of the control groups, has been observed, but the majority of these are lymphoreticular malignancies (Good, 1974). The Denver Tumor Registry contains extremely inter- esting data (Penn, 1974). The iatrogenic immune deficiency states are associated with an increased incidence of malignancy. They do not, however, represent the spectrum of the naturally occurring malignancies, since two-thirds of the cases had epithelial tumors and mesenchymal tumors were encountered in one-third of the cases. The most common group within the mesenchymal tumors were the reticulum cell sarcomas. Not everybody, however, will agree with Prehn (1974) who stated that "Immunologic surveillance, as originally conceived, probably does not exist." The immune system no doubt plays a role, but what role may well depend on many factors, such as the spontaneous rate of occurrence of a given tumor in a given

W. HIJMANS AND
C. F. HOLLANDER

species, the etiology of the tumor, etc. Leibowitz and Schwartz (1971), in a detailed discussion on malignancy as a complication of immunosuppressive therapy in man, state that the influence of immune mechanisms in cancer is beyond doubt, but that they are not persuaded that the development of cancer is a direct consequence of immunosuppression. In a balanced review of the subject, Klein (1975) argues that immune surveillance as a natural defense mechanism against malignancy is a reality, but only in relation to tumor-associated antigen systems, such as viral antigens that have been regularly encountered by most members of the species, at least during their recent evolution. This conclusion agrees with the increased susceptibility of the congenitally thymus-deprived nude mice to virus oncogenesis (Allison *et al.,* 1974), since these animals are not known to develop more tumors spontaneously than control animals, in spite of being immunologically impaired. Immune surveillance for tumors could, therefore, represent a selective mechanism that operates for certain kinds of tumors. A specific disturbance in the immune system could then indicate a loss of control and the development of a specific tumor. Of course, this does not exclude a role of the immunogenicity of the tumor itself. The lack of an immunogenic coat and/or the presence of solubilized tumor cell surface antigen in the blood may provide an immune escape mechanism for tumor cells (Kim *et al.,* 1975).

3.4. Amyloidosis

The existence of a close relationship between amyloidosis and immune processes has been emphasized for many years (see Teilum, 1967). In the clinical situation, the primary form is distinguished from the secondary, which is associated with chronic inflammatory disease. In the latter, one can postulate a continuous antigenic stimulation by the disease process itself, e.g., via the formation of debris. Amyloidosis is also observed in multiple myeloma, a disease with an immune dysfunction by definition. Further evidence comes from the observation that amyloidosis can be induced in experimental animals by repeated administration of antigen. The immunological theory was placed on a solid basis when it was shown that the amyloid substance in patients with primary amyloidosis and in multiple myeloma consists primarily of fragments of immunoglobulin light chains. Another amyloid fibril protein, which can be found in patients with secondary amyloidosis and some familial forms of this disorder, has a unique protein known as amyloid A protein as a major component. This component is also normally present in the serum and it is of interest from the gerontological point of view in that its level increases upon aging (Rosenthal and Franklin, 1975). This supports the conclusion that amyloidosis—which can be observed in over half the male population over 70 years of age—can be considered as the most characteristic immune disorder of aging. The frequency can also be extremely high in the experimental animal, and the absence of amyloidosis in aged animals of some strains of mice is a great exception (Dunn, 1967). Genetic factors probably play a major role here, as they also seem to do in the familial form of amyloidosis in man.

4. Summary and Conclusions

In the first part of this review, the major characteristics of the immune system are mentioned. Included are the diversity within the bone-marrow-derived humoral immune response with its broad repertoire of antibodies, the thymus system, which is responsible for the cellular immunity, and the interaction of the B and T systems, in which the T cells can exert a helper as well as a suppressor effect on the synthesis of antibodies. The existence of other positive and negative feedback mechanisms should also be taken into account, such as has been done by Jerne (1973, 1976) in his multidimensional network model, which thus forms an integral part of a highly complex homeostatic regulatory system.

In the second part, the age-dependent immune dysfunctions are discussed briefly. Immune deficiencies can occur in old age at the B cell as well as at the T cell level. It is not an invariable phenomenon, but rather the expression of a selective defect. The occurrence of this defect may be strongly influenced by genetic factors. The second immune dysfunction in this category leads to an increased occurrence of autoantibodies. Its cause has not yet been elucidated, but the possibility that it is a consequence of decreased activity of the suppressor function of the thymus is entertained. The same defect may also be held responsible for the third group of age-dependent immune dysfunctions, that of the paraproteins. These can be detected in a large percentage of aged persons. They have also been recently reported in aging mice, especially in the C57BL strain.

Finally, age-related immunopathology is reviewed. Infection is still an important cause of death in geriatric cases; however, there is only circumstantial evidence for a role of a specific immune dysfunction. Autoimmune diseases occur more frequently in the older age groups, but this is definitely not a general feature of all autoimmune disorders. Malignancies have been postulated to be subjected to the influence of immune surveillance. The existence of this phenomenon and its effectiveness has been much debated recently. Whatever the outcome, it is most likely that it does not constitute a general defense mechanism against tumors. The last disorder discussed is amyloidosis. It is the most frequent disease of aging and it reflects a disturbed immune function. Its occurrence in mice may very well be genetically determined.

One may conclude that a number of different patterns can be discerned in the biology of aging of the immune system. A dysfunction is often seen, but it is not invariably present, nor is it now possible to predict whether or not abnormalities will occur. Exogeneous and endogenous factors determine the specific pattern. In any study on the precise definition of these abnormalities, it should be borne in mind that the immune system is a complex network of interacting and interdependent subsystems. In old age, subtle lesions can occur in a restricted area. These may lead to selective dysfunctions and, finally, to specific abnormalities.

ACKNOWLEDGMENTS

We are pleased to acknowledge the discussions with Drs. M. J. Blankwater, J. J. Haaijman, J. Rádl, and C. Zurcher from the Institute for Experimental Gerontology of the Organization for Health Research TNO.

References

Allison, A. C., Monga, J. N., and Hammond, V., 1974, Increased susceptibility to virus oncogenesis of congenitally thymus-deprived nude mice, *Nature* **252**:746–747.
Anderson, R. E., 1976, Use of germfree animals to study immunity and aging, in this volume.

Benner, R., Meima, F., Meulen, G. van der, and Ewijk, W. van, 1974, Antibody formation in mouse bone marrow. III. Effects of route of priming and antigen dose, *Immunology* **27**:747–760.

Blankwater, M. J., Levert, L. L., and Hijmans, W., 1975, Age-related decline in the antibody response to *E. coli* lipopolysaccharide in New Zealand Black mice, *Immunology* **28**:847–854.

Boorman, G. A., Lina, P. H. C., Hollander, C. F., and Zurcher, C., 1977, The occurrence of spontaneous tumors following neonatal thymectomy in the WAG/Rij rat, to be published.

Burnet, F. M., 1970, The concept of immunological surveillance, *Prog. Exp. Tumor Res.* **13**:1–27.

Cochrane, C. G., and Koffler, D., 1973, Immune complex disease in experimental animals and man, in: *Advances in Immunology,* (F. J. Dixon and H. G. Kunkel, eds.), pp. 185–264, Academic Press, New York.

Dunn, T., 1967, Amyloidosis in mice, in: *Pathology of Laboratory Rats and Mice* (E. Cotchin and F. J. C. Roe, eds.), pp. 181–212, Blackwell Scientific Publ., Oxford.

Ehrlich, P., 1906, Experimentelle Carcinomstudien an Mäusen, *Arb. Inst. exp. Ther. Frankfurt* **1**:15–102. Reprinted in: Paul Ehrlich: *Gesammelte Arbeiten, Zweiter Band* (F. Himmelweit, ed.), pp. 493–511, 1957, Pergamon Press, London.

Ehrlich, P., 1909, Über den jetzigen Stand der Karzinomforschung. *Ned. Tijdschr. Geneesk.* **53**:273–290. Reprinted in: Paul Ehrlich: *Gesammelte Arbeiten, Zweiter Band* (F. Himmelweit, ed.), pp. 550–562, 1957, Pergamon Press, London.

Elkerbout, E. A. S., and Hijmans, W., 1974, Relative avidity of antibodies towards sheep red blood cells in New Zealand Black mice, *Immunology* **26**:901–907.

Englisova, M., Englis, M., Kyral, V., Kourilek, K., and Dvorak, D., 1968, Changes of immunoglobulin synthesis in old people, *Exp. Gerontol.* **3**:125–127.

Friou, G. J., and Teague, P. O., 1964, Spontaneous autoimmunity in mice: Antibodies to nucleoprotein in strain A/J, *Science* **143**:1333–1334.

Gerbase-DeLima, M., Wilkinson, J., Smith, G. S., and Walford, R. L., 1974, Age-related decline in thymic-independent immune function in a long-lived mouse strain, *J. Geront.* **29**:261–268.

Good, R. A., 1974, The lymphoid system, immunodeficiency, and malignancy, in: *Advances in the Biosciences 12* (G. Raspé and S. Bernard, eds.), pp. 123–159, Pergamon Press, Vieweg.

Goodman, S. A., and Makinodan, T., 1975, Effect of age on cell-mediated immunity in long-lived mice, *Clin. exp. Immunol.* **19**:533–542.

Grossman, J., Baum, J., Gluckman, J., Fusner, J., and Condemi, J. J., 1975, The effect of aging and acute illness on delayed hypersensitivity, *J. Allergy Clin. Immunol.* **55**:268–275.

Hori, Y., Perkins, E. H., and Halsall, M. K., 1973, Decline in phytohemagglutinin responsiveness of spleen cells from aging mice, *Proc. Soc. Exp. Biol. Med.* **144**:48–53.

Jaroslow, B. N. Suhrbier, K. M., and Fritz, T. E., 1974, Decline and restoration of antibody forming capacity in aging beagle dogs, *J. Immunol.* **112**:1467–1476.

Jerne, N. K., 1973, The immune system, *Sci. Am.* **1973**:52–60.

Jerne, N. K., 1976, The immune system: A web of V-domains, in: *The Harvey Lectures, 1975–1976,* Academic Press, New York, 1976.

Katz, F. E., and Steward, M. W., 1975, The genetic control of antibody affinity in mice, *Immunology* **29**:543–548.

Kim, U., Baumler, A., Carruthers, C., and Bielat, K., 1975, Immunological escape mechanism in spontaneously metastasizing mammary tumors, *Proc. Nat. Acad. Sci. U.S.* **72**:1012–1016.

Klein, G., 1975, Immunological surveillance against neoplasia, in: *The Harvey Lectures, 1973–1974,* p. 71, Academic Press, New York.

Konen, T. G., Smith, G. S., and Walford, R. L., 1973, Decline in mixed lymphocyte reactivity of spleen cells from aged mice of a long-lived strain, *J. Immunol.* **110**:1216–1221.

Lawrence, J. S., and Wood, P. H. N., 1966, Criteria for rheumatoid arthritis in population samples, in: *Population Studies of the Rheumatic Diseases* (P. H. Bennett and P. H. N. Wood, eds.), pp. 164–174, Excerpta Medica Foundation, New York.

Leibowitz, S., and Schwartz, R. S., 1971, Malignancy as a complication of immunosuppressive therapy, *Adv. Int. Med.* **17**:95–123.

Makinodan, T., Perkins, E. H., and Chen, M. G., 1971, Immunologic activity of the aged, in: *Advances in Gerontological Research,* Vol. 3 (B. L. Strehler, ed.), pp. 171–198, Academic Press, New York.

Makinodan, T., Heidrick, M. L., and Nordin, A. A., 1975, Immunodeficiency and autoimmunity in aging, in: *Immunodeficiency in Man and Animals* (D. Bergsma, ed.), pp. 193–198, Sinauer Associates Inc., Sunderland, Mass.

Mellors, R. C., and Huang, C. Y., 1966, Immunopathology of NZB/BL mice. V. Viruslike (filtrable) agent separable from lymphoma cells and identifiable by electron microscopy, *J. Exp. Med.* **124**:1031–1038.

Myerowitz, R. L., Medeiros, A. A., and O'Brien, T. F., 1971, Recent experience with bacillemia due to Gram-negative organisms, *J. Infect. Dis.* **124**:239–246.

Penn, I., 1974, Occurrence of cancer in immune deficiencies, *Cancer* **34**:858–866.

Prehn, R. T., 1974, Immunomodulation of tumor growth, *Am. J. Pathol.* **77**:119–122.

Prehn, R. T., 1974, Immunological surveillance: Pro and Con, *Clin. Immunol.* **2**:191–203.

Rádl, J., and Hollander, C. F., 1974, Homogeneous immunoglobulins in sera of mice during aging, *J. Immunol.* **112**:2271–2273.

Rádl, J., Sepers, J. M., Skvaril, F., Morell, A., and Hijmans, W., 1975, Immunoglobulin patterns in humans over 95 years of age, *Clin. exp. Immunol.* **22**:84–90.

Roberts-Thomson, I. C., Wittingham, S., Youngchaiyud, U., and Mackay, I. R., 1974, Ageing, immune response, and mortality, *Lancet II,* **7877**:368–370.

Rosenthal, C. J., and Franklin, E. C., 1975, Variation with age and disease of an amyloid A protein-related serum component, *J. Clin. Invest.* **55**:746–753.

Schreffler, D. C., and Davis, C. S., 1975, The H-2 major histocompatibility complex and the I immune response region: Genetic variation, function and organization, in: *Advances in Immunology* (F. J. Dixon and H. G. Kunkel, eds.), pp. 125–190, Academic Press, New York.

Steward, M. W., Katz, F. E., and West, N. J., 1975, The role of low affinity antibody in immune complex disease. The quantity of anti-DNA antibodies in NZB/W F_1 hybrid mice, *Clin. exp. Immunol.* **21**:121–130.

Stutman, O., 1974, Cell-mediated immunity and aging, *Fed. Proc.* **33**:2028–2032.

Teague, P. O., 1974, Spontaneous autoimmunity and involution of the lymphoid system, *Fed. Proc.* **33**:2051–2052.

Teilum, G., 1967, Origin of amyloidosis from PAS-positive, reticuloendothelial cells in situ and basic factors in pathogenesis, in: *Amyloidosis,* (E. Mandema, L. Ruinen, J. H. Scholten, and A. S. Cohen, eds.), pp. 37–44, Excerpta Medica Foundation, Amsterdam.

Thomas, L., 1959, Reactions to homologous tissue antigens in relation to hypersensitivity, in: *Cellular and Humoral Aspects of the Hypersensitive States* (H. S. Lawrence, ed.), pp. 529–532, Hoeber-Harper, New York.

Walford, R. L., 1969, The immunologic theory of aging, Munksgaard, Copenhagen.

Williams, E. D., and Doniach, I., 1962, The post-mortem incidence of focal thyroiditis, *J. Path. Bact.* **83**:255–264.

Yunis, E. J., and Greenberg, L. J., 1974, Immunopathology of aging, *Fed. Proc.* **33**:2017–2019

4

The Immunoepidemiology of Aging

IAN R. MACKAY, SENGA F. WHITTINGHAM, and JOHN D. MATHEWS

1. Summary

Age-related changes in man are particularly evident, structurally and functionally, in the thymus and thymus-dependent lymphocyte population as judged by several indices of integrity of the T cell system, whereas B cell functions appear to be relatively well preserved.

All reported human population studies point to an incremental increase with aging of various autoantibodies and, since autoantibodies are associated with degenerative vascular disease, particularly in males, vascular degeneration appears to be mediated in part through autoimmune mechanisms. There is also evidence that age-associated failure of the thymus-dependent immune functions predisposes to mortality.

Thus the contribution of thymic failure to aging is determined in several ways, either by defective "helper" and effector functions, so predisposing to infections and emergence of cancer, or by defective suppressor functions, so predisposing to autoimmunity and autoantibody-mediated vascular disease.

2. Introduction

The present title, The Immunoepidemiology of Aging, was selected with three considerations in mind: (a) that aging processes affect the immunological system, and these are manifested both morphologically and functionally; (b) that assessment of functional changes with aging at the population level—immunoepidemiology— provides insight into immunological aging; and (c) that functional deterioration in

IAN R. MACKAY, SENGA F. WHITTINGHAM, and JOHN D. MATHEWS • Clinical Research Unit of The Walter and Eliza Hall Institute of Medical Research, and The Royal Melbourne Hospital, Victoria, Australia.

the immune system has secondary deleterious effects that can accelerate aging processes.

Although no formal classification is at present possible for age-related diseases, certain major categories can be recognized. These include:

1. Atherosclerotic vascular disease with morbidity related to particular distribution areas, brain, heart, kidneys, or periphery;
2. Neoplasia, the age-specific incidence of which is explainable (for most types) by the duration and degree of exposure to a carcinogen, the activity and inherent susceptibility of the exposed tissue, and possibly immunological surveillance;
3. Infections, particularly pulmonary, to which aged persons become increasingly vulnerable;
4. Autoimmunity, which, in age, particularly affects certain endocrine or exocrine tissues;
5. Environmental toxic degradation, exemplified by emphysema in smokers;
6. Cellular degeneration and fall-out, the ultimate failure of aging, best exemplified by neural tissues, and manifested by senile dementia and Parkinson's disease, and by lymphoid tissues for which a "Hayflick limit" may be applicable (Burnet, 1970).

Immunological function can be related in one way or another to almost all these categories.

3. Age-Associated Changes in Primary Lymphoid Organs

In man, the thymus begins its phase of maturation at the eighth to tenth week of fetal life when the organ becomes lymphoid, and thereafter enlarges rapidly. After birth, there is further but slower enlargement until adolescence, when loss of thymic tissue (involution) occurs progressively and particularly affects the lymphoid component. The degree of functional activity of the adult thymus, in terms of export of newly patterned thymic lymphocytes or production of thymic hormone, is uncertain, but from observations on experimental thymectomy in adult mice and therapeutic thymectomy in humans for myasthenia gravis (Vessey and Doll, 1972), there is minimal immunological deficit. This is because of the ample pool of memory T cells "educated" for reactivity with the common environmental antigens and the relatively slow depletion of this pool with time.

In regard to the B cell system, the source tissue is the bone marrow. It is known that there is a decrease with age in the "amount" of hemopoietic marrow, but it would be difficult to quantify this; however, the precursor tissue for B cells does not appear to undergo involution as does the thymus. In aplastic anemia, in which there is loss of functional bone marrow, a deficiency of B cells has been reported (Morley et al., 1974).

4. Age-Associated Changes in Indices of Immunity

Age-associated studies on populations or groups of normal human subjects have been made with respect to various indices, including amounts of immunoglobulins, numbers of B and T cells, and antibody and delayed hypersensitivity responses.

4.1. B Cell Functions

4.1.1. Levels of B Cells in Blood

Studies on counts of circulating B cells with age show that there is no change in absolute numbers, but the proportion may increase because of a fall in the proportion of T cells (Diaz-Jouanen *et al.*, 1975).

4.1.2. Immunoglobulins

According to Walford (1969), a consensus from earlier studies (with some disagreements) would be that there is an increase in all globulin fractions with increasing age; representative figures for gamma globulin (grams per 100 ml) would be an increase from 0.87 to 1.39 from the third to the seventh decades. Acheson and Jessop, and Kipshidze (cited by Mackay, 1972) reported that mean gamma globulin levels peaked in later life and then fell with a terminal rise in extreme old age. More recently, studies have been reported on changes with age in immunoglobulin classes. Schwick and Becker (1969), in a study on blood donors, found, with aging, a rise in IgG and a significant fall in level of IgM. Buckley and Dorsey (1970) used polynomial analysis of data from a population study and concluded that aging was associated with a gradual decrease in IgG and IgM concentrations. Cassidy *et al.* (1974) reported on a large community-based study of immunoglobulins of 3,213 persons from 3 to 94 years of age, with evaluation of differences by multiple–linear regression on $\log_e$ transformed data. In keeping with earlier data on age-related changes in total gamma globulin, the concentration of IgG and IgA increased with age, whereas IgM did not change. The discrepancies in changes in immunoglobulin levels with age may be accounted for by the fact that population studies are cross-sectional rather than longitudinal in design (Buckley *et al.*, 1974).

Other reports describe a fall, with age, in levels of IgD (Leslie *et al.*, 1975) and of IgE (Grundbacher, 1974; Orren and Dowdle, 1975).

4.1.3. Abnormal Serum Components

M Components. Electrophoretically homogeneous monoclonal (M) components occur with increasing frequency on aging. Two cited incidences are: 3% (Hallen, 1963) and 19% (Rádl *et al.*, 1975). These may be the expression of a clone of B cells that escaped from the normal controlling influences within the immunological system.

Amyloid. Amyloid is a proteinaceous substance with a fibrillar structure deposited in extracellular tissues in certain disease states and in aging. Amyloid fibrils consist of two major proteins that exist either singly or in combination: one is known as AL and consists of fragments of immunoglobulin light chains, and the other, AA, consists of a protein that is unrelated to immunoglobulin (Franklin, 1975–1976). Amyloid deposits increase in number with age as senile plaques in many tissues and are said to be the best single indicator of the aging process (Wright *et al.*, 1969). Moreover, the AA protein, present in the amyloid tissue from patients with secondary amyloidosis, was shown to be present in the serum of 60% of aged people, whereas a younger group of adults, blood donors, had only a 3% frequency (Benson *et al.*, 1975).

Natural Antibody. This term describes antibody that is detectable in serum prior to immunization with the corresponding antigen and arising presumably from immunization with cross-reactive determinants. The best examples of natural antibody are blood group antibodies, and age-related changes in these were described by Somers and Kuhns (1972). These authors remarked on reports that "low levels of blood group immunoglobulins were not uncommon in senescence," and hence investigated 197 patients from 15 to 50 years of age, 91 from 51 to 69 years of age, and 90 from 70 to 98 years of age. Average titers of anti-A and anti-B isoagglutinins decreased progressively from 20 years of age to quite low levels in senescence, and this was attributed to "refractoriness to immune stimuli" (Somers and Kuhns, 1972). In studies conducted by our laboratory (Rowley, 1970), IgM natural antibody to flagellin from *S. adelaide* became detectable in human infants in the first year of life; mean peak titers were reached at 30 years of age, with a slow decline thereafter, although the range of values at all ages was wide.

4.1.4. Previously Evoked Antibodies

Attention has been drawn by Schwick and Becker (1969) to lower levels of antibody to various bacterial and viral antigens in subjects 55 to 65 years of age than in those from 20 to 30 years of age. However, this could be no more than an expression of clonal decay in the absence of boosting, rather than an age-attributable cellular failure.

4.1.5. Stimulated Antibody, Primary Responses

The ideal study to assess antibody-producing responsiveness in human aging would require use of a range of antigens in a population study to detect random losses of capacity to react, but this is hardly feasible. There are data available from our laboratory (Rowley and Mackay, 1969; Roberts-Thomson *et al.*, 1974) on responses at different ages to immunization with 5 μg of flagellin, a potent immunogen in man. Mean titers of total antibody (IgM and IgG) and IgG antibody were similar, and the levels of total antibody were well sustained, but there was a failure in the older subjects to maintain levels of IgG antibody at 10 weeks, attributed to impaired "helper" activity of T cells *(vide infra)*. Preservation of humoral immune responses in the aged were reported for influenza vaccine (Feery *et al.*, 1976) and for tetanus toxoid (Solomonova and Vizev, 1973).

4.1.6. Stimulated Antibody, Secondary Responses

Studies in our laboratory (Mackay and Whittingham, 1976) on the secondary response to 5μg of flagellin showed first that preimmunization levels of total and IgG antibody were lower in subjects over 60 than in those under 50 years of age, indicating that the level of antibody raised by primary challenge had been less well maintained. After secondary challenge, the older subjects attained lower titers of total antibody (IgM + IgG), and IgG antibody at the time of peak response (two weeks) and also throughout the response to ten weeks.

4.2.1. Levels of T Cells in Blood

There have been several studies on levels of T cells in human blood at differing ages, using, for enumeration, cells forming rosettes with sheep erythrocytes (E rosettes). A decline with age in counts of E rosettes is the usual finding (Carosella *et al.*, 1974; Diaz-Jouanen *et al.*, 1975), but this was not observed in one study (Weksler and Hütteroth, 1974).

4.2.2. Functional Activities of T Cells

The several procedures that have been used to measure function of the T lymphocyte system have included (a) responsiveness to a range of ubiquitous antigens (candidin, mumps, trichophyton, tuberculin, and varidase are used); (b) capacity to be sensitized to dinitrochlorobenzene (DNCB); (c) responsiveness of blood lymphocytes *in vitro* to mitogens, particularly phytohemagglutinin (PHA); (d) capacity for stimulation–response to allogeneic lymphocytes in mixed lymphocyte culture (MLC); and (e) capacity to provide "help" in humoral immune responses.

As shown in Table 1, there was a decline with age in responsiveness to ubiquitous antigens (Toh *et al.*, 1973). The capacity to become sensitized to DNCB does fall, but only in advanced age, beyond 70 years (Waldorf *et al.*, 1968). Impaired mitogenic responsiveness to PHA with aging has been frequently documented (Mackay, 1972); data from our laboratory are shown in Figure 1. Reports on responsiveness of lymphocytes in MLC do not indicate marked changes with age (Heine *et al.*, 1969–1970; Carosella *et al.*, 1974), which is at variance with findings in the mouse (Konen *et al.*, 1973).

After immunization with flagellin, subjects show less well-sustained levels of IgG antibody in the primary responses (Figure 2) which is indicative of poorer T-cell-helper function, as judged by this presumably "thymus-dependent" antigen (Roberts-Thomson *et al.*, 1974).

TABLE 1. Incidence (and Percentage) of Positive Delayed-Type Hypersensitivity Reactions to Five Antigens[a]

Antigen	Controls	Advanced age
Candidin	32 (73%)	15 (33%)
Mumps	35 (80%)	15 (33%)
Trichophyton	14 (32%)	2 (5%)
Tuberculin	33 (75%)	12 (27%)
Varidase	34 (77%)	9 (20%)
All antigens	148 (70%)	53 (24%)

[a]In 45 subjects over 80 years of age compared with 44 controls ranging in age from 19 to 75 years.

IAN R. MACKAY
ET AL.

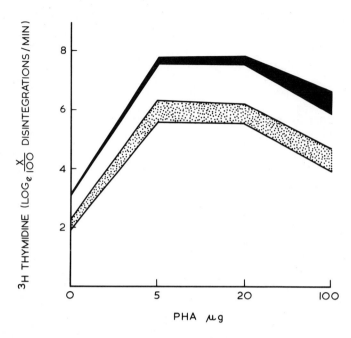

Figure 1. Lymphocyte response to phytohemagglutinin (PHA) in young and old people. The mean lymphocyte response ($\pm$ standard error) to various concentrations of PHA was significantly less for 20 subjects over 60 years of age (dotted line) than for 20 subjects less than 25 years of age (solid line). (Reproduced with permission of the Editor of *Lancet*.)

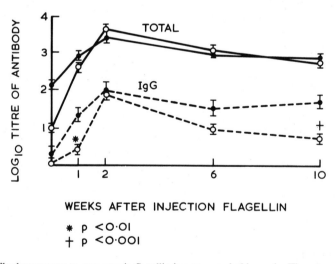

Figure 2. Antibody response to monomeric flagellin in young and old people. The geometric mean titer of total antibody ($\pm$ standard error) was the same in 44 subjects over 60 years of age (O) as in 27 subjects less than 25 years of age ($\bullet$); however, titers of IgG antibody were lower before and after the peak titer, and there was a more rapid fall-off with time. (Reproduced with permission of the Editor of *Lancet*.)

In several studies on populations (Serafini *et al.*, 1964; Whittingham *et al.*, 1969; Couchman *et al.*, 1970; Hooper *et al.*, 1972; Shu *et al.*, 1975), it has been shown that there is, with increasing age of the population, an increase in prevalence of most of the routinely measured autoantibodies.

This unit has been participating in an ongoing project relating to the population prevalence of autoantibodies in collaboration with a study group based on the town of Busselton in Western Australia (Hooper *et al.*, 1972; Mathews *et al.*, 1973; Mathews *et al.*, 1976). In 1969, sera were obtained from over 90% of the adult population (some 3,500 persons), and correlations were made between various autoantibody reactions, carcinoembryonic antigen (CEA), and other health variables tested for at the time of blood sampling; the population has been kept under close health surveillance over subsequent years, and the causes of death have been ascertained. The findings can be summarized as follows:

1. There was a general increase with age in prevalence for most autoantibodies. This held for antibodies to thyroglobulin and thyroid epithelial cell antigen, parietal cell antigen, cell nuclei, and antigens of the gamma globulin molecule (rheumatoid factor), but could not be shown for smooth muscle antibody or mitochondrial antibody, possibly because the population frequency of these autoantibodies is low or because of induction of autoantibody (e.g., smooth muscle antibody) by endemic infection, thus masking the age-related increase. It was of interest that the prevalence of a heteroantibody (for rat tissues) demonstrable in some 3% of human subjects did not change with age (Strickland and Hooper, 1972), thus differing from autoantibody that increases with age and natural antibody that decreases with age, *vide supra*.

2. There was a dip in prevalence of most autoantibodies at 70 years of age, possibly attributable to increased mortality in autoantibody positive subjects (Hooper *et al.*, 1972).

3. There was a highly significant tendency for such older persons to be positive for autoantibodies of more than one specificity, partly because of the higher prevalences of most autoantibodies in older persons.

4. However, within each five year age group, subjects positive for thyroid autoantibodies had a much increased prevalence of gastric autoantibodies (and vice versa), reflecting the association that occurs in patients with thyroid and gastric autoimmune disease.

5. There was also, for ages up to 60 years, a marginally increased prevalence of nuclear autoantibodies in subjects positive for thyroid or gastric autoantibodies, but this did not hold for older subjects.

6. There was a progressive increase with age in the prevalence of raised levels of CEA, which was independent of the effects of smoking and sex (Figure 3), and the presence of autoantibodies (Cullen *et al.*, 1976).

These observations may have important implications; first, the dependence of autoantibody prevalences on age suggests that autoantibodies may be determined by intrinsic age-related changes in the immune system and/or by the cumulated effects of environmental noxae over the life span. Second, as the associations of

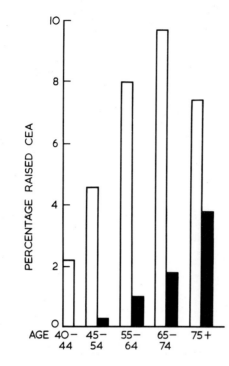

Figure 3. Associations of carcinoembryonic antigen (CEA) with age and smoking. In Busselton subjects over 40 years of age there was an age-related increase in prevalence of CEA, shown as percent of subjects with raised levels, in both nonsmokers ■ and smokers □, and among smokers there was an increased prevalence at all ages. (Reproduced with permission of the Editor of the *Australian and New Zealand Journal of Medicine.*)

thyroid with gastric autoantibodies and of thyrogastric with nuclear autoantibodies were not completely explained as effects of chronological age, it appears that there may be more specific determinants of loss of tolerance to one or more autoantigens. These determinants may be genetic, as evidenced by the familial aggregation of thyroid, gastric, and other autoantibodies, or environmental, as evidenced by the observation that for all age groups of men, nuclear autoantibodies were more prevalent in smokers than in ex-smokers, and more prevalent in ex-smokers than in those who never smoked (Table 2). Third, the association of thyrogastric autoantibodies with nuclear autoantibodies in younger but not in older subjects suggests that mortality is increased among subjects with multiple autoantibodies. Fourth, the independence of CEA and autoantibodies suggests that autoantibodies are not attributable to damaging effects of carcinogenic influences.

TABLE 2.   **Percentage of Men with Positive Nuclear Autoantibody Reactions According to Age and Smoking Habit**

Age	Smoking habit		
	Never smoked	Ex-smoker	Current smoker
21–40	1[a]	1[a]	1
41–60	3	4	4
61+	5	9	15
All ages	2	5	7

[a]By extrapolation in view of small numbers of men.

5.1. Consequences of Age-Related Changes in Immunological Function

It is important to consider whether the age-related changes in the structure and function of the immunological system in man are merely secondary to aging *per se,* or whether they provide any evidence for the view that immunological effector mechanisms contribute to the pathogenesis of age-related diseases in man. For the second possibility to be true, a necessary (but not sufficient) condition is that the age-related diseases measuring the biological rate of aging should be more closely related to the immunological changes than they are to chronological age. In other words, if the causal hypothesis were true, then at any chronological age, immunological indices would still be correlated with biological age as measured by the presence of age-related disease and by the risk of death.

We have pursued two lines of enquiry in assessing possible effects of age-related immunological dysfunction, namely, T-cell failure and mortality in octogenarians, and the association of autoantibodies with mortality and morbidity in the Busselton population.

5.1.1. T Cell Failure and Mortality

It was shown in a population study by Roberts-Thomson *et al.* (1974) on 199 persons over 60 years of age that there was less reactivity, as compared with younger subjects, in three indices of T cell function: (a) capacity to express DTH responses to ubiquitous antigens, (b) lymphocyte response to the T cell mitogen, PHA, and (c) maintenance of the IgG response to flagellin, which requires T cell help. In the course of this study, 52 subjects over 80 years of age were assessed in relation to DTH responses to five ubiquitous antigens and mortality over the subsequent two years. It was found that those with nil or one positive response had a significantly greater mortality than those within our normal range of two or more responses. The recorded causes of death were nondescript, bronchopneumonia and vascular accidents, but an impaired immune response to a relatively banal infection may have made a major contribution.

For example, as shown in Table 3, those octogenarians with impaired T cell activity died sooner than those with normal T cell activity. This suggests that the level of T cell activity is more sensitive than chronological age as an index of biological age; although this finding is consistent with the hypothesis that immunological mechanisms contribute to aging, it cannot discriminate the causal hypothesis from the alternative hypothesis that there are prior causes of aging that (coincidentally) also cause the immunological changes. The causal hypothesis would be more strongly supported if it were shown that intervention to reverse the immunological concomitants of aging was also able to reduce the death rate and the rate of progression of age-related diseases.

5.2. Autoantibodies and Disease at the Population Level

As autoantibodies increase in prevalence with age, they are necessarily concomitants of age-related diseases; this finding could mean that both autoantibodies and disease are merely secondary to chronological age. To proceed further, it is necessary to examine the relationship of autoantibodies to indices of disease independently of the association of both with chronological age.

TABLE 3. Delayed Type Hypersensitivity Skin
Reactions and Deaths Over 2 Years in People >80
Years of Age[a]

Number of positive reactions	Number of people	Number dead after 2 years
0	21	17 } 80%
1	14	11
2	10	2
3	3	2 } 35%
4	4	2
5	0	0
	52	34

[a]Reproduced with permission from the Editor of *Lancet*.

Table 4 summarizes the prevalence relationship of certain disease indices with autoantibodies in the Busselton population. In men, angina was associated with tissue autoantibodies (thyroid, gastric, nuclear, and/or smooth muscle autoantibodies) and this was independent of the confounding effects of chronological age. In women, angina was associated with rheumatoid factor, but not with tissue autoantibodies. Both men and women showed some association of hypertension with the presence of rheumatoid factor, and in women there was a striking association of dyspnea (shortness of breath) with rheumatoid factor. The relationship of autoanti-

TABLE 4. Observed and Expected Numbers of Subjects with Autoantibodies
and Various Indices of Disease

Index	Sex	Numbers of subjects with index and	
		Any tissue autoantibody	Rheumatoid factor only
Angina	M	41 (28.80)[c]	7 (10.85)
	F	47 (53.00)	17 (9.86)[b]
History suggestive of myocardial infarction	M	26 (27.08)	8 (8.08)
	F	36 (44.19)	11 (8.46)
Ischemic changes on ECG	M	41 (41.41)	15 (16.67)
	F	66 (75.86)	17 (12.14)
Cerebrovascular symptoms	M	49 (41.10)	15 (16.28)
	F	75 (84.95)	23 (16.29)[b]
Mean blood pressure >120 mm	M	92 (87.91)	42 (33.42)[a]
	F	152 (161.07)	36 (26.62)[b]
Dyspnea	M	72 (72.67)	28 (26.79)
	F	161 (167.54)	42 (30.86)[d]

Expected numbers in parentheses (corrected for confounding effects of age).
[a]$P < 0.10$
[b]$P < 0.05$
[c]$P < 0.01$
[d]$P < 0.001$

bodies to a history of myocardial infarction, to cerebrovascular symptoms, and to ischemic changes on the electrocardiograph were unremarkable.

One striking feature of the findings in Table 4 is that tissue autoantibodies are associated with indices of disease in men but not in women, whereas the reverse pattern is seen for rheumatoid factor. Another feature of the associations was their age dependence. As shown in Table 5, the association of angina with tissue autoantibodies (independent of chronological age) was more evident in younger men than in older men, but more evident in older women than in younger women. This pattern is complex, and could have arisen by chance. On the other hand, it could reflect important sex differences in adaptation to autoimmunity.

Elsewhere we have reported that autoantibodies are associated with obesity in younger men, but not in older men, and that thyrogastric autoantibodies are associated with frank diabetes mellitus and with higher 1-hr blood glucose levels in men up to 60 years of age (Mathews, Rodger, and Stenhouse, 1976).

These prevalence findings are of interest; they suggest that autoantibodies may be associated with disease in a way that does not merely reflect the association of both with chronological age. However, there are two important reservations: the first is that in any statistical comparison involving multiple variables, statistically "significant" findings are to be expected by chance alone; the second is that the associations of autoantibodies with disease indices in prevalence data may not reflect their value in predicting disease in incidence studies. In particular, if there is selective mortality of autoantibody positive subjects, this may distort the associations of autoantibodies with indices of disease in prevalence studies.

To assess whether autoantibodies were predictive of mortality in the Busselton population, we related autoantibody status as determined in 1969 to mortality in Busselton up to September 1975. Causes of death were categorized as cancer (rubrics 140 to 199, ICD, 8th revision), degenerative vascular disease (rubrics 400 to 448) or other causes (residual rubrics). There were 198 deceased subjects, 118 men and 80 women, whose records could be linked back to their autoantibody status in 1969.

The relationship between causes of death and autoantibody status is shown in Table 6. Presented in the table are the observed number of deaths from particular causes (*vide infra*) and the numbers "expected" on the null hypothesis of no association between autoantibody status and death. Considering all deaths, there were 85 in subjects with a positive test for autoantibody or rheumatoid factor as opposed to an expected 63, whereas there were 113 deaths among those with

TABLE 5. Ratios of Observed to Expected Numbers of Subjects with Angina According to Autoantibody Grouping, Sex, and Age[a]

Autoantibody	Men				Women			
	21−	41−	61−	All	21−	41−	61−	All
Tissue autoantibody	2.68	1.81	1.10[b]	1.42	0.85	1.19	1.44[b]	0.89
Rheumatoid factor only	0	0.53	0.79	0.65	2.79	0.89	1.92	1.73

[a]All ratios corrected for confounding effects of age. Difference between man and women $P < 0.001$.
[b]Age trend for tissue autoantibodies: men $P < 0.03$; women $P < 0.03$.

TABLE 6.   Numbers of Busselton Deaths (1970–1975) According to Autoantibody Status in 1969

| Cause of death | Sex | Autoantibody status | | | | Total deaths |
		Any tissue autoantibody (A)	Rheumatoid factor only (B)	Either A or B	None	
Vascular	M	18 (10.19)[a]	4 (4.14)	22 (14.34)	32 (39.66)	54
(I. C. D. 400–448)	F	19 (13.79)	2 (2.78)	21 (16.58)	21 (25.42)	42
Cancer	M	9 (5.85)	6 (2.37)	15 (8.22)	16 (22.78)	31
(I. C. D. 140–199)	F	7 (5.91)	1 (1.19)	8 (7.10)	10 (10.90)	18
Other	M	6 (6.23)	3 (2.53)	9 (8.76)	24 (24.24)	33
	F	8 (6.57)	2 (1.33)	10 (7.90)	10 (12.10)	20
All causes	M	33 (22.27)	13 (9.04)	46 (31.32)	72 (86.68)	118
	F	34 (26.27)	5 (5.30)	39 (31.58)	41 (48.42)	80

[a]In parentheses are given the numbers of deaths expected on the null hypothesis of no association between autoantibody status and death.

negative tests as opposed to an expected 135. Thus autoantibodies appeared to be associated with excess mortality.

Considering the sexes independently, there were 46 men who were positive for one or more autoantibodies or for rheumatoid factor, whereas 31.32 would have been "expected" ($\chi_1^2 = 9.26$, $P < 0.005$). The effect in men was even more striking when deaths from other causes (including accidents) were excluded (observed, 37; expected, 22.56; $\chi_1^2 = 12.5$, $P < 0.001$). This yielded a relative risk of 2.1 for the association of autoimmunity with death from vascular causes or cancer. In women there were 39 deaths with autoantibodies or with rheumatoid factor in 1969, whereas the expected number was 31.58, but this excess was not statistically significant ($\chi_1^2 = 2.82$, $P = 0.10$).

The expected numbers in Table 6 are not corrected for the associations of both autoimmunity and risk of death with chronological age; Table 7 examines the age-dependence of the association of autoimmunity with risk of death in men. Although the small numbers preclude rigorous statistical testing, it appears that over most age

TABLE 7.   Numbers of Deaths in Busselton Men According to Age and Autoantibody Status in 1969

| Age in 1969 | Cause of death | | | |
| | Vascular disease | | Cancer | |
	Any tissue autoantibody	Rheumatoid factor only	Any tissue autoantibody	Rheumatoid factor only
< 50	0 (0.27)[a]	0 (0.13)	0 (0.27)	0 (0.13)
50–59	4 (2.03)	0 (0.75)	0 (0.68)	1 (0.25)
60–69	7 (5.24)	1 (1.70)	6 (4.19)	2 (1.36)
70–79	6 (4.66)	2 (1.70)	3 (2.17)	3 (0.80)
80+	1 (1.50)	1 (1.00)	0 (0.56)	0 (0.38)

[a]Expected numbers in parentheses.

groups there is an excess mortality of men with autoantibodies from vascular causes and of men with rheumatoid factor from cancer. These limited follow-up data suggest that in men, but not in women, autoantibodies are predictive of death from vascular causes, and rheumatoid factor is predictive of death from cancer; both observations appear independent of the confounding effect of chronological age.

In regard to these findings from the Busselton population, it is accepted that vascular disease is multifactorial and would not be wholly accounted for by autoantibodies, which may be one of several risk factors. It is clear that females are less vulnerable than males to autoantibody-related vascular disease, explained by Mathews *et al.* (1974) on the basis of the IgM class of autoantibody and protective effects of rheumatoid factor in females. The ways in which autoantibody may be pathogenic include lodgement of immune complexes in vessel walls and damaging reactions with antigens of the arterial intima (Mathews *et al.*, 1974).

6. Conclusions

Numerous studies indicate that aging in man is accompanied by altered indices of immunological activity. This is most evident for T-cell-dependent functions that are decreased in aged persons. In regard to B-cell-dependent functions, the results of population studies are less decisive, particularly in regard to changes with age in the major immunoglobulin classes G and M. The capacity to produce specific antibody is well preserved in aged persons, although the thymus-dependent component (sustained IgG production) appears to falter. There is an increase with aging in abnormal serum components, including monoclonal immunoglobulins, the AA protein of amyloid, and CEA. All reported population studies indicate that aging is associated with an increased prevalence of various autoantibodies.

It is evident that the thymus-based immunological system follows other bodily systems in suffering a loss of vigor with aging. Waning function of helper or effector T cells could accentuate the deficits of aging through increased susceptibility to and impaired recovery from infection and by impaired activity of the presumed T-cell-dependent surveillance over emergence of cancer.

Many immunological abnormalities are now being examined in terms of functions of "suppressor" T cells, e.g., autoimmunity in which functional failure of such T cells allows emergence of autoreactive B cells. Indeed, studies in man by Waldorf *et al.* (1968) and Diaz-Jouanen *et al.* (1975) show that depressed T cell function with aging is associated with a concomitant increase in circulating autoantibodies, although in the latter study there was no correlation between T cell decrease and autoantibodies in individual patients. Thus the proposition that autoimmunity in B cells represents a "release" from suppression remains *sub judice* pending methods of characterizing suppressor T cells in man.

ACKNOWLEDGMENTS

I.R.M., S.F.W., and J.D.M. are in receipt of grants from the National Health and Medical Research Council of Australia, and express appreciation to the Busselton Population Studies Group for their continuing collaboration.

References

IAN R. MACKAY
ET AL.

Benson, M. D., Skinner, M., Lian, J., and Cohen, A. S., 1975, "A" protein of amyloidosis. Isolation of a cross-reacting component from serum by affinity chromatography, *Arthr. Rheum.* **18**:315–322.

Buckley, C. E., and Dorsey, F. C., 1970, The effects of aging on human serum immunoglobulin concentrations, *J. Immunol.* **105**:964–972.

Buckley, C. E., Buckley, E. G., and Dorsey, F. C., 1974, Longitudinal changes in serum immunoglobulin levels in older humans, *Fed. Proc.* **33**:2036–2039.

Burnet, F. M., 1970, An immunological approach to ageing, *Lancet* **2**:358–360.

Carosella, E. D., Mochanko, K., and Braun, M., 1974, Rosette-forming T cells in human peripheral blood at different ages, *Cell. Immunol.* **12**:323–325.

Cassidy, J. T., Nordby, G. L., and Dodge, H. J., 1974, Biologic variation of human serum immunoglobulin concentrations: sex–age specific effects, *J. Chron. Dis.* **27**:507–516.

Couchman, K. G., Wigley, R. D., and Prior, I. A. M., 1970, Autoantibodies in the Carterton population survey. The prevalence of thyroid and gastric antibodies, antinuclear and rheumatoid factors, in a probability based population sample, *J. Chron. Dis.* **23**:45–53.

Cullen, K. J., Stevens, D. P., Frost, M. A., and Mackay, I. R., 1976, Correlations between carcinoembryonic antigen, smoking and cancer in a population study, *Aust. N.Z. J. Med.* **6**:279–283.

Diaz-Jouanen, E., Strickland, R. G., and Williams, R. D., 1975, Studies of human lymphocytes in the newborn and the aged, *Am. J. Med.* **58**:620–628.

Feery, B. J., Morrison, E. I., and Evered, M. G., 1976, Antibody responses to influenza virus subunit vaccine in the aged, *Med. J. Aust.* **1**:540–542.

Franklin, E. C., 1975–1976, Amyloidosis, *Bull. Rheum. Dis.* **26**:832–837.

Grundbacher, F. J., 1974, Causes of variation in serum IgE levels in normal populations, *J. Allergy Clin. Immunol.* **56**:104–111.

Hallen, J., 1963, Frequency of 'abnormal' serum globulins (M-components) in the aged, *Acta Med. Scand.* **173**:737–744.

Heine, K. M., Stobbe, H., Klatt, R., Sahi, J., and Herrmann, H., 1969–1970, Lymphocyte function in the aged, *Helv. Med. Acta.* **35**:484–489.

Hooper, B., Whittingham, S., Mathews, J. D., Mackay, I. R., and Curnow, D. H., 1972, Autoimmunity in a rural community, *Clin. Exp. Immunol.,* **12**:79–87.

Konen, T. G., Smith, G. S., and Walford, R. L., 1973, Decline in mixed lymphocyte reactivity of spleen cells from aged mice of a long-lived strain, *J. Immunol.* **110**:1216–1221.

Leslie, G. A., Lopez Correa, R. H., and Holmes, J. N., 1975, Structure and biological functions of human IgD, *Int. Arch. Allergy,* **49**:350–357.

Mackay, I. R., 1972, Ageing and immunological function in man, *Gerontologia* **18**:285–304.

Mathews, J. D., Hooper, B. M., Whittingham, S., Mackay, I. R., and Stenhouse, N. S., 1973, Association of autoantibodies with smoking, cardiovascular morbidity, and death in the Busselton population, *Lancet* **2**:754–758.

Mathews, J. D., Whittingham, S., and Mackay, I. R., 1974, Autoimmunity and human vascular disease—Hypothesis, *Lancet* **2**:1423–1427.

Mathews, J. D., Rodger, B. M., and Stenhouse, N. S., 1976, The significance of the association of tissue autoantibodies and rheumatoid factor with angina in the Busselton population, *J. Chron. Dis.* **29**:345–353.

Morley, A., Holmes, K., and Forbes, I., 1974, Depletion of B lymphocytes in chronic hypoplastic marrow failure (aplastic anaemia), *Aust. N. Z. J. Med.* **4**:538–541.

Orren, A., and Dowdle, E. B., 1975, The effects of sex and age on serum IgE concentrations in three ethnic groups, *Int. Arch. Allergy* **48**:824–835.

Rádl, J., Sepers, J. M., Skvaril, F., Morell, A., and Hijmans, W., 1975, Immunoglobulin patterns in humans over 95 years of age, *Clin. Exp. Immunol.* **22**:84–90.

Roberts-Thomson, I. C., Whittingham, S., Youngchaiyud, U., and Mackay, I. R., 1974, Ageing, immune response and mortality, *Lancet* **2**:368–370.

Rowley, M. J., 1970, 'Natural' antibody in man to flagellar antigens of *Salmonella adelaide, Aust. J. Exp. Biol. Med. Sci.* **48**:249–252.

Rowley, M. J., and Mackay, I. R., 1969, Measurement of antibody-producing capacity in man. I. The normal response to flagellin from *Salmonella adelaide, Clin. Exp. Immunol.* **5**:407–418.

Schwick, H. G., and Becker, W., 1969, Humoral antibodies in older humans, in: *Current Problems in Immunology,* (Westphal, Bock, and Grundmann, eds.), Bayer-Symp. **1**:253–257.

Serafini, U., Torrigiani, G., and Masala, C., 1964, The evidence of autoantibodies in the normal population, in: Proceedings of the Vth International Congress of Allergology, Madrid, October, pp.527–539.

Shu, S., Nisengard, R. J., Hale, W. L., and Beutner, E. H., 1975, Incidence and titers of antismooth muscle and other autoantibodies in blood donors, *J. Lab. Clin. Med.* **86**:259–265.

Solomonova, K., and Vizev, St., 1973, Immunological reactivity of senescent and old people actively immunised with tetanus toxoid, *Z. Immun-Forsch.* **146**:81–90.

Somers, H., and Kuhns, W. J., 1972, Blood group antibodies in old age, *Proc. Soc. Exp. Biol. Med.* **141**:1104–1107.

Strickland, R. G., and Hooper, B. M., 1972, The parietal cell heteroantibody in human sera: Prevalence in a normal population and relationship to parietal cell antibody, *Pathology* **4**:259–263.

Toh, B. H., Roberts-Thomson, I. C., Mathews, J. D., Whittingham, S., and Mackay, I. R., 1973, Depression of cell mediated immunity in old age and the immunopathic diseases, lupus erythematosus, chronic hepatitis and rheumatoid arthritis, *Clin. Exp. Immunol.* **14**:193–202.

Vessey, M. P., and Doll, R., 1972, Thymectomy and cancer: a follow-up study, *Brit. J. Cancer* **26**:53–58.

Waldorf, D. S., Willkens, R. F., and Decker, J. L., 1968, Impaired delayed hypersensitivity in an aging population. Association with antinuclear reactivity and rheumatoid factor, *J. Amer. Med. Assoc.* **203**:831–834.

Walford, R. L., 1969, *The Immunologic Theory of Aging,* Munksgaard, Copenhagen.

Weksler, M. E., and Hütteroth, T. H., 1974, Impaired lymphocyte function in aged humans, *J. Clin. Invest.* **53**:99–104.

Whittingham, S., Irwin, J., Mackay, I. R., Marsh, S., and Cowling, D. C., 1969, Autoantibodies in healthy subjects, *Aust. Ann. Med.* **18**:130–134.

Wright, J. R., Calkins, E., Breen, W. J., Stolte, G., and Schultz, R. T., 1969, Relationship of amyloid to aging. Review of the literature and systematic study of 83 patients derived from a general hospital population, *Medicine (Baltimore)* **48**:39–60.

5

The Thymus and Aging

1. Introduction

The thymus was an organ of mystery until about 15 years ago when Miller (1961), Good *et al.* (1962), and Jankovic *et al.* (1962), through their neonatal thymectomy studies of experimental animals, revealed that it plays a major role in the development of the immune system. Since then, the thymus has been extensively examined by many investigators. Thus we now know that (a) it is one of the central lymphoid tissues with the ability of transforming bone marrow precursor cells into thymus-derived T cells, and (b) the T cells that migrate out into the various peripheral lymphoid tissues play a major role in immunological surveillance (Burnet, 1970) by participating in (1) the delayed hypersensitivity reaction, (2) foreign graft rejection, (3) resistance against viruses, fungi, and intracellular bacteria, (4) tumor cell immunity, and (5) regulation of immune responses (Good and Gabrielson, 1964).

The thymus begins to involute around the time of sexual maturity in humans and mice (Good and Gabrielson, 1964). Not long thereafter, certain normal immunologic activities will begin to decline (Makinodan *et al.*, 1971), and associated with the decline is an increase in the incidence of certain types of infection, autoimmunity, and cancer (Walford, 1969). These reciprocal phenomena (i.e., fall in immune activity and rise in disease incidence) have prompted many to characterize the cellular nature of age-related decline in immune functions. Their results show that the decline is due primarily to changes in the T cell population (Adler *et al.*, 1971; Konen *et al.*, 1973; Hori *et al.*, 1973; Kishimoto *et al.*, 1969; Goodman and Makinodan, 1975). These age-related sequential events would suggest that thymus involution may be responsible for the decline and, if so, one likely possibility is that as the thymus involutes, it may be losing its ability to transform precursor cells into T cells (Bach *et al.*, 1973; Hirokawa and Makinodan, 1975a).

In view of the above consideration, I wish to focus on age-related morphological and functional changes of the thymus in this chapter. First, there will be a brief discussion on some of the endocrine organs, since hormonal changes extrinsic to

KATSUIKU HIROKAWA • Department of Pathology, Medical Research Institute, Tokyo Medical and Dental University, Yushima, Bunkyo-ku, Tokyo, Japan.

the thymus can be responsible for its involution (Section 2). This will be followed by discussions on morphological and functional changes associated with thymic involution (Sections 3 and 4), since such information is necessary before we can consider the possibility that involution may be due to causes intrinsic to the thymus. The final section will be devoted to the relationship of the thymus, stem cells, and humoral factors to immunologic activities of the aged (Section 5) and consideration that the immune system of the aged experimental animals can be revitalized through cellular therapy.

2. Thymus and Endocrine Organs

The thymus has been assumed to be an endocrine organ for a long time, mainly because of its ontogenetic development from the branchial pouches in a manner similar to that of the parathyroid and the thyroid. However, unlike the parathyroid and the thyroid, definitive evidence that it is, in fact, an endocrine organ has been lacking until recently, in spite of the energetic efforts of many.

Regarding the relationship of the thymus to other endocrine organs, Fabris *et al.* (1972) recently presented convincing evidence that there is an intimate relationship between the thymus and the pituitary in very short-lived hypopituitary dwarf mice. They showed that the abnormal condition of these prematurely aging mice can be corrected by injecting either growth hormone and thyroxin or lymph node cells from normal heterozygous donors. However, it was not effective when the thymus was removed before the injection. These results strongly suggest that thymic function depends on normal production of growth hormone and thyrotropic hormone by the pituitary gland, and thymic involution is closely related to age-related changes in the pituitary and possibly the hypothalamus. Consistent with this view is the observation that the serum level of growth hormone is extremely high in newborn humans when the thymus is growing rapidly and low in adults (Catt, 1971). There are also data suggesting that the thymus may be interacting with the gonads (Nishizuka *et al.,* 1971; Pantelouris, 1972; Vasilakis *et al.,* 1974) and other steroid hormone secreting organs (Dougherty, 1952). However, most of the findings suggest that the growth and involution of the thymus are closely interrelated with the normal function of the endocrine system.

Osoba and Miller (1963) were the first to present convincing evidence that a humoral thymic factor is responsible for T cell maturation. They showed that the impaired immune system of neonatally thymectomized mice can be restored by implanting cell-impermeable Millipore diffusion chambers containing a thymic tissue intraperitoneally. Subsequently, there have been more refined studies demonstrating that the thymus secretes a hormone-like substance that can transform precursor cells to T cells and drive immature T cells further along in their differentiation (see Trainin, 1974).

More recently, a number of laboratories have attempted to extract, purify, and characterize the thymus hormone-like substance; i.e., thymosin (Goldstein *et al.,* 1966), thymic humoral factor (Trainin *et al.,* 1966; Bach *et al.,* 1973) and thymopoietin (Goldstein, G., 1974). However, the biochemical as well as the biological properties of the thymic preparation differ between laboratories.

Studies in aging individuals have been limited to those of Bach *et al.* (1975). They reported that the level of serum thymic activity, measured by the rosette inhibition assay, declines with advancing age in mice, and the decline is accelerated in autoimmune prone mice. These results are quite consistent with morphologic changes associated with aging which will be described in the following sections. However, in our recent studies, injection of thymosin was ineffective in restoring the impaired mitogenic responsiveness of lymphoid cells of old mice (Hirokawa *et al.*, unpublished). This is quite consistent with the observation that the newborn thymus graft alone cannot restore the reduced antisheep RBC response in old mice, which will be discussed in Section 5.

3. Morphology of the Aging Thymus

3.1. Histological Changes

The general pattern of age-related thymus weight change is about the same in mice and humans (Boyd, 1932; Shisa *et al.*, 1971). Thus the thymus of female BC3F$_1$ mice increases in mass very rapidly after birth from 10 mg to its peak of 70 mg at six weeks of age. It then decreases rapidly until six months of age and gradually thereafter throughout life, such that at 36 months of age the thymus weighs only about 5 mg (Figure 1). Weight change can be mainly ascribed to a decrease in the cortex. Histologically, the cortex of an involuted thymus is sparsely populated with lymphocytes and replaced by numerous macrophages filled with lipoid granules (Figure 2). In addition, infiltration of plasma cells and mast cells can be observed in the medulla as well as the cortex. These are characteristic findings in old atrophic thymuses of mice 24 months or older.

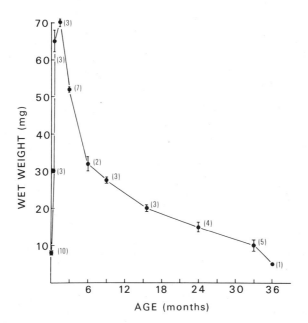

Figure 1. Age-related changes of thymus weight of BC3F$_1$ female mice. Vertical bars, one standard error. Number in parenthesis, sample size. (From Hirokawa and Makinodan, 1975a.)

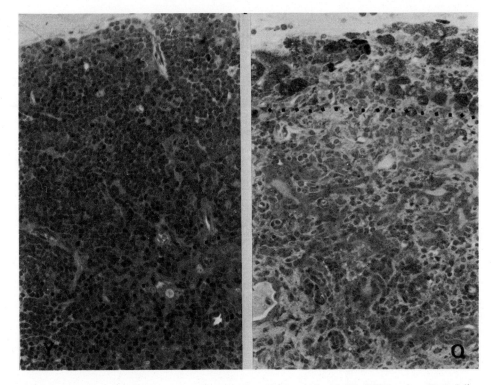

Figure 2. Histology of thymus of 3-month-old (Y) and 33-month-old (O) BC3F$_1$ mice. Dotted line, corticomedullary border. Note the distinct decrease of lymphoid cells and increase of lipoid-laden macrophages in the cortex of old thymus.

In order to determine to what extent an age-related decrease in cortical mass is related to the proliferative activity of the thymocytes, the number of ^{3}H-thymidine pulse-labeled thymocytes was assessed in newborn, 3-, 16-, and 33-month-old mice. The relative number of labeled thymocytes, located primarily in the outer periphery of the cortex, was comparable among newborn, 3-, and 16-month-old thymuses. These findings confirm those of Andreasen *et al.* (1949) and Blau (1972). An additional observation is the sharp reduction in the number of labeled thymocytes in the extremely atrophic thymus of 33-month-old mice. Two explanations can be offered for the latter observation. One is that in very old mice the thymic epithelial cells have lost their ability to produce the T-cell-transforming thymic hormone. The other is that in very old mice the precursor cells in bone marrow are not responsive to the T-cell-transforming thymic hormone.

3.2. Electron Microscopic Changes

The secretory activity of mouse thymic epithelial cells was first suggested by Clark (1966) and Hoshino (1963), who found vesicles containing electron dense granules in them that are electron microscopically characteristic of secretory cells. Similar observations have been made subsequently in other strains and species (Kohnen and Weiss, 1964; Kameya and Watanabe, 1965; Hirokawa, 1969; Mandel,

1970). To test the notion of whether age affects the secretory activity of thymic epithelial cells, newborn to 33-month-old thymuses were examined electron microscopically. The basic structure of young thymus (Figure 3) is a spongy meshwork composed of epithelial cells, dense in the medulla, coarse in the cortex, and packed with thymocytes. At the periphery and around the vascular areas, the thymic parenchyma is separated by a thin basement membrane. Such a basic structure is well maintained until 16 months of age. However, in the atrophic thymus at 24 months and older, distinct structural changes occur (Figure 3), i.e., splitting of the meshwork of epithelial cells into small nests by infiltrating macrophages, plasma cells, lymphocytes, and fibroblasts. Most of these epithelial cellular nests do not contain thymocytes, and they are still separated from the infiltrating cells by a basement membrane. In addition, each nest contains intercellular cysts bordered with microvilli (Figure 4), which could be reflective of the branchial origin of the thymus. Thus the intimate contact between thymocytes and epithelial cells, characteristic of a young thymus, is absent in the old atrophic thymus, and in its place we find small clusters of membrane-bordered epithelial cells devoid of or with limited numbers of thymocytes.

The secretory epithelial cells can be classified into two types. One possesses vesicles (0.3–1.0 μm in diameter) with cilia-like or microvillous structures packed with a fine granular substance of moderate electron density (Figure 5). The other

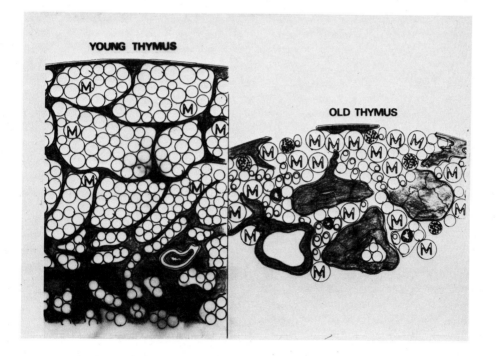

Figure 3. Electron microscopic schema of young and old thymus. ◯, lymphoid cells; M, macrophages; dotted circles, mast cells; ovals, plasma cells. Note disruption of meshwork of epithelial cells in the old thymus.

KATSUIKU
HIROKAWA

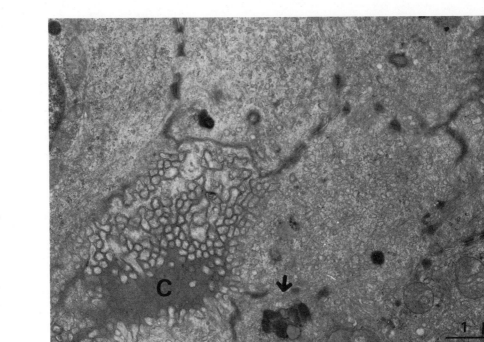

Figure 4. Electron microscopy of thymic epithelial cells of a 33-month-old BC3F₁ female mouse. Note that the cells are interconnected with each other through many desmosomes and are rich in small vesicles. Two intercellular cysts (C) with microvilli and lysosomal bodies (arrow) are observed (× 18,000).

also possesses vesicles of the same size, but they contain a small amount of coarse granular or membranous substance of moderate electron density (Figure 6). The former type is almost exclusively observed in the medulla of newborn thymus when the thymic activity is most active, for it is rarely seen in the thymus after one month of age. The latter type, which is found mainly in the cortex, is observed in thymus of all ages, but the quantity is reduced in atrophic thymus of 24 months and older. At around 16 months, irregular vesicles packed with coarse granular substance of high electron density emerge (Figure 7), increasing in number with advancing age. Occasionally, electron-dense microbodies or crystals can be seen, some of which are coalesced with lipoidal substances in the old atrophic thymus (Figure 8). Ordinary secretory organelles, like the Golgi apparatus and smooth-surfaced small vesicles, do not seem to change markedly with age.

The thymic epithelial cell of the first type, which is, in many respects, very similar to the cystic cell of Mandel (1970) and the inclusion cell of Smith (1965), is the most likely candidate as the hormone secreting cell. Since old atrophic thymus still possesses a limited immunological potential (as will be discussed later) the possibility exists that the second type of epithelial cell may also possess hormone secreting capacity; if so, it should be less efficient than the first type. It is my suspicion that vesicles with electron dense granules and crystals, which are found only in the atrophic thymus, are storage sites for denatured thymic hormones or their precursors. It is of interest to note that a similar type of crystal has been

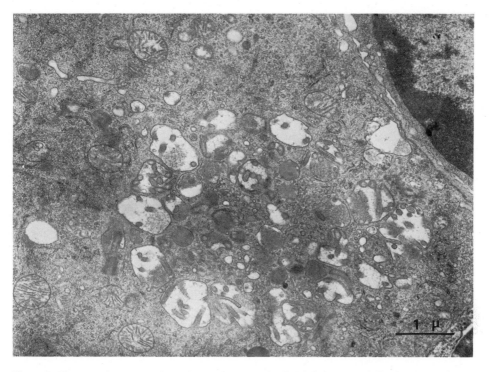

Figure 5. Electron microscopy of putatively secretory epithelial cells in the medulla of newborn thymus (× 18,000).

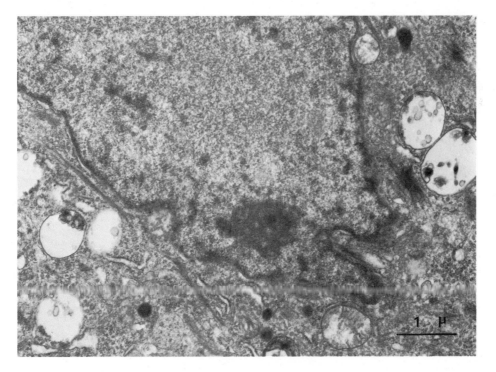

Figure 6. Electron microscopy of epithelial cell in the cortex of the newborn thymus. Note vesicles containing a small amount of coarse granular or membranous substance (× 18,000).

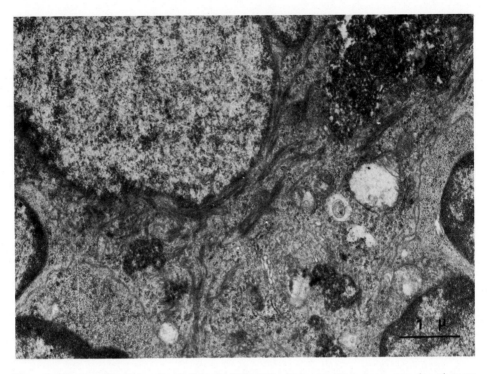

Figure 7. Electron microscopy of epithelial cell of 29-month-old thymus. Note coarse granular substance in the cytoplasm (× 18,000).

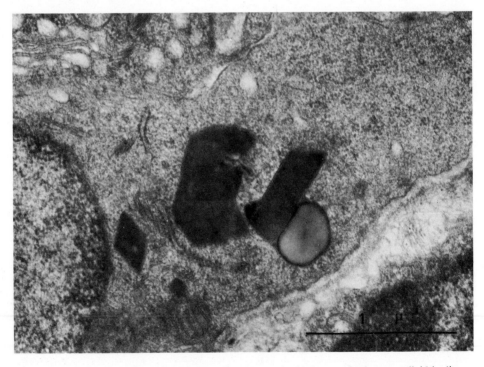

Figure 8. Electron microscopy of epithelial cell of 33-month-old thymus, having crystalloid bodies (× 45,000).

observed in the thymus of autoimmune prone Swan mice, whose thymic function is known to decline earlier in life than normal mice (Schmitt *et al.*, 1974).

4. The Differentiation Potential of Thymus of Aging Individuals

Until recently, there have been only a few brief reports on the functional capacity of aged thymus. Thus Davies (1969), in his review of the thymus, commented that old thymus grafts can facilitate immunologic recovery of X-irradiated animals. A few years later, Yunis *et al.* (1972), in their review on autoimmunity and aging, reported that the allogeneic skin graft rejecting capacity of neonatally thymectomized mice, reconstituted with an old thymus graft, is less than those reconstituted with a young thymus graft. They further reported that the relative restorative capacity of an old thymus graft is in part dependent upon the strain of mice; e.g., it is lower in autoimmunity prone strains than in nonautoimmunity prone strains (Yunis *et al.*, 1973).

The purpose of this section is to determine to what extent age-related degenerative changes of the thymus affect its capacity to influence the maturation of precursor cells into T cells.

4.1. Methods of Assessment

One thymic lobe from donor mice, ranging in age from one day to 33 months, was implanted under the kidney capsule of a T-cell-deprived, syngeneic, young adult recipient mouse (thymectomized, X-irradiated, and reconstituted with bone marrow cells), which will be referred to hereafter as a TXB mouse. The emergence of T cells was assessed kinetically by various morphological and functional indices, which may be reflective of different T cell subpopulations (Figure 9).

The grafted thymus undergoes necrosis within a few days after the implantation, but within a week regeneration of thymic epithelial cells of donor origin can be detected. Donor thymocytes present in the grafted thymus can also regenerate but they seem to possess only a limited proliferative potential, for it has been shown that they are completely replaced by host cells within three weeks (Dukor *et al.*, 1965). This means that donor lymphocytes cannot contribute to the T cell population one or more months after thymic implantation. Thus it is clear that in the studies to be discussed, the number and functional activity of T cells one to three months after thymic implantation are reflective of T cells of host bone marrow origin that have emerged under the influence of the grafted donor thymic epithelial cells.

4.2. Morphology of the Thymus Graft

The size of the grafted thymus lobe is mainly dependent on the number of thymocytes, and the number of thymocytes is assumed to be dependent on the relative activity of thymic epithelial cells. If so, the difference in size of the grafts should be proportional to the difference in the activity of thymic epithelial cells.

Twelve weeks after the implantation, the size of the transplanted thymic tissue from donors ranging in age from one day to 33 months tends to be smaller as the age of the donor increases (Figure 10). This would suggest that the activity of thymic

KATSUIKU
HIROKAWA

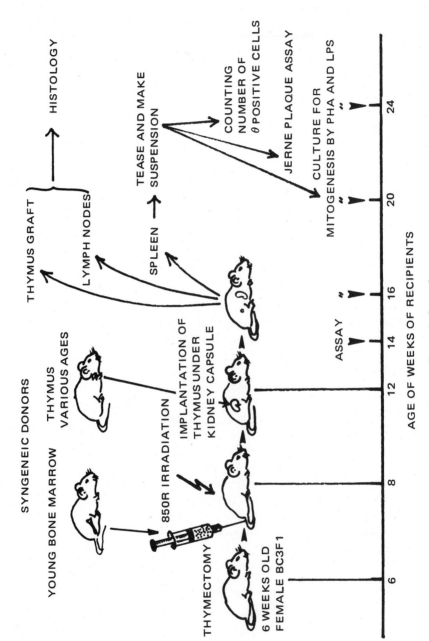

Figure 9. Protocol of experiment.

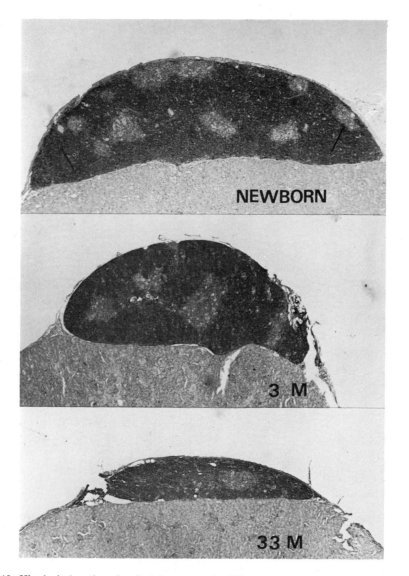

Figure 10. Histological section of grafted thymuses under kidney capsule. Top, newborn; middle, three-month-old thymus; bottom, 33-month-old thymus.

epithelial cells is declining with age. Nevertheless, it is apparent that even grafts from 33-month-old donor mice are reasonably well repopulated with many thymocytes. This indicates that the degenerated thymic stroma from old mice, when transplanted in a young environment, can become active. To verify this notion that epithelial cells of the old thymic graft are being revitalized in the young host environment, some of the old thymic grafts were observed under the electron microscope. Irregular vesicles, packed with coarse granular substances of high electron density, a characteristic landmark of an old atrophic thymus, disappeared and were replaced by more regular secretory vesicles containing a granular sub-

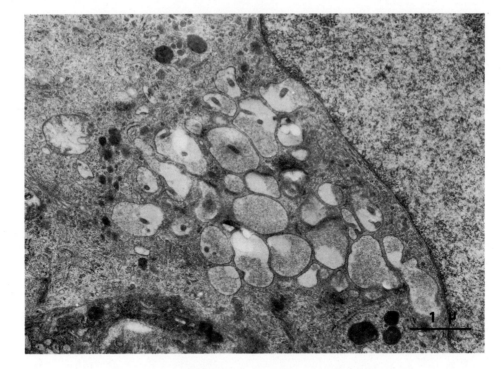

Figure 11. Electron microscopy of epithelial cell of 24-month-old thymus grafted in young TXB mouse. Note a cluster of vesicles with microvilli projections, surrounded by dense bodies of various size (× 18,000).

stance of moderate electron density, which may be characteristic of a putatively active secretory cell (Figure 11).

4.3. Repopulation of the Spleen and Lymph Nodes

The T-cell-dependent areas (Parrott *et al.,* 1966) of the spleen and lymph nodes of TXB mice were histologically examined 4, 8, and 12 weeks after the implantation of thymic tissues from donors of various ages. The periarteriolar areas of spleen were repopulated with lymphocytes by four weeks, and distinct differences were not apparent with respect to the age of thymus donors. In contrast, the paracortical areas of mesenteric and subcutaneous lymph nodes were repopulated with lymphocytes only in those TXB recipients bearing a newborn thymus graft; i.e., the thymus of mice three months and older have apparently lost their capacity to generate lymph-node-seeking T cells (Figure 12), but not spleen-seeking T cells. Some irreversible changes could have occurred in the thymic epithelial cells sometime between one day and three months of age such that they could no longer secrete a differentiation factor(s) that endows T cells with the ability to home into the peripheral lymph nodes. It is of interest to note that cellular characteristics of thymocytes, such as electrophoretic mobility (Dumont, 1974) and responsiveness to Con A (Stobo and Paul, 1972) and PHA (Byrd *et al.,* 1973), were reported to undergo quantitative changes shortly after birth or during the juvenile growth phase of life. In any event, the findings reported here are compatible with the view that

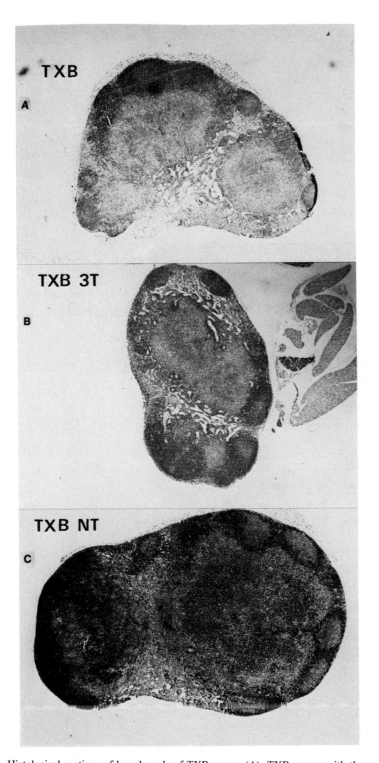

Figure 12. Histological sections of lymph node of TXB mouse (A), TXB mouse with three-month-old thymus graft (B), and TXB mouse with newborn thymus graft (C).

peripheralization of lymphocytes from the thymus occurs during the very early phase of life when the thymus is most active (Linna, 1968; Joel *et al.*, 1972) and, moreover, can explain why wasting syndrome occurs when thymectomy is performed shortly after the birth but not later.

4.4. Splenic θ^+ Lymphocytes

Kinetic assessment of the total number of splenic θ^+ cells revealed that newborn thymus grafts are most effective in generating θ^+ cells as judged by the indirect immunofluorescence method of Cerottini and Brunner (1967). Overall, the results (Figure 13) indicate that the capacity of the thymus graft to transform precursor bone marrow cells into spleen-seeking T cells decreases with advancing age, but that even the very atrophic old thymus graft of 33-month-old mice still possesses this capacity.

4.5. Splenic Antisheep RBC Response

A preliminary experiment was performed to determine what donor age interval would be most desirable to study the effect of age of graft on T-cell-dependent

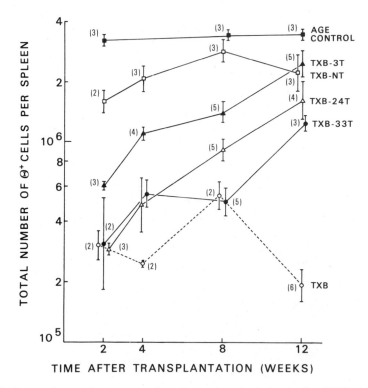

Figure 13. Influence of age of the thymus graft on the number of splenic θ^+ cells of TXB recipient mice at various intervals after transplantation. Vertical bars, one standard error; number in parenthesis, sample size; age control, sham-thymectomized unirradiated mice; TXB-NT, TXB mice with newborn thymus graft; TXB-3T, TXB mice with three-month-old thymus graft; TXB-24T, TXB mice with 24-month-old thymus graft; TXB-33T, TXB mice with 33-month-old thymus graft.

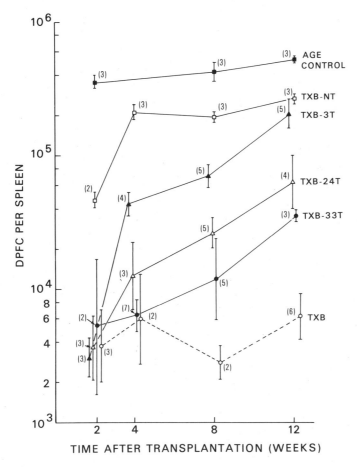

Figure 14. Influence of age of the thymic graft on the recovery rate of splenic T-cell-dependent antisheep RBC response of TXB recipient mice. Thymus-grafted TXB mice were given 10^9 sheep RBC i.p. at various intervals after transplantation and their spleens were assessed for DPFC 4.5 days later. Vertical bars, one standard error; number in parenthesis, sample size.

antisheep red blood cells (RBC) humoral response (Hirokawa and Makinodan, 1975a). It was found that antibody response decreases with an increase in age of the thymus donor such that only a minimal difference is noted among TXB recipient mice bearing a thymus graft from 3-, 6-, and 12-month-old donors. Consequently, in the subsequent experiment, thymus grafts from newborn, 3-, 24-, and 33-month-old donors were tested at varying intervals after thymic implantation. The results revealed that the pattern of recovery of T-cell-dependent humoral immune activity (Figure 14) is remarkably similar to that of the total number of θ^+ splenic T cells, with a coefficient of correlation of 0.79. However, it should be emphasized that a significant rise in activity was detected at 12 weeks even in TXB mice bearing the 33-month-old atrophic thymus graft.

Two explanations can be offered as to why the number of splenic θ^+ cells and the splenic T-cell-dependent humoral immune activity failed to reach the level of the control in 12 weeks. One possibility is that a single lobe is not adequate to reconstitute TXB mice (Davies, 1969). Another is that lethal X-irradiation may have irreversibly altered certain tissue functions that are essential for full restoration of splenic T cells. Obviously, recovery patterns extending beyond 12 weeks would be desirable.

4.6. Mitogenic Response of Splenic T Cells to PHA, s-Con A, and Allogeneic Lymphocytes

Two experiments were carried out. In the first experiment, a portion of the spleen used in the T-cell-dependent humoral immune response study was processed for mitogenic activity in response to PHA and s-Con A; i.e., spleens that had been removed 4.5 days after SRBC injection at each of the four time intervals (2, 4, 8, and 12 weeks) after thymic implantation. The results (Figure 15) show that recovery pattern of splenic T cells responsive to T-cell-specific mitogens are quite different from those of the total number of splenic θ^+ cells and T-cell-dependent humoral immune response. Full recovery of mitogenic responsiveness is seen only in TXB-NT mice, while in all other groups recovery after 12 weeks is only 10–20% of the control. Moreover, the magnitude of recovery in these latter groups appears to be inversely related to the age of thymic graft donors.

Because there is the possibility that splenic T cells stimulated *in situ* with SRBC beforehand may not respond maximally to PHA and s-Con A *in vitro* 4.5 days later, a second experiment was carried out involving the use of spleens of thymus-grafted TXB mice that had not been exposed previously to SRBC. In this experiment, TXB-NT, TXB-3T, and TXB-33T mice, in addition to control TXB and sham-thymectomized, nonirradiated mice, were tested eight weeks after thymic implantation. Five indices were assessed of individual spleens: PHA, s-Con A, LPS, MLC, and *in vitro* DPFC. The results (Figure 16) show that the age-related decline in PHA and s-Con A indices is comparable to that of mice that had been previously exposed to SRBC, indicating the *in situ* SRBC stimulation 4.5 days beforehand had a minimal effect on the *in vitro* mitogenic responsiveness of T cells. In contrast to the age-related decline in mitogenic response of splenic T cells to plant lectins, the mitogenic response to allogeneic lymphocytes is comparable to the control, regardless of the age of thymic graft donors. These same spleens show a decrease with age in their *in vitro* DPFC response index, which is comparable to that observed *in vivo*. The LPS index, which is reflective of a B cell mitogenic activity, is the same in all five groups, indicating that the B cell population can be fully reconstituted in TXB mice without further treatment (Peavy *et al.*, 1974). This would indicate that the T cells, and not the B cells, are the limiting cells in thymus-grafted mice undergoing anti-SRBC response. So far as T cells are concerned, these thymus-grafted TXB mice are comparable to normal adult mice (Groves *et al.*, 1970).

The correlation is poor between the recovery patterns of the number of splenic θ^+ lymphocytes and the responsiveness of splenic lymphocytes to T-cell-specific mitogens and to allogeneic lymphocytes (or MLC reaction) on the one hand, and good between the recovery patterns of the number of splenic θ^+ cells and the splenic T-cell-dependent humoral immune response on the other hand. Two explanations can be offered for these relationships. One possibility is that each of the functional indices may reflect a unique, or overlapping, functional property of T cells. That is,

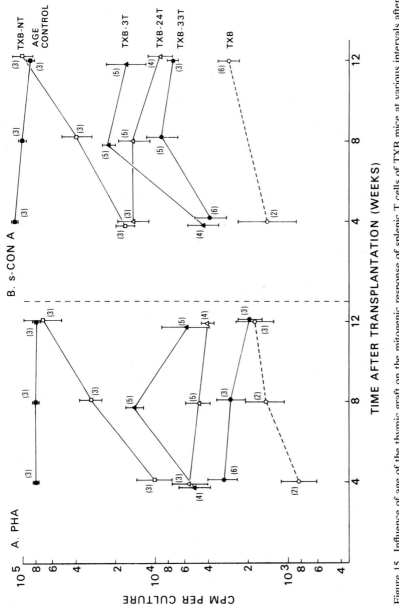

Figure 15. Influence of age of the thymic graft on the mitogenic response of splenic T cells of TXB mice at various intervals after transplantation. Vertical bars, one standard error; number in parenthesis, sample size.

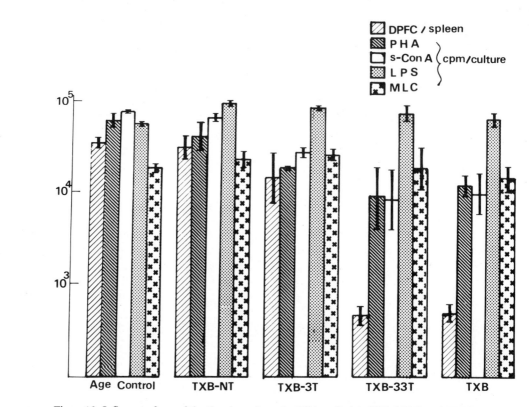

Figure 16. Influence of age of the thymic graft on the PHA, s-Con A, LPS, MLC, and DPFC response indices of TXB recipient mice eight weeks after transplantation. Vertical bars, one standard error.

proliferation is not obligatory in certain types of functions, such as response to SRBC, but is obligatory in other functions, such as response to PHA and s-Con A. If so, these results would suggest that as far as spleen-seeking T cells are concerned, the thymus is losing certain thymic transforming capacities with age. Another possibility, which is not necessarily mutually exclusive of the first explanation, is that suppressor cells (Gershon *et al.*, 1972) are being generated under the influence of the thymus whose activity varies, depending upon the immunologic function. With regard to the MLC index of splenic cells, it should be noted that while T cells are essential for the initiation of the reaction, B and "null" (non-B and non-T lymphocytes) cells present in the culture also could have undergone mitosis (Adler *et al.*, 1970; Harrison *et al.*, 1973) in response to stimulants released by the activated T cells. This could account for the minimal age dependency of this index, since the stimulator cells interacting with the responder spleen cells would be minimally effected by age.

The results presented in this section show that the generation of functional T cells by grafted thymic tissues in TXB mice generally decreased with the age of the graft. The differences in the patterns of recovery of various functional activities of thymus-grafted TXB mice suggest that the extent to which T cells can mature is related to the degree of thymic involution. In particular, thymic tissues lose, with advancing age, the ability to influence the following T-cell-differentiation steps:

first, the influence on T cells to home into T-cell-dependent areas of lymph nodes; second, the influence on splenic T cells to respond mitogenetically to T-cell-specific mitogens, PHA and s-Con A; third, the influence on splenic T cells to "help" B cells in their response to SRBC; and fourth, the influence on splenic T cells to respond mitogenetically to allogeneic lymphocytes.

Based on these initial kinetic findings, it is clear that the problem on the underlying nature of age-related thymic involution appears most formidable. Nevertheless, it is encouraging that atrophic thymus from 33-month-old mice can be rejuvenated, at least partially, when transplanted into young recipients, indicating that there may be a reasonable approach to this problem.

5. The Thymus, Bone Marrow, and Humoral Factors in Aging

In the preceding sections, discussion was focused on the T-cell-differentiation capacity of aging thymus in a young humoral environment with young precursor cells; i.e., a TXB mouse. In contrast to the T cells whose PHA and s-Con A induced proliferative activity falls off dramatically with age (e.g., Hori *et al.*, 1973), the total number of stem cells in the bone marrow remains relatively constant throughout life (Chen, 1971). Therefore it would be desirable to know what role the age of T cell precursors plays in the differentiation of T cells. Accordingly, young female $BC3F_1$ mice (three months old) were x-irradiated (850 R) and reconstituted with equivalent numbers of stem cells from young (three months old, 5×10^6 bone marrow cells) and old (24 months old, 10×10^6 bone marrow cells) (Hirokawa and Makinodan, 1975b). Splenic antisheep RBC response was examined at 2, 4, 8, and 12 weeks after the treatment and a fraction of the spleens was processed for mitogenic activity in response to PHA and LPS.

Preliminary results suggest that B cells arising from old bone marrow cells still possess defects even after they were cultured in a young host environment, but T cells arising from old bone marrow cells under the influence of young thymus and young host environment are quite active.

The next issue to resolve was to what extent age of the host humoral environment influences immune responses. Accordingly, a preliminary study with limited numbers of 27-month-old female $BC3F_1$ mice were separated into four groups and treated as follows: (a) old mice without any treatment as control; (b) old mice implanted with one lobe of newborn thymus under the kidney capsule; (c) old mice, sublethally irradiated and reconstituted with 5×10^6 three-month-old bone marrow cells; and (d) old mice, sublethally irradiated and reconstituted with three-month-old bone marrow cells, followed one month later by implantation of one lobe of newborn thymus. In addition, three-month-old intact, normal mice were used as another control. *In situ* T-cell-dependent antisheep RBC response was determined three months after the irradiation (Hirokawa and Makinodan, 1975b). The results suggested the following:

1. If the thymus is old, the immunological response is generally low, even in a young host environment and in the presence of young bone marrow stem cells.
2. If the thymus and host environment are young, the response is generally high, even in the presence of old bone marrow stem cells.

3. The low response in old host environment can be enhanced by the combined presence of young thymus and young bone marrow stem cells.

The results are obviously still preliminary and many other immunological indices need to be examined.

Previously, Metcalf *et al.* (1961) reported that single or multiple thymus grafts in old A/J mice failed to prevent the age-related decline in responsiveness to SRBC. This is quite consistent with the result of group (b), which revealed that a newborn thymus graft alone could not enhance the low response in old mice. Several authors (Yunis *et al.,* 1972; Kysela and Steinberg, 1973) reported that thymus grafting could improve the diseased condition of autoimmune, disease-prone, short-lived NZB mice, but only temporarily and increase their survival only slightly. The preliminary findings reported here indicate that thymus grafting alone may not be adequate to fully restore the immune activity of these short-lived immunodeficient mice.

6. Summary

The thymus of long-lived BC3F$_1$ mice involutes progressively throughout life, beginning at about six weeks of age. This involution process does not seem to be an independent phenomenon, but rather it is dependent on other endocrine organs. Morphological and functional findings were obtained, indicating that the T cell transforming influence of thymic tissues generally decreases as the thymus involutes. Morphologically, the most active secretory structure seemed to be limited exclusively to the newborn thymus. Certain structural changes, reflective of a decline in secretory function, can also be detected early in life and they become more pronounced with age.

Functionally, the magnitude of decline in thymic influence on T cell differentiation depends on the immunologic index. In particular, thymic tissue loses its capacity to influence the following functions with advancing age: (a) lymphocyte repopulation of the T-cell-dependent areas of lymph nodes; (b) mitogenic reactivity of splenic cells to T-cell-specific mitogens (PHA and s-Con A); (c) splenic T cell helper function in a humoral response; and (d) mitogenic reactivity of splenic T cells to allogeneic lymphocytes. It should be emphasized that even the very old and atrophic thymus still possesses certain T cell transforming potential.

The three key factors which determine the magnitude of immunologic activity of the aged are the thymus, the bone marrow, and the humoral environment. Of these, the thymus is the most limiting factor in the aged.

Finally, studies in progress indicate that the immunologic activities of old mice can be enhanced effectively by the combined grafting of the young thymus and young bone marrow stem cells.

References

Adler, W. H., Takiguchi, T., Marsh, B., and Smith, T. T., 1970, Cellular recognition by mouse lymphocytes in vitro. 2. Specific stimulation by histocompatibility antigens in mixed cell culture, *J. Immunol.* **105**:948–1000.
Adler, W. H., Takiguchi, T., and Smith, T. T., 1971, Effect of age upon primary alloantigen recognition by mouse spleen, *J. Immunol.* **107**:1357–1362.
Adler, W. H., 1974, personal communication.

Andreasen, E., and Christensen, S., 1949, Rate of mitotic activity in lymphoid organs of rat, *Anat. Record* **103**:401–412.

Bach, F. J., Dardenne, M., and Salomon, J. C., 1973, Studies on thymus products. IV. Absence of serum thymic activity in adult NZB and (NZB × NZW)F1 mice, *Clin. Exp. Immunol.* **14**:247–256.

Bach, F. J., Dardenne, M., Pleau, J. M., and Bach, M. A., 1975, Isolation, biochemical characteristics, and biological activity of a circulating thymic hormone in the mouse and in the human, *Ann. N.Y. Acad. Sci.* **249**:186–210.

Blau, J. N., 1972, DNA synthesis in the adult and ageing guinea pig thymus, *Clin. Exp. Immunol.* **11**:461–468.

Boyd, E., 1932, The weight of the thymus gland in health and in disease, *Amer. J. Diseases Children* **43**:1162–1214.

Burnet, F. M., 1970, *Immunological Surveillance,* Pergamon Press, Oxford, England.

Byrd, W. J., von Boehmer, H., and Ponse, B. T., 1973, The role of the thymus in maturational development of phytohemagglutinin and pokeweed mitogen responsiveness, *Cellular Immunol.* **6**:12–24.

Catt, K. J., 1971, *An ABC of Endocrinology,* Little, Brown and Company, Boston.

Cerottini, J. C., and Brunner, K. T., 1967, Localization of mouse isoantigens on the cell surface as revealed by immunofluorescence, *Immunology* **13**:395–403.

Chen, M. G., 1971, Age-related changes in hematopoietic stem cell populations of a long-lived hybrid mouse, *J. Cellular Physiol.* **78**:225–232.

Clark, S. L., Jr., 1966, Cytological evidences of secretion in the thymus, in: *Thymus: Experimental and Clinical Studies* (Ciba Fdn. Symp.), pp. 3–29, Churchill, London.

Davies, A. J. S., 1969, The thymus and the cellular basis of immunity, *Transplant. Rev.* **1**:43–91.

Dougherty, T. F., 1952, Effect of hormones on lymphatic tissue, *Physiol. Rev.* **32**:379–401.

Dukor, P., Miller, J. F. A. P., House, W., and Allman, V., 1965, Regeneration of thymus graft. 1. Histological and cytological aspects, *Transplantation* **3**:639–668.

Dumont, F., 1974, Electrophoretic analysis of cell subpopulation in the mouse thymus as a function of age, *Immunology* **26**:1051–1057.

Fabris, N., Pierpaoli, W., and Sorkin, E., 1972, Lymphocytes, hormones and ageing, *Nature* **240**:557–559.

Gershon, R. K., Cohen, P., Honcin, R., and Liebhaber, S. A., 1972, Suppressor T cells, *J. Immunol.* **108**:586–590.

Goldstein, A. L., Slater, F. D., and White, A., 1966, Preparation, assay and partial purification of thymic lymphocytopoietic factor (thymosin), *Proc. Nat. Acad. Sci. U.S.* **56**:1010–1017.

Goldstein, G., 1974, Isolation of bovine thymin: a polypeptide hormone of the thymus, *Nature* **247**:11–14.

Good, R. A., and Gabrielson, A. B., (eds.), 1964, *Thymus in Immunobiology,* Hoeber-Harper, New York.

Good, R. A., Dalmasso, A. P., Martinez, C., Archer, O. K., Pierce, J. C., and Papermaster, B. W., 1962, The role of the thymus in development of immunologic capacity in rabbits and mice, *J. Exp. Med.* **116**:773–796.

Goodman, S. A., and Makinodan, T., 1975, Effect of age on cell-mediated immunity in long-lived mice, *Clin. Exp. Immunol.* **19**:533–542.

Groves, D. L., Lever, W. E., and Makinodan, T., 1970, A model for the interaction of cell types in the generation of hemolytic plaque forming cells, *J. Immunol.* **104**:148–165.

Harrison, M. R., and Paul, W. E., 1973, Stimulus response in the mixed leucocyte response, *J. Exp. Med.* **138**:1602–1607.

Hirokawa, K., 1969, Electron microscopic observation of the human thymus of the fetus and the newborn, *Acta Pathol. Japonica* **19**:1–13.

Hirokawa, K., and Makinodan, T., 1975a, Thymic involution: Effect on T cell differentiation, *J. Immunol.* **114**:1659–1664.

Hirokawa, K., and Makinodan, T., 1975b, Role of thymus, bone marrow stem cells, and humoral factors on age-associated decline in normal immune response, *Proceedings of the 10th International Congress of Gerontology,* **2**:19.

Hori, Y., Perkins, E. H., and Halsall, M. K., 1973, Decline in phytohemagglutinin responsiveness of spleen cells from aging mice, *Proc. Soc. Exp. Biol. Med.* **144**:48–53.

Hoshino, T., 1963, Electron microscopic studies of the epithelial reticular cells of the mouse thymus, *Z. Zellforsch.* **59**:513–529.

Jankovic, B. D., Waksman, B. H., and Arnason, B. G., 1962, Role of the thymus in immune reactions in rats. I. The immunologic response of bovine serum albumin (antibody formation, Arthus reactivity, and delayed hypersensitivity) in rats thymectomized or splenectomized at various times after birth, *J. Exp. Med.* **116**:159–176.

Joel, D. D., Hess, M. W., and Cottier, H., 1972, Magnitude and pattern of thymic migration to neonatal mice, *J. Exp. Med.* **135**:907–923.

Kameya, T., and Watanabe, Y., 1965, Electron microscopic observations on human thymus and thymona, *Acta Pathol. Jap.* **15**:223–246.

Kishimoto, S., Tsuyuguchi, I., and Yamamura, 1969, Immune response in aged mice, *Clin. Exp. Immunol.* **5**:525–530.

Kohnen, P., and Weiss, L., 1964, An electron microscopic study of thymic corpuscles in the guinea pig and the mouse, *Anat. Record* **148**:29–58.

Konen, T. G., Smith, G. S., and Walford, R. L., 1973, Decline in mixed lymphocyte reactivity of spleen cells from aged mice of a long-lived strain, *J. Immunol.* **110**:1216–1221.

Kysela, S., and Steinberg, A. D., 1973, Increased survival of NZB/W mice given multiple syngeneic young thymus grafts, *Clin. Immunol. Immunopath.* **2**:133–136.

Linna, T. J., 1968, Cell migration from the thymus to other lymphoid organs in hamsters of different ages, *Blood* **31**:727–746.

Makinodan, T., Perkins, E. H., and Chen, M. G., 1971, Immunologic activity of the aged, *Adv. Gerontol. Res.* **3**:171–198.

Mandel, T., 1970, Differentiation of epithelial cells in mouse thymus, *Z. Zellforsch.*, **106**:498–515.

Metcalf, D., Sparrow, N., Nakamura, K., and Ishidate, M., 1961, The behavior of thymus grafts in high and low leukemia strains of mice, *Aust. J. Exp. Biol.* **39**:441–454.

Miller, J. F. A. P., 1961, Immunological function of the thymus, *Lancet* **2**:748–749.

Nishizuka, Y., and Sakura, T., 1971, Ovarian dysgenesis induced by neonatal thymectomy in the mouse, *Endocrinology* **89**:886–893.

Osoba, D., and Miller, J. F. A. P., 1963, Evidences for a humoral thymus factor responsible for the maturation of immunological faculty, *Nature* **199**:653–654.

Pantelouris, E. M., 1972, Thymic involution and ageing: a hypothesis, *Exp. Gerontol.* **7**:73–81.

Parrott, D. M. W., de Sousa, M. A. B., and East, J., 1966, Thymus dependent areas in the lymphoid organs of neonatally thymectomized mice, *J. Exp. Med.* **123**:191–204.

Peavy, D. L., Adler, W. H., Shands, J. W., and Smith, R. T., 1974, Selective effects of mitogens on subpopulations of mouse lymphoid cells, *Cellular Immunol.* **11**:86–98.

Schmitt, D., and Monier, J. C., 1974, Crystalline inclusions observed in the cytoplasm of thymic epithelial cells of Swan mice with high anti-nuclear autoantibody titers, *J. Int. Res. Comm.* **2**:1250.

Shisa, H., and Nishizuka, Y., 1971, Determining role of age and thymus in pathology of 7-12-dimethyl-benzanthracene-induced leukemia in mice, *Gann* **62**:407–412.

Smith, C., 1965, Studies on the thymus of the mammal. XIV. Histology and histochemistry of embryonic and early postnatal thymuses of C57BL/6 and AKR strain mice, *Am. J. Anat.* **116**:611–621.

Stobo, J. D., and Paul, W. E., 1972, Functional heterogeneity of murine lymphoid cells. II. Acquisition of mitogen responsiveness and of theta antigen during the ontogeny of thymocytes and "T" lymphocytes, *Cellular Immunol.* **4**:367–380.

Trainin, N., 1974, Thymic hormones and the immune response, *Physiol. Rev.* **54**:272–315.

Trainin, N., Bejerano, A., Strahelevitch, M., Goldring, D., and Small, M., 1966. A thymic factor preventing wasting and influencing lymphopoiesis in mice, *Israel J. Med. Sci.* **2**:549–559.

Yunis, E. J., Fernandes, G., Teague, P. O., Stutman, O., and Good, R. A., 1972, Thymus, autoimmunity and the involution of the lymphoid system, in: *Tolerance, Autoimmunity and Aging* (M. M. Siegel and R. A. Good, eds.), pp. 62–119, Charles C Thomas, Springfield, Illinois.

Yunis, E. J., Fernandes, G., Smith, J., Stutman, O., and Good, R. A., 1973, Involution of thymus dependent lymphoid system, *Adv. Exp. Med. Biol.* **29**:301–306.

Vasilakis, G., Kunz, H. W., and Gill, T. J., III, 1974, The effect of gonadectomy on antibody production by inbred rats, *Int. Arch. Allergy Appl. Immunol.* **47**:730–736.

Walford, R. L., 1969, *The Immunologic Theory of Aging,* Munksgaard, Copenhagen.

6

Hormones and Aging

NICOLA FABRIS

1. Life Expectancy and Hormonal Environment

A number of investigations, reviewed in other chapters of this book, have documented the decline in immune function that occurs with advancing age.

The use of different mitogens as probes of lymphocyte function in terms of cell division and different antigens to evaluate the integrity of some multicellular processes has produced results that suggest that the age-related decline of immunological vigor is particularly evident at the level of the thymus-dependent system. Furthermore, the "overseer" role played by the T cell through the modulation of its helper or suppressor activity in its interaction with B cells (Gershon, 1974), as well as the B-dependent suppression of potentially self-reactive cells (Phillips and Wegman, 1973), have offered an explanation of the link between immunological failure and increased autoimmune phenomena observed in aged individuals (Rowley and MacKay, 1969; Walford, 1969).

These findings are consistent with the idea of a progressive reduction with age either of the number of immunocompetent units or of proliferative capacity and/or differentiated lymphoid cells (Price and Makinodan, 1972a; Heidrick and Makinodan, 1972; Gerbase-DeLima et al., 1974; Walford, 1974; Goodman and Makinodan, 1975). Such an age-dependent immunodeficiency may stem from a genetic program (Yunis et al., 1975), which may express itself through either a programmed limited number of doublings of a dividing cell population (Hayflick, 1966; Williamson and Askonas, 1972) or through any one of the different hypotheses proposed to explain basic aging phenomena (Spiegel, 1972), although the majority of these lack immunological evidence.

While it is likely that longevity is genetically determined, it is not equally proved that the time needed to exhaust its own quota of genetic programming is chronologically defined. Some particular macroenvironmental conditions, such as caloric undernutrition during early life in rats (McCay, 1952; Stuchlíková et al., 1975) and mild lowering of body temperature in poikilothermic animals, especially during the last half of life (Liu and Walford, 1972, 1975), prolong life span and delay

NICOLA FABRIS   •   Experimental Gerontology Center, INRCA, Ancona, Italy.

the age-related decline of some immunological functions (Walford *et al.,* 1973, 1974).

Even at tissue level it has been proven that some tissue or cells may survive beyond their normal life expectancy, provided, however, that these cells or tissues are serially transplanted into syngeneic young recipients (Krohn, 1966; Hoshino and Gardner, 1967). Also, lymphocytes can survive well beyond the normal life span of the species from which they derive, again, provided that these cells are serially transplanted into syngeneic young recipients (Barnes *et al.,* 1959). On the other hand, if we consider the actual potentiality of lymphoid cells from old individuals, it seems well demonstrated that they may perform better when inoculated into a young environment (Price and Makinodan, 1972b) or treated *in vivo* with polyribonucleotides (Braun *et al.,* 1970) or *in vitro* with a "thymic hormone" preparation (Friedman *et al.,* 1974).

These findings suggest that the life expectancy and the actual performance of some cells, lymphocytes included, can be appreciably modified and that such a modification may be markedly dependent on internal environmental conditions.

In the light of these considerations, the physiological neuroendocrine homeostatic mechanisms, which affect the proliferation and/or differentiation of the lymphoid system may well be involved in the progressive decline of immunological functions with advancing age. Although the experimental evidence indicates that relatively little change occurs in endocrine function with age in terms of the secretory capacity of endocrine glands and metabolism of hormones (Timiras, 1972), it is to be taken into account that, as homeostatic mechanisms are complex and involve integration at several levels, even a minor alteration in these integrative mechanisms will lead to significant impairment of adaptive response. Yet the synthesis of some hormones, such as insulin, steroids, and pituitary gonadotropins, is definitely altered in aged individuals (Timiras and Meisami, 1972). A progressive reduced synthesis of the still undefined thymus derived hormone-like factor also has been reported (Bach and Dardenne, 1973).

On the other hand, the degree of responsiveness to hormonal stimuli exhibited by cell and tissue from old individuals is frequently altered, either increased or decreased, and may reflect age-related changes in hormone binding to specific receptors of target cells, this initial step being required to elicit the response (Roth and Adelman, 1975).

With regard to the interrelationship between lymphoid cell proliferation and/or differentiation and hormonal balance during aging, very little is experimentally proved and too much is left to speculation. Such a lack of knowledge is partially due to the general difficulty of following quantitative and/or qualitative changes in adaptative responsiveness of cells to hormones either during developmental stages or maturity or in a given age in dependence of the extra cellular concentration of hormones (Gavin *et al.,* 1974).

Nevertheless, a considerable body of evidence has accumulated in the past ten years, indicating that the different hormones deeply affect proliferation and/or differentiation of lymphoid cells and that some of them may control the aging processes of the immune system.

The interrelationship between these hormones and the immune system will be briefly summarized, and the impact of such observations with aging processes will be discussed later on.

The reader is cautioned, however, that hormone-dependent lymphocyte modulations have been measured, with few exceptions, at a systemic rather than at cell or target tissue level, thus leaving open the possibility that more than one hormonal dependency or regulatory mechanism in each experimental model might be involved.

2. Hormones and the Lymphoid System

2.1. Growth Hormone

The relevance of growth hormone (GH) for the ontogenetic development of the lymphoid system and primarily of thymus-dependent functions has been demonstrated by using different experimental models. Thymus-dependent immunodeficiencies have been found in mice treated with antipituitary antisera (Pierpaoli and Sorkin, 1969) as well as in congenitally hypopituitary Snell (dw) dwarf mice (Fabris *et al.*, 1970, 1971a). The dwarf mice immunodeficiency develops after weaning and is characterized by hypoplasia of the thymus-dependent areas, by impaired transplantation immunity, and by slightly reduced humoral immune responses to thymus-dependent antigens (Fabris *et al.*, 1971a), while serum immunoglobulin levels are within normal range (Wilkison *et al.*, 1970). These findings have been confirmed by other authors (Duquesnoy and Good, 1971; Duquesnoy 1975) in another strain of hypopituitary dwarf mice, the Ames (df) strain.

The immunological deficiency of dwarf mice may be corrected by treating them daily for 30 days with bovine GH, provided, however, the thymus was not previously removed (Fabris *et al.*, 1971b, 1972).

The high sensitivity of the thymus-dependent system to growth hormone is further supported by the observation that GH may influence DNA synthesis of thymocytes (Pandian and Talwar 1971). Moreover, the presence of membrane receptors for GH on thymocytes has been recently demonstrated (Arrembrecht, 1974).

The GH requirements of the thymus-dependent system are not limited to developmental stages, but last during the whole life of the animal, as shown by the deficient immunological recovery from X-irradiation in hypophysectomized adult rats (Duquesnoy *et al.*, 1969) as well as by the increased graft vs. host reaction mounted by adult spleen cells when injected into growth-hormone-treated hybrid F_1 recipients (Pierpaoli *et al.*, 1970).

Finally, the impact of GH with the lymphoid system is supported also by the observations that daily injections of GH in rats and mice increase the incidence of spontaneous lymphosarcomas (Moon *et al.*, 1952), whereas hypophysectomy prevents the emergence of Gross-virus-induced leukemia (Bentley *et al.*, 1974) and treatment with antipituitary antiserum decreases the incidence of X-ray or DMBA-induced lymphosarcomas in mice (Pierpaoli and Haran-Ghera, 1975).

2.2. Insulin

Little is known about the effect of insulin on the immune system. A role in inflammatory and immunological responses has been suggested (Thompson, 1967; Lundin and Angervall, 1970; Pierpaoli *et al.*, 1971).

Indeed, insulin receptors are present on the membrane of human circulating lymphocytes (Archer *et al.*, 1973) and of human lymphoid lines (Gavin *et al.*, 1974). Moreover, the concentration of insulin receptors on peripheral lymphocytes increases during blastic transformation (Krug *et al.*, 1972).

Such a binding of insulin on lymphocytes may well have a biological significance, since an insulin-dependent stimulation of membrane ATPase activity and glucose uptake has been observed (Hadden *et al.*, 1972).

More recent results (Fabris and Piantanelli, submitted for publication) have shown that young rats, made diabetic by either surgical removal of the pancreas or treatment with alloxan, are immunologically crippled. In particular, the ability to synthesize antibody against different antigens is normal, whereas cell-mediated immune reactions, such as PHA response, MLC reactivity, and allogeneic skin-graft rejection capacity are significantly impaired. The lymphoid tissues show a reduced cellularity, particularly evident in the thymus and in the thymus-dependent areas. Moreover, the recovery of transplantation immunity in heavily cortisonized animals is greatly impaired. Complete immunological reconstitution is achieved by treating diabetic rats with exogenous insulin (Fabris and Piantanelli, submitted for publication).

Although data are few and not uniform, they suggest, however, that insulin acts more on the T-dependent function than on the B-dependent system. The reason for such behavior is still unknown, but it is surprising that the immunological deficiencies observed in insulin-deprived animals are quite similar to those shown by hypopituitary animals. Since insulin and GH are physiologically linked by different direct and indirect relationships, the observed similarity may not be casual and may reflect a common underlying mechanism.

Data on a possible relationship between insulin and lymphoid tumors are not available, at least to our knowledge, although insulin receptors on the membrane of leukemic lymphoblast have been found in high concentration (Krug *et al.*, 1972).

2.3. Thyroxine

A strong effect of thyroxine on the lymphoid system was suggested a long time ago from the observation that hyperthyroid patients show an increased level of serum immunoglobulin, lymphoid hyperplasia, and strong allergic reactions. Experimentally, it has been demonstrated that the removal of the thyroid gland induces hypotrophy of the lymphoid system (Lundin, 1958). On the other hand, administration of exogenous thyroxine to otherwise normal animals results in enlargement of both central and peripheral lymphoid organs; in particular, the outflow of lymphocytes from the thymus increases during treatment with thyroxine (Ernstrom and Larsson, 1966).

From a functional point of view, thyroxine-deprived animals, either by propyl-tiouracil (PTU) injection (Pierpaoli *et al.*, 1970), by surgical removal of the gland (Fabris, 1973a) or by ^{131}I administration (Fabris, unpublished experiments) show a generalized immunodepression. Both antibody synthesis and cell-mediated immunity are, in fact, strongly decreased in hypothyroid mice and rats. Such an immunological deficiency is fully restored by daily injection with exogenous thyroxine (Fabris, 1973a).

Experiments performed either in neonatally or in adult thyroidectomized rats have shown that thyroxine is needed during the whole life of the animal in order to maintain the efficiency of the immune system, although the requirement seems to be higher during the ontogenetic development (Fabris, 1973a). It is of interest to point out here that the peak response of PFC against SRBC in physiological conditions is not the maximal peak obtainable. Treatment with exogenous thyroxine in otherwise normal mice and rats can increase the peak response three- to fourfold in spite of the augmented thyroxine-dependent release of corticosteroids (N. Fabris, unpublished experiments).

With regard to lymphoid tumor incidence, it has been reported that the incidence of malignant lymphomas is higher in hyperthyroid patients than in randomly chosen patients suffering from diseases not involving the thyroid gland (Ultman *et al.*, 1963) and in mice carrying thyrotropic tumors (Sproul *et al.*, 1963).

2.4. Corticosteroids

The effect of adrenal cortical hormones on lymphoid tissues has been extensively investigated, since Kendall succeeded in isolating them (Dougherty, 1952). Corticosteroids, and particularly those of the cortisol type can suppress antibody response (Eliott and Sinclair, 1968) as well as cell-mediated immunity (Gunn *et al.*, 1970). The effects of adrenalectomy have been less extensively studied, although an overproliferation of lymphatic tissues, including the thymus, after adrenalectomy is well documented in mice and rats (Dougherty, 1952; Ambrose, 1964; Gunn *et al.*, 1970).

These observations would imply that even at physiological levels, adrenal cortical hormones inhibit the immunological responses, or at least antagonize the proliferative stimuli exerted by other hormones (Fabris, *et al.*, 1970). Recent experiments, however, have demonstrated that some immunological responses are absolutely dependent on corticosteroids for their induction.

Thus it has been shown that physiological levels of corticosteroids are required either during the inductive phase of *in vitro* antibody response (Ambrose, 1970) or during an *in vitro* lymphocyte antifibroblast reaction (Stavy, 1974).

Moreover, it has been shown that adrenalectomy, which entails a higher antibody synthesis in adult animals, causes a depression of humoral immune responses when performed on lactating mice (Fabris, in preparation).

These findings suggest, therefore, that, although physiological levels of corticosteroids may represent a limiting factor for the magnitude of immunological responses, they are needed, nevertheless, for some steps of ontogenetic maturation of the lymphoid system and for the actual performance of lymphocytes.

2.5. Sexual Hormones

The capacity of the female to outperform the male in terms of immune responsiveness has been documented in various mammalian species, including man (Rowley and Mackay, 1969; Terres *et al.*, 1968). The reasons for these differences have not been adequately defined, although the role of sex hormones seems to be preeminent for differentiation either of T or B cell, the effect being more impressive on B-lymphocyte responses (Eidinger and Garrett, 1972).

Due to the complexity of the hormonal feedback mechanisms related to sex, it is difficult at present to define which one among the sexual hormones is directly involved in the immunopotentiating effect of female or of castrated male environment. Both pituitary gonadotropins and target gland hormones may well mediate this effect. Androgens (Szemberg, 1970), estrogens (Waltman *et al.,* 1971), and progestagens (Munroe, 1971), or combinations of them, such as those used for contraceptive treatment (Barnes *et al.,* 1974), may act as immunodepressive agents. This observation, however, cannot be generalized either because some hormones, such as progesterone, may actually enhance some antibody response—PFC response for instance—while depressing cell-mediated immunity (Rembiesa *et al.,* 1974) or because all the above mentioned hormones, when injected *in vivo,* selectively modify the secretion of pituitary gonadotropines through a feedback mechanism, which in turn may affect immunological response in a different direction (Fabris and Piantanelli, 1976). The interrelationship between pituitary and target gland hormones suggests that in some peculiar endocrinological situations, such as menstrual cycle or pregnancy, it is the day-by-day readjustment of hormonal balance that determines the level of immunological reactions (Fabris *et al.,* submitted for publication). Although our knowledge is very poor in this field, the overall impression is, however, that the hormonal balance of feminity, including pregnancy, may favor antibody response (Nossal *et al.,* 1970; Fabris, 1973b) over cell-mediated immunity, thus offering a working hypothesis on the high frequency of autoantibodies in women during the last decades of their lives (Rowley and Mackay, 1969; Walford, 1969).

Sex is also an important factor in leukemogenesis, although findings on the subject are controversial (Toh, 1973). While the incidence of spontaneous leukemia is higher in men than in women, the frequency of spontaneous, carcinogen, or X-ray-induced leukemias in experimental animals is sex dependent in some strains, whereas in others there is little or no sex difference (Kaplan *et al.,* 1954; Toh, 1973).

It has also been reported that pituitary gonadotropins and testosterone enhance the incidence and the growth rate of mineral-oil-induced myeloma in mice, while progesterone may reduce them (Hollander *et al.,* 1968).

2.6. Thymic Factors

Since the observation that thymus grafts in a Millipore chamber partially reconstitute neonatally thymectomized animals (Osoba and Miller, 1963), a considerable body of evidence has been accumulated, indicating that the thymus does secrete one or more humoral factors acting on the development of the lymphoid system and, maybe, on apparently unrelated organs and functions.

Notwithstanding the fact that isolation procedures of such factors from crude thymus extracts need to be further defined, some clear effects on the lymphoid system seem to be established, although the biological significance is still controversial. Thymosine (White and Goldstein, 1970), thymic factor (Trainin and Small, 1970), and thymine or thymopoietin (Goldstein, 1974) are three of the seemingly best preparations of humoral factors secreted by the thymus. Although such preparations differ from one another either in the isolation procedure or in some particular nonimmunological effects, they are all capable, in defined experimental conditions, of promoting the development and the expression of T cell characteristics and functions (Goldstein *et al.,* 1972; Dardenne and Bach, 1973; Komuro and

Boyse, 1973; Trainin *et al.*, 1973; Dauphinee *et al.*, 1974). Moreover, the presence of thymosine-like material has been recently demonstrated in human serum (Bach *et al.*, 1972) and in normal mouse serum (Bach and Dardenne, 1973).

In spite of these recent achievements, the whole picture of thymic hormones or of thymus-dependent activities remains to be explored. Besides the effect on neuromuscular transmission exerted by the "thymine" preparation or, more precisely, by the two closely related polypeptides that have been isolated (Goldstein, 1974), there is consistent experimental evidence that the thymus may, directly or indirectly, affect nonimmunological functions. It has been observed, in fact, that neonatal thymectomy and the thymusless *Nu/Nu* mutation cause delayed sexual maturation (Nishizuka and Sakakura, 1969; Besedowski and Sorkin, 1974), and impaired DNA synthesis in submandibular glands in response to isoproterenol (Piantanelli and Fabris, 1975; Fabris and Piantanelli, in press, the latter test being indicative of a peculiarity shown by old animals (Roth and Adelman, 1975). Moreover, both thymectomy and the nude mutation induce alterations in other endocrine glands, such as hypophysis (Pierpaoli and Sorkin, 1967), adrenals, and thyroid (Pierpaoli and Besedowski, 1975), although some of these observations are still controversial (Wortis, 1975). Nevertheless, these findings give further evidence of the existence of thymic factors, since one of the typical features of hormones is that they are mutually balanced insofar as any modification of the synthesis of one hormone will entail a new balance for the others.

2.7.   Other Hormones

In recent years it has been demonstrated that hormones, besides those taken into consideration here, may exert their action on the lymphoid system. Vasopressin and parathyroid hormones induce proliferation of thymocytes (Whitfield, 1970); epinephrine acts on thymocytes and presumably also on lymphocytes through the cyclic AMP system (Lichtenstein and Henney, 1974). Finally, prostaglandins seem also to be involved in some functional aspect of the immune system (Stockman and Humford, 1974). Yet many more hormones or humoral factors are probably involved in the homeostasis of the lymphoid system, but only further investigation in this direction will reveal their action.

3.   The Impact of Hormones on Aging of the Immune System

From the previous considerations, it can be deduced that hormones do play a major role in the homeostasis of the lymphoid system, although present knowledge does not allow us to draw a comprehensive picture of all existing interrelationships. Such a complexity suggests that any impact hormones may have on aging is supported more by a modified balance among different hormones or between hormones and the lymphoid system than by a single hormonal deficiency.

With these premises, the relevance of hormones to aging of the immune system may be visualized at different levels.

First, the age-dependent hormonal environment may modify either the actual performance of mature lymphocytes or their differentiation from precursor cells. Although direct experimental evidence for such interrelationships is still lacking, the possibility of achieving in "old" cells either an *in vitro* reactivation of immunocompetence by thymus factors (Friedman *et al.*, 1974), an increased immunocompetence *in vivo* by mercaptoethanol (T. Makinodan, personal communication), or by thyroxine (Piantanelli and Fabris, 1976) suggests that the better performance shown by "old" cells when inoculated into a "young" environment (Price and Makinodan, 1972b) may, at least partially, depend on hormonal factors.

Moreover, that some hormones are essential for the maintenance of a threshold pool of precursor cells is demonstrated by the fact that adult pancreatectomy prevents immunological recovery from heavy cortisonization (Fabris and Piantanelli, submitted for publication). The fact, however, that either hypophysectomized or insulin-deprived or thyroxine-deprived (Fabris, 1973a) animals do not show immunological deficiencies shortly after the operation, whereas other biological functions are impaired, demonstrates that the action of those hormonal imbalances is exerted at levels that precede antigenic stimulation.

The constant requirement of the right hormonal balance to maintain a threshold pool of precursor cells should be taken into account in all young-to-old or old-to-young transfer experiments, since the short-term effect of a given environment may not be comparable to one resulting from prolonged exposure.

An interesting, although speculative, point comes from the observation that, on one hand, the progressive immunological deterioration with advancing age seems to affect the thymus-dependent rather than the B-dependent system (Burnet, 1970; Roberts-Thomson *et al.*, 1974; Gerbase-DeLima *et al.*, 1974), on the other hand, the known age-related hormonal changes, particularly of those hormones which act preferentially only on one kind of cell, either T or B, give rise to an overall hormonal balance that may better support B cell than T cell proliferation. Suffice it to reiterate here that insulin deficiency and the hormonal pattern of sexual decline tip the balance in favor of humoral immunity and allow development of aberrancies, which might account for the observation of a greatly increased incidence of autoantibody with age (Fabris and Piantanelli, in press).

Second, the hormones can affect the aging of the immune system by acting during rather early stages of ontogenetic development, in the course of which they may induce permanent modifications of target cell functions. This assumption has been suggested by some observation on nonimmunological functions.

Thus exposure of the neonatal female to androgenic influence during the first week of life, but not thereafter, causes an alteration in the development of the hypothalamus so that at adulthood, male behavior is observable (Jost *et al.*, 1973). Even treatment during pregnancy, e.g., with GH induces a higher learning ability in the pups when adult (Sara and Lazarus, 1974).

On the other hand, some macroenvironmental factors, whose biological effect may be mediated by hormones, can change the future performance of cells if they exert their action in a given critical period. For example, rats handled daily before weaning show an increased immunological responsivness in adulthood (Solomon *et al.*, 1968). Moreover, caloric restriction at a young age, which extends life span (McCay, 1952) and delays age-related deterioration of the immune system (Walford *et al.*, 1973/1974) seems, from experiments in progress (W. Pierpaoli, personal communication), to induce modifications of the hormonal balance that are maintained throughout life, even after food restriction stops. Some hormonal treatments, starting early in life, may also prolong life span in short-lived strains of mice (Bellamy, 1968).

In a more direct way, it has been shown that treatment of "early aging" dwarf mice (Fabris *et al.,* 1972) with GH during the first 30 days after weaning significantly prolongs the life span of these animals (from 4 months to 15–18 months), provided the thymus is not removed before the hormonal treatment. More recently, we have shown that the efficiency of the hormonal therapy depends on the period of life at treatment (Figure 1). Hormonal treatment from 30 to 60 days of life results in 90% survival up to 15 months; treatment from 60 to 90 days of life, to 10 months; whereas treatment after 90 days does not modify life span at all. The relationship may not be casual that the age at which hormone treatment of dwarf mice is most effective is identical to the age at which neonatally thymectomized mice can be restored with thymic humoral factors (Stutman, personal communication). This would suggest that the action of GH and thyroxine on dwarf mice is mediated through the release of thymic hormones, which should therefore be considered as factors actively participating in the general endocrinological homeostasis.

Independent of the hormones involved, these observations suggest that a particular hormonal balance is present during a critical period of development which is essential for the maturation and efficiency of the lymphoid system during adulthood and old age. This deduction could explain the failure of neonatal thymus, when grafted in old mice, in reconstituting their deficient immunological response (Metcalf, 1966) while, apparently, thymic factors do. It is likely, in fact, that the hormonal balance in old age is qualitatively different, being, therefore, unable to sustain maturation. For given functions, the critical period may even be quite short, as suggested by the fact that the prevention of the delay of vaginal opening in nude mice may be achieved by neonatal thymus grafts performed during the first week of

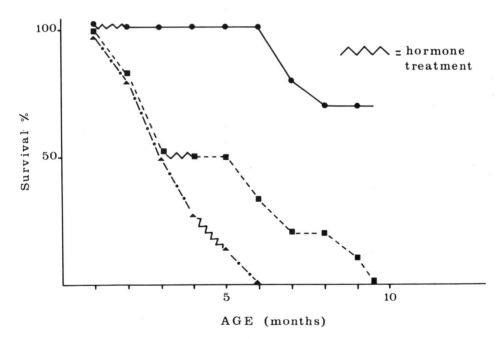

Figure 1. Relevance of the timing of a 30-day hormonal therapy for survival of hypopituitary immunodeficient dwarf mice. Bovine growth hormone and L-thyroxine were given respectively at the daily dosage of 100 μg and 1 μg.

life, but not thereafter (Besedowski and Sorkin, 1974; Pierpaoli and Besedowski, 1975).

In order to analyze these thoughts schematically we (Piantanelli and Fabris) have tried to express them graphically in Figure 2, which is a plot of range of resistance to different insults (and/or recovery from) vs. age.

A stage in early life represents a critical period during which differentiative and proliferative processes, whose rate may depend on either the genetic background or environmental conditions, take place in order to reach the maximal range of resistance observed in a normal population (e.g., in phenotypically normal Snell or haired $Nu/+$ mice).

Following this period of life, there is a progressive decline in the level of such a resistance, and death ensues when the level drops below threshold.

The curve of a genetically deficient animal (dwarf or nude mouse) reaches a lower range of resistance with a higher rate of decline than does one for normal mice. The reconstitutive therapy (by endocrine glands, or hormones, or cell replacement, whose efficiency is indicated by angle α) causes both an increased range of resistance and a reduced rate of decline, so that the curve of reconstituted animals approaches that of a normal population. A full reconstitution is not indicated on the figure because, although theoretically possible, it is experimentally difficult to achieve.

Any improvement during the critical period amplifies the range of resistance to insults and/or recovery therefrom and consequently reduces the rate of its decline with age. This is graphically expressed by using a right angle to link the two portions of the curve (note that this is compatible with the life spans expected at the limiting conditions, i.e., when the range approaches zero or infinity).

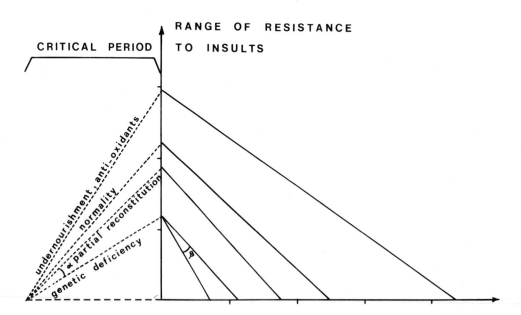

Figure 2. Graphical representation of the range of resistance to insults and the life expectancy undergone when favorable or unfavorable conditions occur early in life (critical period). For explanation, see the text.

The length of the critical period is arbitrarily indicated, because it may last from one to two months, as in the case of the timing of hormonal treatment of dwarf mice (Figure 1), to several months, as in the case of caloric undernourishment in rodents (McCay, 1952; Stuchlíková *et al.*, 1975). According to our schematic, animals undernourished during early life should reach a higher range of resistance, which, consequently, causes a decrease in the rate of decline in resistance with age.

The greater relevance of the critical period, when compared with subsequent periods of life, stems from the fact that any experimental manipulation undertaken during this period gives rise to quite different effects when compared to those induced with the same manipulation at later periods of life. Due to these considerations, the hormonal treatment of dwarf mice, undertaken too late in life (angle β), may only slow the rate of decline of resistance without any great modification on longevity, whereas a similar treatment performed early in life (angle α) induces permanent modification of the range of resistance itself, with a reduction in the rate of decline even when hormonal treatment is not protracted throughout life. It is an obvious oversimplification that the difference among the levels of the range of resistance reached by various populations is indicated in Figure 2 in quantitative terms, while it may also reflect different homeostatic equilibria, which, for longevity, but not obligatory for other performances, offer some advantages.

4. The Impact of Hormone–Lymphocyte Relationship on the Aging Processes

Both hormonal changes (Dilman, 1971) and lymphoid system modifications (Walford, 1969; Burnet, 1970) have been taken into consideration as pathogenetic, if not etiological, factors in basic aging phenomena. That the lymphoid system may interfere with some aging processes is supported, in addition to the evidence mentioned previously (Walford, 1969; Burnet, 1970), by the observations that postthymectomy wasting disease is accompanied by a number of nonimmunological consequences, such as degranulation of GH-producing cells in the adenohypophysis (Bianchi *et al.*, 1970), sexual retardation (Nishizuka and Sakakura, 1969), impairment of liver regeneration (Fachet *et al.*, 1963) and general body growth defects. Moreover, *Nu/Nu* mice show alterations of hormonal levels (Pantalouris, 1973; Pierpaoli and Sorkin, 1972), of liver enzyme activity, of the ratio of soluble/insoluble collagen (Pantalouris, 1973), of sexual maturation (Besedowski and Sorkin, 1974), and of isoproterenol-induced DNA synthesis by submandibular glands (Piantanelli and Fabris, 1975; Fabris and Piantanelli, in press), which, together with the previous observations, suggest that the lymphoid system and particularly the thymus may be linked to the general hormonal homeostatic mechanisms and directly, or through them, may control the function of other body tissues.

The relevance of such a relationship for some age-related processes has been suggested (Fabris *et al.*, 1972; Fabris and Sorkin, 1975; Fabris and Piantanelli, in press) by the observation that both hypopituitary dwarf and thymusless nude mice (Pantalouris, 1973) are affected by a kind of early aging syndrome, and that both hormonal and immunological recoveries are required in order to prevent the early appearance of age-related symptoms.

While these findings suggest that there may be means of preventing the age-related deterioration of certain functions, it seems unlikely that maintenance of the integrity of either the hormonal balance or the lymphoid system can prevent the multifaceted deteriorating aging process.

The relationship between hormonal balance and immunological function may, however, represent a relevant factor for controlling some particular age-related processes, especially those characterized by abnormal growth patterns. In addition to the effect on immunological efficiency and, therefore, on immunological surveillance on cancer, hormones do act also on tumor growth itself. It has been reported by many authors (Gardner, 1953; Toh, 1973) that some tumors, in addition to the well-known hormone-sensitive tumors, may grow only if the hormonal balance is satisfactory. Thus spontaneous sarcomas (Moon *et al.*, 1952), MCA-induced sarcomas, DMBA carcinomas, and aminofluorene-induced hepatomas are absent or show a reduced frequency in hypophysectomized rats (Gardner, 1953). Moreover, Gross-virus leukemia is not inducible in hypophysectomized rats (Bentley *et al.*, 1974), whereas chronic treatment with GH induces lymphosarcomata in rats (Moon *et al.*, 1952).

On the other hand, the incidence and the growth rate of MCA-induced sarcomas (Bielschowsky and Bielschowsky, 1959; Fabris, unpublished experiments), of aminofluorene-induced papillomas (Bielschowsky and Bielschowsky, 1960), and of the Erlich ascites tumor or sarcoma 180 (Turolla, 1960) in hypopituitary dwarf mice is similar to that observed in normal littermates. These conflicting findings may be explained by taking into consideration that, although hormonal imbalance in adult hypophysectomized rats is similar to that in dwarf mice, their immunological efficiencies are quite different, since adult hypophysectomy does not cause immunological impairment, at least shortly after the operation (Duquesnoy *et al.*, 1969), whereas congenital hypopituitarism does (Fabris *et al.*, 1971a, 1972). It is therefore likely that the incidence of tumors as well as their growth pattern stem more from the balance existing in a given animal between hormonal condition and immunological efficiency. One may speculate that during the life of an organism such a balance changes, giving rise to a favorable condition for tumor growth only during a particular period of life.

With regard to the tumors of the lymphoid system, another consideration is that the hormonal sensitivity of leukemic cells may well be higher than that of normal lymphoid cells. In fact, a higher concentration of insulin receptor has been found in lymphoblastoid cells than in peripheral lymphocytes (Krug *et al.*, 1972), thus giving some tumor lines a "hormonal" advantage over the normal cells. If so, it is not inconceivable that other age-related diseases, characterized by abnormal cloning of cells, such as some autoimmune disorders, may be favored by an advantageous hormonal sensitivity or by a particular age-related hormonal balance.

5. Conclusions

The hormonal homeostatic system constitutes one of the most relevant "pillars" of life, the stability of which may largely determine the normal aging processes. Since the lymphoid system is particularly sensitive to hormonal changes, its deterioration with age may depend to a great extent on age-related modifications of the hormonal homeostatic control, due as much to alteration in sensitivity of target lymphoid cell as to changes in the activity of endocrine glands. Even more relevant is the role played by hormonal control during early stages of life, when the range of future performance of lymphocytes is determined concomitantly by their genetic program and by the environmental conditions.

Due to these considerations, any trial to experimentally prolong the efficiency of lymphoid system throughout life will be more fruitful if conducted in early stages of development than in adult life. Such a perspective needs, however, to deeply investigate the effect of hormones on dissected immunological functions in order to assess the hormonal sensitivity of functionally distinct subpopulations of either T or B cells or of other immunological cells, such as macrophages.

The achievement and the maintenance of the optimal ratio among functionally distinct subpopulations of lymphocytes, as well as of their efficiency throughout life, might well depend on the fitness between the immunological and the endocrinological "orchestra."

References

Ambrose, C. T., 1964, The requirement for hydrocortisone in antibody-forming tissue cultivated in serum free medium, *J. Exp. Med.* **119:**1027–1049.

Ambrose, C. T., 1970, The essential role of corticosteroids in the induction of the immune response in vitro, in: *Hormones and Immune Response,* Ciba Study Group No. 36 (G. E. W. Wolstenholme and J. Knight, eds.), pp. 100–116, Churchill, London.

Archer, J. A., Gorden, P., Gavin III, J. R., Lesniak, M. A., and Roth, J., 1973, Insulin receptors in human circulating lymphocytes: application to the insulin resistance in man, *J. Clin. Endocrinol. Metab.* **36:**627–633.

Arrembrecht, S., 1974, Specific binding of growth hormone to thymocytes, *Nature* **252:**255–257.

Bach, J. F., and Dardenne, M., 1973, Studies on thymus products. II. Demonstration of a circulating thymic hormone, *Immunology* **25:**353–366.

Bach, J. F., Dardenne, M., Papiernik, M., Barois, A., Lavasseur, P., and Le Brigand, H., 1972, Evidence for a serum-factor secreted by the human thymus, *Lancet* **ii:**1056–1058.

Barnes, D. W. H., Ford, C. E., and Loutit, J. E., 1959, Grèffes en serie de moélle osseuse chez des souris irradiées, *Sang.* **30:**762–765.

Barnes, E. W., Loudon, N. B., MacCuish, A. C., Jordan, J., Irvine, W. J., 1974, Phytohaemagglutinin-induced lymphocyte transformation and circulating autoantibodies in women taking oral contraceptives, *Lancet* **i:**898–900.

Bellamy, D., 1968, Long-term action of prednisolone phosphate on a strain of short-lived mice, *Exp. Gerontol.* **3:**327–334.

Bentley, H. P., Hughes, E. R., and Peterson, R. D. A., 1974, Effect of hypophysectomy on a virus-induced T-cell leukaemia, *Nature* **252:**747–748.

Besedowski, H. O., and Sorkin, E., 1974, Thymus involvement in female sexual maturation, *Nature* **249:**356–358.

Bianchi, E., Pierpaoli, W., and Sorkin, E., 1970, Cytological changes in the mouse anterior pituitary after neonatal thymectomy: a light and electron microscopcal study, *J. Endocrin.* **51:**1–6.

Bielschowsky, F., and Bielschowsky, M., 1959, Carcinogenesis in the pituitary dwarf mouse. The response to methylcholanthrene injected subcutaneously, *Brit. J. Cancer* **13:**302–305.

Bielschowsky, F., and Bielschowsky, M., 1960, Carcinogenesis in the pituitary dwarf mouse. The response of 2-aminofluorene, *Brit. J. Cancer* **14:**195–199.

Braun, W., Yajima, Y., and Ishizuka, T., 1970, Synthetic polynucleotides as restorers of normal antibody forming capacity in aged mice, *RES* (N.Y.), **7:**418–424.

Burnet, M., 1970, *Immunological Surveillance,* Pergamon Press, Australia.

Dauphinee, M. J., Talal, N., Goldstein, A. L., and White, A., 1974, Thymosine corrects the abnormal DNA synthetic response of NZB mouse thymocytes, *Proc. Nat. Acad. Sci.* **71:**2637–2641.

Dardenne, M., and Bach, J. F., 1973, Studies on thymus products. I. Modification of rosette-forming cells by thymic extracts. Determination of target RFC subpopulation, *Immunol.* **25:**343–352.

Dilman, V. M., 1971, Age-associated elevation of hypothalamic threshold to feed-back control, and its role in development, ageing, and disease, *Lancet* **i:**1211–1217.

Dougherty, T. F., 1952, Effect of hormones on lymphatic tissue, *Physiol. Rev.* **32:**379–401.

Duquesnoy, R. J., 1975, The pituitary dwarf mouse: a model for study of endocrine immunodeficiency disease, in: *Immunodeficiency in Man and Animals,* Birth Defects, Original Article Series, Vol. XI, No. 1 (D. Bergsma, ed.) pp. 536–543, Sinauer Assoc. Inc., Sunderland, Mass.

Duquesnoy, R. J., and Good, R. A., 1971, Prevention of immunologic deficiency in pituitary dwarf mice by prolonged nursing, *J. Immunol.* **6:**1553–1558.

Duquesnoy, R. J., Mariani, T., and Good, R. A., 1969, Effect of hypophysectomy on the immunological recovery from X-irradiation, *Proc. Soc. Exp. Biol. Med.* **132:**1176–1178.

Eidinger, D., and Garrett, T. J., 1972, Studies on the regulatory effects on the sex hormones on antibody formation and stem cell differentiation, *J. Exp. Med.* **136:**1098–1116.

Eliott, E. V., and Sinclair, C., 1968, Effect of cortisone acetate on 19s and 75s haemolysin antibody. A time course study, *Immunology* **15:**643–652.

Ernström, U., and Larsson, B., 1966, Thymic and thoracic duct contribution to blood lymphocytes in normal and thyroxin treated guinea-pig, *Acta Physiol. Scand.* **66:**189–195.

Fabris, N., 1973a, Immunodepression in thyroid-deprived animals, *Clin. Exp. Immunol.* **15:**601–611.

Fabris, N., 1973b, Immunological reactivity during pregnancy in the mouse, *Experientia* **29:**610–612.

Fabris, N., and Sorkin, E., 1975, Relation of lymphoid system and hormones to aging, in: *Immunodeficiency in Man and Animals,* Birth Defects Original Article Series, Vol. XI, No. 1 (D. Bergsma ed.) pp. 533–536, Sinauer Assoc., Mass.

Fabris, N., and Piantanelli, L., 1976, Effect of chorionic gonadotropins on humoral and cell-mediated immunity, in: *Immune Reactivity of Lymphocytes* (M. Feldman and A. Globerson, eds.), pp. 635–638, Plenum Press, New York.

Fabris, N., and Piantanelli, L., Contributions of hypopituitary dwarf and athymic nude mice to the study of the relationships among thymus, hormones, and aging, in: *Genetic Effects on Aging* (D. E. Harrison, ed.), Birth Defects Original Article Series, Sinauer Assoc., Sunderland, Mass., in press.

Fabris, N., and Piantanelli, L., Differential effect of pancreatectomy on humoral and cell-mediated immunity, *Clin. Exp. Immunol.,* submitted for publication.

Fabris, N., Pierpaoli, W., and Sorkin, E., 1970, Hormones and the immune response, in: *Developmental Aspects of Antibody Formation and Structure* (J. Sterzl and I. Riha, eds.) pp. 79–87, Czechoslovak Academy Press, Prague.

Fabris, N., Pierpaoli, W., and Sorkin, E. 1971a, Hormones and the immunological capacity. III. The immunodeficiency diseases of the hypopituitary Snell-Bagg dwarf mouse, *Clin. Exp. Immunol.* **9:**209–225.

Fabris, N., Pierpaoli, W., and Sorkin, E., 1971b, Hormones and the immunological capacity. IV. Restorative effects of developmental hormones or of lymphocytes on the immunodeficiency syndrome of the dwarf mouse, *Clin. Exp. Immunol.* **9:**227–240.

Fabris, N., Pierpaoli, W., and Sorkin, E., 1972, Lymphocytes, hormones and ageing, *Nature* **240:**557–559.

Fabris, N., Piantanelli, L., and Muzzioli, M., Differential effect of pregnancy and gestagens on humoral and cell-mediated immunity, *Clin. Exp. Immunol.,* submitted for publication.

Fachet, J., Stark, E., Palkovits, M., and Vallent, K., 1963, Der Einfluss der Thymectomie auf die Leberregeneration nach partielle Hepatektomie, *Z. Zellforsch.* **60:**609–614.

Friedman, D., Keiser, V., and Globerson, A., 1974, Reactivation of immunocompetence in spleen cells of aged mice, *Nature* **251:**545–547.

Gardner, W. U., 1953, Hormonal aspects of Experimental Tumorigegenesis, in: *Advances in Cancer Research,* Vol. 1 (J. P. Greenstein and A. Haddow eds.), pp. 173–232, Academic Press, N. Y.

Gavin III, J. R., Roth, J., Neville, D. M., DeMeyts, P., and Buell, D. N., 1974, Insulin-dependent regulation of insulin receptors concentrations: a direct demonstration in cell culture, *Proc. Nat. Acad. Sci. U.S.A.* **71:**84–88.

Gerbase-DeLima, M., Wilkinson, J., Smith, G. S., and Walford, R. L., 1974, Age-related decline in thymic-independent immune function in a long-lived mouse strain, *J. Geront.* **29:**261–268.

Gershon, R. K., 1974, T cell control of antibody production, in: *Contemporary Topics in Immunobiology* (M. D. Cooper and N. L. Warner, eds.), pp. 1–40, Plenum Press, New York.

Goldstein, G., 1974, Isolation of bovine thymin: a polypeptide hormone of the thymus, *Nature* **247:**11–14.

Goldstein, A. L., Guha, A., Zatz, M. M., Hardy, M. A., and White, A., 1972, Purification and biological activity of thymosin, a hormone of the thymus gland, *Proc. Nat. Acad. Sci.* **69:**1800–1803.

Goodman, S. A., and Makinodan, T., 1975, Effect of age on cell-mediated immunity in long-lived mice, *Clin. Exp. Immunol.* **19:**533–542.

Gunn, A., Lance, E. M., Medawar, P. B., and Nehlsen, S. L., 1970, Synergism between *cortisol* anti antilymphocyte serum, in: *Hormones and Immune Response,* Ciba Study Group, No 36 (G. E. W. Wolstenholme and J. Knight, eds.) pp. 66–95, Churchill, London.

Hadden, J. W., Hadden, E. M., Wilson, E. E., Good, R. A., and Coffey, R. G., 1972, Direct action of insulin on plasma membrane ATPase activity in human lymphocytes, *Nature N.B.* **235:**174–176.

Hayflick, L., 1966, Cell culture and the aging phenomenon, in: *Topics in the Biology of Aging* (P. L. Krohn, ed.), pp. 83–100, Interscience, New York.

Heidrick, M. L., and Makinodan, T., 1972, Nature of cellular deficiencies in age-related decline of the immune system, *Gerontologia* **18:**305–320.

Hollander, U. P., Takakura, K., and Yamada, H., 1968, Endocrine factors in the pathogenesis of plasma cell tumors, *Recent Progress Horm. Res.* **24:**81–137.

Hoshino, K., and Gardner, W. U., 1967, Transplantability and life-span of mammary gland during serial transplantation in mice, *Nature* **213:**193–195.

Kanugo, M. S., Patnaik, S. K., and Koul, O., 1975, Decrease in 17-β-oestradiol receptor in brain of ageing rats, *Nature* **253:**366–367.

Kaplan, H. S., Nagareda, C. S., and Brown, M. B., 1954, V. The role of hormones in blood and blood-forming organs. Endocrine factors and radiation-induced lymphoid tumors of mice, *Recent Progress Horm. Res.* **10:**293–333.

Komuro, K., and Boyse, E. A., 1973, *In vitro* demonstration of thymic hormone in the mouse by conversion of precursor cells into lymphocytes, *Lancet* **i:**740–743.

Krohn, P. L., 1966, Transplantation and aging, in: *Topics in the Biology of Aging* (P. L. Krohn, ed.) pp. 125–173, Interscience, New York.

Krug, U., Krug, F., and Cuatrecasas, P., 1972, Emergence of insulin receptors on human lymphocytes during *in vitro* transformation, *Proc. Nat. Acad. Sci. U.S.A.* **9:**2604–2608.

Jost, A., Vigier, B., Prepin, J., and Perchellet, J. P., 1973, Studies on sex differentiation in mammals, *Rec. Progr. Hormone Res.* **29:**1–36.

Lichtenstein, L. M., and Henney, C. S., 1974, Adenylate cyclaselinked hormone receptors: an important mechanism for the immunoregulation of leucocytes, in: *Progress in Immunology,* Vol 2 (L. Brent and J. Holborrow, eds.), pp. 73–83, North-Holland Publ. Co., Amsterdam.

Liu, R. K., and Walford, R. L., 1972, The effect of lowered body temperature on life-span and immune and nonimmune processes, *Gerontologia* **18:**363–388.

Liu, R. K., and Walford, R. L., 1975, Mid-life temperature-transfer effects on life-span of annual fish, *J. Geront.* **30:**129–131.

Lundin, P. M., 1958, Anterior pituitary gland and lymphoid tissue growth, *Acta Endocrinol.,* Suppl. Vol. 40.

Lundin, P. M., and Angervall, L., 1970, Effect of insulin on rat lymphoid tissue, *Path. Europ.* **3:**273–278.

McCay, C. M., 1952, Chemical aspects of aging and the effect of diet upon aging, in: *Cowdry's Problems of Ageing* (L. I. Lansing, ed.), pp. 139–202, Williams and Wilkins Co., Baltimore.

Metcalf, D., 1966, The thymus, in: *Recent Result in Cancer Research* Monog. No 5, Springer-Verlag, N.Y.

Moon, H. D., Simpson, M. E., Li, C. H., and Evans, H. M., 1952, Effect of pituitary growth hormone in mice, *Cancer Res.* **12:**448–450.

Munroe, J. S., 1971, Progesteroids as Immunosuppressive agents, *J. Reticuloendothelial Society* **9:**361–375.

Nishizuka, Y., and Sakakura, T., 1969, Thymus and reproduction: sex-linked dysgenesia of the gonad after neonatal thymectomy in mice, *Science* **166:**753–755.

Nossal, J. V., Bussard, A. E., Lewis, H., and Mazie, J. C., 1970, Formation of hemolitic plaques by peritoneal cells *in vitro.* I: a new technique enabling micromanipulation and yielding higher plaque numbers, in: *Developmental Aspects of Antibody Formation and Structure* (Riha and Sterzl, eds.), p. 655–670 Czecoslovak Academic Press, Prague.

Osoba, D., and Miller, J. F. A. P., 1963, Evidence for a humoral thymus factor responsible for maturation of immunological faculty, *Nature* **199:**653–656.

Pandian, M. R., and Talwar, G. P., 1971, Effect of growth hormone on the metabolism of thymus and on the immune response against sheep erythrocytes, *J. Exp. Med.* **134:**1095–1113.

Pantalouris, E. M., 1973, Athymic development in the mouse, *Differentiation* **1:**437–450.

Phillips, S. M., and Wegman, T. G., 1973, Active suppression as a possible mechanism of tolerance in tetraparental mice, *J. Exp. Med.* **137**:291–300.

Piantanelli, L. and Fabris, N., 1975a, Decreased rate of DNA synthesis in submandibular glands of thymusless nude mice after isoproterenol stimulation, in: *FEBS Abstract,* 10th FEBS meeting, Abs. No. 1595, Société de Chimie Biologique, Paris.

Pierpaoli, W., and Besedowski, H. O., 1975, Role of the thymus in programmation of neuroendocrine functions, *Clin. Exp. Immunol.* **20**:323–338.

Pierpaoli, W., Fabris, N., and Sorkin, E., 1970, Developmental hormones and immunological mutura-tion, in: *Hormones and the immune response,* Ciba Study Group No. 36 (G. E. W. Wolstenholme and J. Knight, eds.), pp. 126–143, Churchill, London.

Pierpaoli, W., Fabris, N., and Sorkin, E., 1971, The effects of hormones on the development of the immune capacity, in: *Cellular Interactions in the Immune Response,* 2nd Int. Convoc. Immunol., Buffalo, pp. 25–30, Karger, Basel.

Pierpaoli, W., and Haran-Ghera, N., 1975, Prevention of induced leukaemia in mice by immunological inhibition of adenohypophysis, *Nature* **254**:334–335.

Pierpaoli, W., and Sorkin, E., 1967, Relationship between thymus and hypopysis, *Nature* **215**:834–837.

Pierpaoli, W., and Sorkin, E., 1969, A study on anti-pituitary serum, *Immunol.* **16**:311–318.

Pierpaoli, W., and Sorkin, E., 1972, Alterations of adrenal cortex and thyroid in mice with congenital absence of the thymus, *Nature N. B.* **28**:282–284.

Price, G. B., and Makinodan, T. 1972a, Immunologic deficiencies in senescence. I. Characterization of intrinsic deficiencies, *J. Immunol* **108**:403–412.

Price, G. B., and Makinodan, T., 1972b, Immunologic deficiencies in senescence. II. Characterization of extrinsic deficiencies, *J. Immunol.* **108**:413–417.

Rembiesa, R., Ptak, W., and Bubak, M., 1974, The immuno-suppressive effects of mouse placental steroids, *Experientia* **30**:82–83.

Roberts-Thomson, I. C., Whittingham, S., Youngchaiyud, U., and Mackay, I. R., 1974, Ageing, immune response and mortality, *Lancet* **ii**:368–370.

Roth, G. S., and Adelman, R. C., 1975, Age related changes in hormone binding by target cells and tissues; possible role in altered adaptive responsiveness, *Exp. Geront.* **10**:1–11.

Rowley, M. J., and Mackay, I. R., 1969, Measurement of antibody-producing capacity in man. I. The normal response to flagellen from Salmonella adelaide, *Clin. Exp. Immunol.* **5**:407–418.

Sara, V. R., and Lazarus, L., 1974, Prenatal action of growth hormone on brain and behaviour, *Nature* **250**:257–258.

Solomon, G. F., Levine, S., and Kraft, J. K., 1968, Early experience and immunity, *Nature* **220**:821–822.

Spiegel, P. M., 1972, Theories of aging, in: *Developmental Physiology and Aging* (P. S. Timiras, ed.), pp. 564–580, MacMillan Co., N.Y.

Sproul, E. E., Grinberg, R., and Werner, S. C., 1963, Lymphoid hyperplasia and neoplasia associated with a mouse pituitary thyrotropic tumor, *Cancer Res.* **23**:1090–1096.

Stavy, L., 1974, Stimulation of rat lymphocyte proliferation by hydrocortisone during the induction of cell-mediated immunity *in vitro, Transplantation* **17**:173–179.

Stockmann, G. D., and Humford, D. H., 1974, The effect of prostaglandins on the *in vitro* blastogenic response of human peripheral blood lymphocytes, *Exp. Hematol.* **2**:65–79.

Stuchlíková, E., Juríková-Horáková, M., and Deyl, Z., 1975, New aspect of dietary effect on life prolongation in rodents. What is the role of obesity in aging?, *Exp. Gerontol.* **10**:141–144.

Szemberg, A., 1970, Influence of testosterone on the primary lymphoid organs of the chicken, in: *Hormones and Immune Responses,* Ciba Study Group No. 36, (G. E. W. Wolstenholme and J. Knight, eds.), pp. 42–45, Churchill, London.

Terres, G., Morrison, S. L., and Habicht, G. S., 1968, A quantitative difference in the immune response between male and female mice, *Proc. Soc. Exp. Biol. Med.* **127**:664–673.

Thompson, G., 1967, Enhancing effect of insulin on the tuberculin reaction of the albino rat, *Nature* **215**:748–749.

Timiras, P. S., 1972, Decline in Homeostatic regulation, in: *Developmental Physiology and Aging* (P. S. Timiras, ed.), pp. 542–563, MacMillan Co., N.Y.

Timiras, P. S., and Meisami, E., 1972, Changes in gonadal function in: *Developmental Physiology and Aging* (P. S. Timiras, ed.) pp. 527–541, MacMillan Co., N.Y.

Toh, Y. C., 1973, Physiological and biochemical reviews of sex differences and carcinogenesis with particular reference to the liver, in: *Advances in Cancer Research* (G. Klein and S. Weinhouse, eds.) pp. 155–209, Academic Press, N.Y.

Trainin, N., Carnaud, C., and Ilfeld, D., 1973, Inhibition of *in vitro* autosensitization by a thymic humoral factor, *Nature N.B.* **245:**253–255.

Trainin, N., and Small, M., 1970, Conferment of immunocopetence on lymphoid cells by a thymic humoral factor, in: *Hormones and Immune Responses* (G. E. W. Wolstenholme and J. Knight, eds.), pp. 24–36, Churchill, London.

Turolla, E., 1960, Attecchimento e sviluppo del tumore di Ehrlich e del Sarcoma 180 in topi con nanismo ipofisario, *Tumori* **46:**20–27.

Ultman, J. E., Hyman, G. A., and Burton Calder, G. A., 1963, The occurrence of lymphoma in patients with long-standing hyperthyroidism, *Blood* **21:**282–293.

Walford, R. L., 1969, *The Immunological Theories of Aging,* Munksgaard, Copenhagen.

Walford, R. L., 1974, The immunological theory of aging: current status, *Fed. Proc.* **33:**2020–2027.

Walford, R. L., Liu, R. K., Mathies, M., Gerbase-DeLima, M., and Smith, G. S., 1973, 1974, Long term dietary restriction and immune function in mice, Response to sheep red blood cells and to mitogens, *Mech. Ageing Develop.* **2:**447–454.

Waltman, S. R., Burde, R. M., and Berrios, J., 1971, Prevention of corneal homograft rejection by estrogens, *Transplantation* **11:**194–196.

White, A., and Goldstein, A. L., 1970, Thymosin, a thymic hormone influencing lymphoid cell immunological competence, in: *Hormones and Immune Responses,* Ciba Study Group No. 36 (G. E. W. Wolstenholme and J. Knight, eds.), pp. 3–18, Churchill, London.

Whitfield, J. F., 1970, Potentiation by antidiuretic hormone (vasopressin) of the ability of parathyroid hormone to stimulate the proliferation of rat thymic lymphocytes, *Horm. Metab. Res.* **2:**233–237.

Wilkinson, P. C., Singh, H., and Sorkin, E., 1970, Serum immunoglobulin levels in thymus deficient pituitary dwarf mice, *Immunol.* **18:**437–441.

Williamson, A. R., and Askonas, B. A., 1972, Senescence of an antibody-forming cell clone, *Nature* **238:**337–339.

Wortis, H. H., 1975, Pleiotropic effects of the nude mutation, in: *Immunodeficiency in man and animals,* Birth Defects Original Article Series, vol. XI, No. 1 (D. Bergsma, ed.), pp. 528–530, Sinauer Assoc., Sunderland, Mass.

Yunis, E. J., Fernandes, B. S., and Greenberg, L. J., 1975, Immune deficiency, autoimmunity and aging, in: *Immunodeficiency in Man and Animals,* Birth Defects, original Article Series, vol XI, No. 1 (D. Bergsma, ed.), pp. 185–192, Sinauer Assoc., Sunderland, Mass.

7

Genetic, Developmental, and Evolutionary Aspects of Life Span

JORGE J. YUNIS, LEONARD J. GREENBERG,
and EDMOND J. YUNIS

1. Introduction

In a broad sense, life span and aging can be defined as the length of survival and the collective changes that occur during the period between conception and death (Buerger, 1957). Like most biological phenomena, there is ample evidence to support both genetic and environmental approaches to the study of life span and aging (Comfort, 1974). Although life, aging, and death are generally accepted as essential to the evolutionary process, little is known about the factors controlling the life span of a species at the phenotypic level. As a consequence, numerous theories have been proposed to explain the aging process. These theories have implicated biological clocks (Landahl, 1959; Burnet, 1973), the waning of immunologic vigor (Ram, 1967; Walford, 1969; Greenberg and Yunis, 1972), the finite lifetime of cells (Strehler, 1966; Novelli, 1970; Hayflick, 1965, 1974), crosslinking of macromolecules (Bjorksten, 1968), somatic mutation (Mole, 1963; Jones and Kimmeldorf, 1964), accumulation of random errors (Orgel, 1963, 1973), dietary caloric intake (Ross, 1959; McIntyre *et al.*, 1964), and many others.

In this chapter we will examine evidence, both old and new, which supports the idea that the life-span and aging of a species is under genetic regulation. It should be kept in mind, however, that this is an extremely complicated process, involving numerous interactions which change throughout life and which are exquisitely sensitive to the environment. Furthermore, the problem becomes more complex in the case of man because of restrictions in experimentation and the multiplicity of changes that occur over a long life span. In what follows we will first consider the

JORGE J. YUNIS, LEONARD J. GREENBERG, and EDMOND J. YUNIS • Department of Laboratory Medicine and Pathology, University of Minnesota, Minneapolis, Minnesota. Present address of E. J. Y. is Sidney Farber Cancer Institute, Harvard Medical School, Boston, Massachusetts.

JORGE J. YUNIS,
LEONARD J.
GREENBERG, AND
EDMOND J. YUNIS

influence of evolutionary aspects on longevity; then we will examine factors acting during embryogenesis and development and others during senescence; next, we will discuss genetic factors controlling life-shortening disease states manifested in some during neonatal, young, and adult life; and finally, we will examine the role of the immune system in the pathogenesis of aging.

2. Evolutionary Aspects of Longevity

Investigation of constitutional factors in mammalian longevity was initiated by Rubner (1908a,b) and Friedenthal (1910) and taken up by Sacher, who has recently suggested that the rate of growth of brain tissue governs the length of gestation time of a species and that, in general, big-brained animals live longer than small-brained animals of similar body size (Sacher and Staffeldt, 1974; Sacher, 1976). Sacher (1976) has also observed that an increase of approximately 12% in brain size took place between the period of evolution of man from *Australopithecus africanus* to *Homo sapiens* over a period of about 200,000 years. During this period, fossil records suggest that there was a concomitant 40-year increase of maximum life span. The genetic basis of such a rapid rate in evolution is not clear, but they alert us to the possibility that those considerable increases in brain size and longevity were accomplished by allelic substitution at a comparatively small number of gene loci.

In addition to the importance of brain size on the length of gestation and life span, it appears that the determination of metabolic entropy of a species also yields a predictive longevity value, since longevity varies inversely as the square root of entropy. This inverse relationship means that an increase of metabolic rate at constant temperature, or a decrease of body temperature at constant metabolic rate, is associated with shorter life, while an increase of body temperature for a constant metabolic rate is associated with longer life (Sacher, 1975). The estimation of metabolic entropy enables one to reconcile a discrepancy previously observed between the longevities of small mammals and like-sized passerine birds, since perching birds as a group outlive mammals of comparable size and have higher body temperatures (2° to 5°C) (Altman and Dittmer, 1972). The consistency between these taxonomically remote classes of vertebrates suggests that the metabolic entropy factor may be found to hold for all vertebrates (Sacher, 1975).

3. Morphogenesis, Cell Program, and Life Span

Although little is known about the pathogenesis of senescence, and little agreement exists regarding the true nature of the aging process, generally there is no difficulty including, as a part of the aging process, conditions such as graying of hair, wrinkling of skin, and arteriosclerosis while excluding embryogenesis and maturation. And yet, both groups of phenomena are clearly interdependent since aging and death of individual cells occur at all stages of development and organs involute according to a specific timetable. For example, the placenta involutes during the gestational period, the thymus involutes during childhood, and the ovary involutes after five decades in normal females. Perhaps the major distinction that can be identified between the processes of development and aging is that during the latter, no proteins, matrices, or organs with essentially new structures or functions arise, and there is a progressive decline of function associated with increased vulnerability (Goldstein, S., 1971a).

Mammalian cells and tissues normally follow a defined schedule of growth. During embryogenesis, all organs increase in size by cell division. By the time of adolescence, the growth of virtually all organs ceases as the somatic proportions of adulthood are attained. Thereafter, in general, much less mitotic activity is required to maintain the steady state. The defined time table of organ development and involution in a species, as well as the limits reflected by a preordained proliferative capacity of cells after birth (Hayflick, 1965, 1974) strongly suggest that the life span of a species is under genetic control and factors involved in cell differentiation and growth are critical to the understanding of longevity and aging.

The study of the differential proliferative capacity of cell types from birth to death suggest that cells and organs are programmed in a precise manner of specific functions in a finite lifetime. For example, nervous tissue and muscle cells lose virtually all mitotic capacity during early adulthood; fibroblasts, hepatic cells, renal tubular cells, and bone cells turn over slowly under normal conditions and regenerate less rapidly in older animals, and gastrointestinal and hematopoietic cells divide at a plateau level through adult life, except for a tendency to decline under senescence (Post and Hoffman, 1968; Goldstein, S., 1971a). Recently, Gelfant and Grove (1974) suggested that the general decline in immunological surveillance that occurs with age is basically related to the age-associated decrease in proliferative capacity observed in immunocompetent T and B cells (Price and Makinodan, 1972; Hori et al., 1973). Since most immunocyte precursors are in the noncycling state (cells blocked in G_1 and G_2 which are capable of moving through the cell cycle upon specific stimulation) and the immune response depends upon proliferation of T and B lymphocytes, it is possible that a critical rate-limiting step may be the impairment of release of noncycling cells to the cycling stage with age. In this context, Burnet (1973) has suggested that the thymus may act as a biological clock which is genetically programmed to operate at a rate consistent with the optimal lifetime of the species.

There appears to be a similar program for the neuroendocrine system, which in turn influences both the differentiative and proliferative functions of body cells during embryogenesis, development, and senescence. For example, there is a precise sequence of biochemical and cell differentiation events that take place during the reproductive cycle of females (Bellamy, 1967); there is an age-dependent loss of proliferative capacity of parotid glands (Adelman et al., 1972); the kidneys' response to antidiuretic hormones is significantly decreased with age (Miller and Shock, 1953); and there is an age-associated reduction in glucose tolerance (Silverstone et al., 1957) that can be explained on the basis of a lower number of beta cells and a reduction in the sensitivity of beta cells of the pancreas to blood sugar levels (Shock and Andres, 1968; Shock, 1974).

Another interesting example of endocrine control can be found in the case of the pituitary dwarf mouse in which a defect, transmitted as an autosomal disease, involves both the endocrine and the immune systems. In these animals, growth is markedly retarded, there is low muscular activity and sterility, and the endocrine system is underdeveloped. Of importance is the fact that the dwarf mouse is affected by an immunodeficiency syndrome, which is characterized by hypotrophy of the thymus with progressive loss of small cortical lymphocytes, hypotrophy of the spleen and nodes, partial impairment of humoral immunity, marked depression of cellular immunity, and, finally, an extremely reduced life span. All these defects can be prevented by administration of growth hormone and thyroxine for 30 days

JORGE J. YUNIS,
LEONARD J.
GREENBERG, AND
EDMOND J. YUNIS

during the post-weaning period (Fabris, 1975). In man, there is no known counter-part for the dwarf mouse except for ataxia telangiectasia in which it is possible that degeneration of the central nervous system affects the hypothalamic control of pituitary function, causing abnormal secretion of growth hormone and resulting in a profound influence on the thymus and immune function (Duquesnoy, 1975). Hypo-thalamic control of endocrine function has been studied by Dilman (1971), who proposed that the hypothalamic activity threshold undergoes an age-associated elevation of feedback suppression. It is possible that this phenomenon results in irreversible changes in the internal environment of the animal which contribute greatly to a breakdown of body functions and become expressed as diseases of aging.

4. Life Shortening Disease States

The central importance of genetic factors on life span become self-evident when it is realized that different species, such as the mouse, dog, horse, and man have differential life spans of 3, 20, 40, and 110 years, respectively, in spite of the fact that they live in a basically similar environment (Makinodan, Chapter 1). In man, there is a positive correlation between parental age and filial life span (Lansing, 1959; Kallman and Jarvik, 1959; Hawkins *et al.*, 1965); monozygotic twins have a similar life span more often than dizygotic twins; and causes of death in monozygotic twins have been found to be similar more than twice as often as in dizygotic twins (Kallman and Sander, 1948; Kallman and Jarvik, 1959; Goldstein, S., 1971a). Although this type of evidence clearly indicates genetic regulation of longevity, it should be kept in mind that the differential life span among individuals of a species, as well as the final aging process, should be viewed in terms of the enormous biochemical variability that exists among members of a species and the exquisite interaction that permeates between environmental and genetic factors. For instance, in man and in *Drosophila,* it is known that up to 30% of their loci are polymorphic (Childs and Der Kaloustian, 1968; Harris and Hopkinson, 1972) and some of these traits respond differently to factors such as diet. Rather striking examples of genetic–environmental interaction come to light in the study of the common type of diabetes and atherosclerosis, in which the onset and the severity of clinical manifestations depend on the interaction of one or several allelic genes in close relation to environmental factors (Goldstein, S., 1971b; Goldstein, J. L., 1973; Ostrander *et al.*, 1974).

Based on actuarial statistics in Europe and North America, it is known that approximately 2% of the population dies before 1 year of age, 5% before 40 years of age, 15% before 60 years of age, 65% before 80 years of age, 90% before 90 years of age, and very few individuals survive the 100-year mark (Makinodan, Chapter 1). At least 40% of all infant mortality results from genetic factors, while congenital malformations are the second leading cause of death of children under 1 year of age (Childs, 1975). Although it is difficult to assign specific genetic defects as a cause of death in the other age categories, the fact is that approximately 20% of the general population have genetic defects which are known to shorten life span (Scriver *et al.*, 1973; Goldstein, J. L., 1973; Ostrander *et al.*, 1974) and must contribute signifi-cantly to the death of individuals below 60–70 years of age. By way of example, we might consider diabetes, which is one of the most common diseases in the general adult population and whose prevalence reaches 2% among men below 40 years of age, 9% before 60 years of age, and 11% before 70 years of age (Ostrander *et al.*, 1974). The significance of diabetes in aging studies comes from its high frequency, the fact that it shortens life span significantly (Garcia *et al.*, 1974), and that it is also one of the most common and significant denominators of the final decline and death of long-lived individuals.

The familial nature of diabetes has long been known (Harris, 1950) and its prevalence increases among parents and siblings of diabetic individuals (Rimoin, 1967). Studies show a significantly greater concordance among monozygotic twins when compared to dizygotic twins (Gottlieb and Root, 1968). Until recently, there has been some confusion as to the precise mode of genetic transmission. It appears now that diabetes mellitus is a heterogeneous group of disorders that can be at least divided into a juvenile form (Danowski *et al.*, 1969; Rosenbloom, 1970), an autosomal dominant mild juvenile diabetes (Tattersall, 1974), and the adult onset or common type of diabetes that is generally believed to be multifactorial and possibly heterogeneous in inheritance (Simpson, 1962; Neel *et al.*, 1965; Goldstein, S., 1971b).

In the case of atherosclerosis and coronary death, family studies have consistently shown that there is a 2½-fold increase in risk of coronary death among first-degree relatives of coronary patients (Gertler and White, 1954; Rose, 1964). Employing life tables to take into account the increasing risks in the population with age, Slack and Evans (1966) found that the increased risk to relatives is greater among younger patients and greatest for relatives of young female patients. In this study there was a five-fold increase in the risk of coronary death before 55 years to male relatives of the younger female patients. Also, twin studies showed that there is a higher concordance rate among monozygotic than among dizygotic twins of like sex and that the difference is greater among female than male pairs. These findings are explained best by polygenic inheritance in which liability for the common type of atherosclerosis can be greatly modified by sex and environmental factors (Harvald and Hauge, 1970; Slack, 1974). In addition to the multigenic type of disease state, at least three types of hyperlipidemia, which is conducive to coronary death have been found to segregate in families as single gene defects. These disorders affect 0.6–0.75% of individuals in the general population and can be listed among the main risk factors for heart attacks early in middle life (Goldstein, 1973).

Another example of a single gene defect is provided by the role of alpha$_1$-antitrypsin deficiency in obstructive emphysema (Talamo, 1975). Alpha$_1$ trypsin inhibitor is a serum protein that exists in the population in multiple forms of which two rather common ones, S and Z, are associated with severe emphysema that develops early in adult life. Since the Z allele has a population frequency of about 2% and the S, of about 4%, the most important problem is not so much the homozygous diseases, which have a frequency of approximately one per 1000, but whether the Z or S alleles in combination or with a normal allele would help explain why some heavy smokers develop emphysema while others do not (Childs, 1975). In this connection, it has recently been shown that the heterozygotes for these alleles have a slightly decreased lung capacity when compared to normal individuals (Cooper *et al.*, 1974).

A final example of single gene defects deals with the relationship between aryl hydrocarbon hydroxylase and the development of bronchogenic carcinoma. This emzyme exists in two forms in the human population, one of which is easily inducible by carcinogens and the other is not. The readily inducible form exists in perhaps 10% of people, the least inducible form in about 45%, with the remainder being heterozygotes with intermediate induction (Kellerman *et al.*, 1973a). When Kellerman *et al.* studied 50 patients with lung cancer, they found the distribution reversed with 30% being highly inducible, 4% poorly inducible, and 66% intermediate (Kellerman *et al.*, 1973b). Also, they observed that all the patients with lung cancer were heavy smokers. More work needs to be done to confirm the conclusion that this study seems to suggest; namely, that there is a relationship between a genetically determined enzyme quality, heavy smoking, and bronchogenic carcinoma.

5. Immunogenetic Aspects of Aging

In an exhaustive treatise, Walford (1969) has proposed an immunologic theory of aging which he claims provides a link between the etiologic theories and actual aging in higher animals. According to Walford, aging is due to changes with age of cells that determine self-recognition. Progressive breakdown of this recognition system results in the onset of autoimmunity and other age-associated disease states. It appears to us, however, that this theory must include the cooperative interactions of T cells and B cells and the genetic control of amplification and/or suppression of their function. The basis for this derives from recently acquired knowledge about the involvement of major histocompatibility systems of mouse and man in the regulation of immune responsiveness and association with disease states (McDevitt and Benacerraf, 1969; Walford, 1970; McDevitt and Bodmer, 1974; Ryder *et al.*, 1974).

In the mouse, a region of chromosome 17 has been defined as containing histocompatibility (H_2) and immune response (Ir) genes as well as several defined genetic systems such as the S region, which controls the synthesis of complement (Shreffler and David, 1975; Benacerraf and McDevitt, 1972; Dorf *et al.*, 1975a,b; Frelinger *et al.*, 1975). In addition, studies have shown linkage of the H_2 antigen complex to susceptibility or resistance to virus infection, neoplasia, and autoimmune disease (Lilly, 1968, 1971; Vladutiu and Rose, 1971; Doherty and Zinkernagel, 1975; Yunis *et al.*, 1975; Greenberg and Yunis, 1975).

In man, there is an association between the histocompatibility complex (HLA) and a variety of disease states that can be grouped into three major categories: the HLA-B27 associated arthropathies (ankylosing spondylitis, reactive arthritis, and acute anterior uveitis), the HLA-B8 and DW3 associated "immunopathic disorders" (juvenile diabetes, myasthenia gravis, coeliac disease, dermatitis herpetiformis, and Addison's and Graves' diseases), and HLA-B7 DW2 associated disorders (multiple sclerosis and C_4 deficiency) (Svejgaard *et al.*, 1975). McDevitt and Bodmer (1974) have reviewed this area and have suggested that anomalies in immune-response genes linked to HLA may explain this phenomenon. To date, however, there is no clear-cut evidence linking Ir genes to disease states in man or mouse, nor is it known whether Ir genes will be important in the clinical outcome of exposure to pathogens. The reliability of HLA antigens as markers of disease states depends on the continuous cosegregation of the genes that are involved. Consequently, in some instances, HLA antigens will serve as reliable markers of disease states, while in other instances they may reflect resistance to disease and may provide a potential marker of longevity. A relationship between histocompatibility markers and longevity has already been observed in mice whereby, in three different strains derived from three different stocks, the $H-2^b$ gene appears to be associated with the longest lived strain (Walford, 1974).

In the foregoing discussion, we have alluded to a balance of immune reaction and genetic regulation of immune responsiveness as necessary requirements for resistance to disease and longevity. Numerous studies suggest that the primary age-related effect on the immune system is a decrease in T cell functional capacity (Heidrick and Makinodan, 1972). That this deficiency may be important in the pathogenesis of diseases of the aged in man gains support by the finding that old people with defective cell-mediated immunity have decreased life expectancy as compared to those with normal T cell function (Roberts-Thomson *et al.*, 1974). Thus an immunologic imbalance of T cell and B cell cooperativity may provide the basis for an important pathogenetic influence in the production of autoantibodies and the diseases of aging. An integral part of the T cell and B cell cooperativity involves different subsets of T lymphocytes which have helper or suppressor function (Gershon and Hencin, 1971; Gershon and Liebhaber, 1972; Hoffman and Kappler, 1972; Baker *et al.*, 1974; Rich and Pierce, 1975).

The profound deficiency of T cell function that occurs with aging could be a consequence of a genetically programmed failure of thymic function, which is consistent with the concept of a thymic clock. This clock phenomenon must vary from strain to strain, autoimmune susceptible versus resistant (Yunis and Greenberg, 1974), and from human to human (Roberts-Thomson *et al.*, 1974). It appears that there is a differential decline in different subsets of T lymphocytes which may be under genetic control.

Burnet (1973) recently presented an interpretation of aging which combines genetic programming with the stochastic random error theory proposed by Orgel (1963, 1973). Under this concept, random accumulation of error in cells results from genetically determined degrees of error-proneness in DNA polymerases and other enzymes that are responsible for the fidelity with which DNA is replicated or reconstituted after damage and repair. The accumulation of errors on thymus-derived lymphocytes could result in age-dependent loss of T cell function. Since T-cell-mediated immunity is important in tumor immunity, in the host defense against infection, in the preservation of self-tolerance, and in the general regulation of the level of immune responsiveness, the genetically programmed failure of thymic function could well play a major role in the pathogenesis of autoimmunity, aging, and age-related diseases.

6. Summary

> *By medicine life may be prolonged*
> *Yet death will seize the doctor too.*
> *—Cymbeline, Shakespeare*

In this chapter it has been pointed out that any definition of aging needs to be related to an understanding of the control mechanisms of morphogenesis, differentiation, and metabolism. These control mechanisms, which regulate the internal and external environment of cellular interactions, are mediated by the coordinated activity of the nervous and endocrine systems and change during life from fertilization to senescence in order to maintain a dynamic steady state. A life-long homeostasis depends, to a considerable degree, upon an intact immune system for the maintenance of internal integrity and for protection against the external environment. Since all processes of life are regulated at various levels of a hierarchy, some acting during embryogenesis, differentiation, and growth and others during senescence, it is not surprising that no single theory of aging is adequate in itself to describe the aging process in its entirety. Within the animal kingdom, however, there are numerous examples that suggest a unitary genetic control of long life to explain the presence of cellular and organ clocks, the existence of long-lived strains of mice, and families with long-lived individuals.

From the foregoing discussion, it appears that the optimum lifetime of a species is predetermined by an exquisite interaction of cells, organs, and systems of the body through various phases of growth and senescence, which is genetically regulated. Although life span is affected by environmental factors and can be manipulated in part by medicine, sanitation, and nutrition, the mechanisms are not fully understood and no one knows how long one can prolong life.

References

Adelman, R. C., Stein, G., Roth, G. S., and Englander, D., 1972, Age-dependent regulation of mammalian DNA synthesis and cell proliferation *in vivo,* in: *Mechanisms of Ageing and Development,* Vol. 1, pp. 49–59, Elsevier Sequoia S.A., The Netherlands.

Altman, P. L., and Dittmer, D. S., 1972, *Biology Data Book,* Vol. I, Federation of American Societies for Experimental Biology, Bethesda, Maryland.

Baker, P. J., Stasliak, P. W., Amsbaugh, D. F., and Prescott, B., 1974, Regulation of the antibody response to type III pneumococcal polysaccharide. III. Mode of action of thymic-derived suppressor cells, *J. Immunol.* **1120:**404–409.

Bellamy, D., 1967, Hormonal effects in relation to ageing in mammals, *Symp. Soc. Exp. Biol.* **21:**427–450.

Benacerraf, B., and McDevitt, H. O., 1972, Histocompatibility-linked immune response-genes; a new class of genes that controls the formation of specific tissue responses has been identified, *Science* **175:**273–279.

Bjorksten, J., 1968, The crosslinkage theory of aging, *J. Am. Geriat. Soc.* **16:**408–427.

Buerger, M., 1957, Biomorphose oder Gerontologie?, *Z. Altersforsch* **10:**279–283.

Burnet, F. M., 1973, A genetic interpretation of ageing, *Lancet* **2:**480–483.

Childs, B., 1975, Prospects for genetic screening, *J. Pediat.* **87:**1125–1132.

Childs, B., and Der Kaloustian, V. M., 1968, Genetic heterogeneity, *New Engl. J. Med.* **279:**1205–1212, 1267–1274.

Comfort, A., 1974, The position of aging studies, in: *Mechanisms of Aging and Development,* Vol. 3, pp. 1–31, Elsevier Sequoia S.A., Lausanne, The Netherlands.

Cooper, D. M., Hoeppner, V., Cox, D., Zamel, N., Bryan, A. C., and Levison, H., 1974, Lung function of alpha$_1$-antitrypsin heterozygotes (Pi type MZ), *Am. Rev. Resp. Dis.* **110:**708–715.

Danowski, T. S., Tsai, C. T., Morgan, C-R., Sieracki, J. C., Alley, R. A., Robbins, T. J., Sabeh, G., and Sunder, J. H., 1969, Serum growth hormone and insulin in females without glucose intolerance, *Metabolism* **18:**811–820.

Dilman, V., 1971, Age associated elevation of hypothalamic threshhold to feedback control and its role in development, ageing, and disease, *Lancet* **1:**1211–1219.

Doherty, P. C., and Zinkernagel, R. M., 1975, A. biological role for the major histocompatibility antigens, *Lancet* **1:**1406–1409.

Dorf, M., Balner, H., and Benacerraf, B., 1975a, Mapping of the immune response genes in the major histocompatibility complex of the Rhesus monkey, *J. Exp. Med.* **142:**673–693.

Dorf, M., Stimpfling, J., and Benacerraf, B., 1975b, Requirement for two H-2 complex *Ir* genes for the immune response to the L-GLU, L-LYS, L-PHE Ter polymer, *J. Exp. Med.* **141:**1459–1463.

Duquesnoy, R., 1975, The pituitary dwarf mouse: A model for study of indocrine immunodeficiency disease, in: *Immunodeficiency in Man and Animals* (D. Bergsma, R. A. Good, and J. Finstad, eds.), *Birth Defects Original Series,* **21**(1):536–543.

Fabris, N., 1975, Relation of lymphoid system and hormones to aging, in: *Immunodeficiency in Man and Animals* (D. Bergsma, R. A. Good, and J. Finstad, eds.), *Birth Defects Original Series* 21(1):533–535.

Frelinger, J. A., Niederhuber, J. E., and Schreffler, D. C., 1975, Inhibition of immune responses *in vitro* by specific antiserums to Ia antigens, *Science* **188**:268–270.

Friedenthal, H., 1910, Über die Gultigkeit der Massenwirkung für den Energiemsatz der lebendigen Substanz, *Zentralbl. Physiol.* **24**:321–237.

Garcia, M. J., McNamara, P. M., Gordon, T., and Kannell, W. B., 1974, Morbidity and mortality in diabetics in the Framingham population. Sixteen year follow-up study, *Diabetes* **23**:105–116.

Gelfant, S., and Grove, G. L., 1974, Cycling ⇄ noncycling cells as an explanation for the aging process, in: *Symp. on the Theoretical Aspects of Aging* (M. Rockstein, ed.), pp. 105–177, Academic Press, New York, San Francisco, London.

Gershon, R. K., and Hencin, R. S., 1971, The DNA synthetic response of adoptively transferred thymocytes in the spleens of lethally irradiated mice, *J. Immunol.* **197**:1723–1728.

Gershon, R. K., and Liebhaber, S. A., 1972, The response of T cells to histocompatibility-2 antigens, dose-response kinetics, *J. Exp. Med.* **136**:112–127.

Gertler, M. M., and White, P. D., 1954, *Coronary Heart Disease in Young Adults; A Multidisciplinary Study,* Harvard University Press, Cambridge, Massachusetts.

Goldstein, J. L., 1973, Genetic aspects of hyperlipidemia in coronary heart disease, *Hosp. Practice* (October):53–65.

Goldstein, S., 1971a, The biology of aging, *New Engl. J. Med.* **285**:1120–1129.

Goldstein, S., 1971b, Analytical review: The pathogenesis of diabetes mellitus and its relationship to aging, *Humangenetik* **12**:83–100.

Gottlieb, M. S., and Root, H. F., 1968, Diabetes mellitus in twins, *Diabetes* **17**:693–704.

Greenberg, L. J., and Yunis, E. J., 1972, Immunologic control of aging: A possible primary event, *Gerontologia* **18**:247–266.

Greenberg, L. J., and Yunis, E. J., 1975, Immunogenetic aspects of viral oncogenesis, in: *Molecular Pathology* (R. A. Good, S. Day, and J. J. Yunis, eds.), pp. 328–353, Charles C Thomas, Springfield, Illinois.

Harris, H., 1950, The familial distribution of diabetes mellitus: A study of the relatives of diabetic propositi, *Ann. Eugen.* (London) **15**:95–119.

Harris, H., and Hopkinson, D. A., 1972, Average heterozygosity per locus in man; an estimate based on the incidence of enzyme polymorphisms, *Ann. Hum. Genet.* **36**:9–20.

Harvald, B., and Hauge, M., 1970, Coronary occlusion in twins, *Acta Geneticae Medicae et Gemellologiae* **19**:248–250.

Hawkins, M. R., Murphy, E. A., and Abbey, H., 1965, The familial component in longevity. A study of the offspring of nonagenarians. I. Methods and preliminary report, *Bulletin of the Johns Hopkins Hospital* **117**:24–36.

Hayflick, L., 1965, The limited *in vitro* lifetime of human diploid cell strains, *Exp. Cell Res.* **37**:614–636.

Hayflick, L., 1974, The longevity of cultured human cells, *Am. Geriatrics Soc.* **22**:1–12.

Heidrick, M. L., and Makinodan, T., 1972, Nature of cellular deficiencies in age-related decline of the immune system, *Gerontologia* **18**:305–320.

Hoffman, M., and Kappler, J. W., 1972, The antigen specificity of thymus derived helper cells, *J. Immunol.* **108**:261–263.

Hori, Y., Perkins, E. H., and Halsall, M. K., 1973, Decline of phytohemagglutinin responsiveness of spleen cells from aging mice (37524), *Proc. Soc. Exp. Biol. Med.* **144**:48–53.

Jones, D. C. L., and Kimmeldorf, D. J., 1964, Effect of age at irradiation on life span in the male rat, *Radiat. Res.* **22**:106–115.

Kallman, F. J., and Jarvik, L., 1959, Individual differences in constitution and genetic background, in: *Handbook of Aging and the Individual, Psychological and Biological Aspects* (J. E. Birren, ed.), pp. 216–263, University of Chicago Press, Chicago, Illinois.

Kallman, F. J., and Sander, G., 1948, Twin studies on aging and longevity, *J. Heredity* **39**:349–357.

Kellerman, G., Luyten-Kellerman, M., and Shaw, C. R., 1973a, Genetic variation of aryl hydrocarbon hydroxylase in human lymphocytes, *Am. J. Hum. Genet.* **25**:327–331.

Kellerman, G., Shaw, C. R., and Luyten-Kellerman, M., 1973b, Aryl hydrocarbon hydroxylase inducibility and bronchogenic carcinoma, *New Engl. J. Med.* **289**:934–937.

JORGE J. YUNIS,
LEONARD J.
GREENBERG, AND
EDMOND J. YUNIS

Landahl, H. D., 1959, in: *Handbook of Aging and the Individual; Psychological and Biological Aspects* (J. E. Birren, ed.), pp. 81–118, University of Chicago Press, Chicago, Illinois.

Lansing, A. I., 1959, General biology of senescence, in: *Handbook of Aging and the Individual; Psychological and Biological Aspects* (J. E. Birren, ed.), pp. 119–135, University of Chicago Press, Chicago, Illinois.

Lilly, F. J., 1968, The effect of histocompatibility-2 type on response to the Friend leukemia virus in mice, *J. Exp. Med.* **127:**465–473.

Lilly, F. J., 1971, The influence of H-2 type on gross virus leukemogenesis in mice, *Transplant. Proc.* **3:**1239–1242.

McDevitt, H. O., and Benacerraf, B., 1969, Genetic control of specific immune responses, *Adv. Immunol.* **11:**31–74.

McDevitt, H. O., and Bodmer, W. F., 1974, HL-A immune-response genes and disease, *Lancet* **1:**1269–1275.

McIntyre, K. R., Sell, S., and Miller, J. F. A. P., 1964, Pathogenesis of the post-neonatal thymectomy syndrome, *Nature* (London) **204:**151–155.

Michael, A. F., Drummond, K. N., Good, R. A., and Vernier, R. L., 1966, Acute poststreptococcal glomerulonephritis: Immune deposit disease, *J. Clin. Invest.* **45:**237–248.

Miller, J. H., and Shock, N. W., 1953, Age differences in the renal tubular response to antidiuretic hormone, *J. Gerontol.* **8:**446–450.

Mole, R. H., 1963, in: *Cellular Basis and Aetiology of Late Somatic Effects of Ionizing Radiation* (H. Harris, ed.), pp. 273–276, Academic Press, New York.

Neel, J. V., Fajans, S. S., Conn, J. W., and Davidson, R. T., 1965, Symposium diabetes mellitus, in: *Genetics and the Epidermiology of Chronic Diseases* (J. V. Neel, M. W. Shaw, and W. J. Schull, eds.), pp. 105–132, Public Health Service Publication #1163.

Novelli, G. D., 1970, Regulation at the cellular level, with possible reference to differentiation and possible mechanisms of aging, in: *Symposium on Cellular and Macromolecular Aspects of Aging,* Oak Ridge Nat. Lab., Gatlinburg.

Orgel, L. E., 1963, The maintenance and accuracy of protein synthesis and its relevance to ageing, *Proc. Nat. Acad. Sci. U.S.A.* **49:**517–521.

Orgel, L. E., 1973, Ageing of clones of mammalian cells, *Nature* **243:**441–445.

Ostrander, L. D., Lamphiear, D. E., Block, W. D., Johnson, B. C., and Epstein, F. H., 1974, Biochemical precursors of atherosclerosis, *Arch. Intern. Med.* **134:**224–230.

Post, J., and Hoffman, J., 1968, Cell renewal patterns, *New Engl. J. Med.* **279:**248–258.

Price, G. B., and Makinodan, T., 1972, Immunologic deficiencies in senescence. I. Characterization of intrinsic deficiencies, *J. Immunol.* **108:**403–412.

Ram, J. S., 1967, Aging and immunological phenomena. A review, *J. Gerontol.* **22:**92–107.

Rich, R. R., and Pierce, C. W., 1975, Biological expressions of lymphocyte activation. II. Generation of a population of thymus derived suppressor lymphocytes, *J. Exp. Med.* **137:**649–659.

Rimoin, D. L., 1967, Genetics of diabetes mellitus, *Diabetes* **16:**346–351.

Roberts-Thomson, I. C., Whittingham, S., Youngchaiyud, U., and MacKay, I. R., 1974, Ageing, immune response, and mortality, *Lancet* **2:**368–370.

Rose, G., 1964, Familial patterns in ischaemic heart disease, *Brit. J. of Preventive and Social Medicine* **18:**75–80.

Rosenbloom, A. L., 1970, Insulin responses of children with chemical diabetes mellitus, *New Engl. J. Med.* **282:**1228–1231.

Ross, M. H., 1959, Proteins, calories and life expectancy, *Fed. Proc.* **18:**1190–1207.

Rubner, M., 1908a, Problemes des Wachstums und der Lebensdauer, Gesellschaft fur innere Medizin und Kinderheilkunde, Wien, Mitteilungen, Beiblatt, Vol. 7, 58–81.

Rubner, M., 1908b, Das Problem der Lebensdauer und seine Beziehungen zum Wachstum and Ernahrung, Oldenbourg, Munich.

Ryder, L. P., Staub-Nielsen, L., and Svejgaard, A., 1974, Association between HLA histocompatibility antigens and non-malignant diseases, *Humangenetik* **25:**251–264.

Sacher, G. A., 1975, Maturation and longevity in relation to the cranial capacity in hominid evolution, in: *Antecedents of Man and After. I. Primates: Functional morphology and evolution* (R. Tuttle, ed.), pp. 417–441, Mouton Publishers, The Hague.

Sacher, G. A., 1976, Evaluation of the entropy and information terms governing mammalian longevity, in: *Interdisciplinary Topics of Gerontology* (R. G. Cutler, ed.), Vol. 9, pp. 69–82, Karger, Basel.

101

GENETIC,
DEVELOPMENTAL,
AND EVOLUTIONARY
ASPECTS OF LIFE
SPAN

Sacher, G. A., and Staffeldt, E. F., 1974, Relationship of gestation time to brain weight for placental mammals: Implications for the theory of vertebrate growth, *The Am. Naturalist* **108**:593–615.

Scriver, C. R., Neal, J. L., Saginur, R., and Clow, A., 1973, The frequency of genetic disease and congenital malformation among patients in a pediatric hospital, *Can. Med. Assoc. J.* **108**:1111–1115.

Shock, N. W., 1974, Physiological theories of aging, in: *Theoretical Aspects of Aging,* (M. Rockstein, ed.), pp. 119–136, Academic Press, New York, San Francisco, London.

Shock, N. W., and Andres, R., 1968, in: *Adaptive Capacities of an Aging Organism* (D. F. Chebatarev, ed.), pp. 235–254, Acad. Sci. USSR, Kiev.

Shreffler, D. C., and David, C. S., 1975, The H-2 major histocompatibility complex and the I immune response region: Genetic variation, function, and organization, in: *Advances in Immunology* (W. H. Taliaferro and J. H. Humphrey, eds.), Vol. 20, p. 125, Academic Press, New York.

Silverstone, F. A., Bradfonbrener, M., Shock, N. W., and Yiengst, M. J., 1957, Age differences in the intravenous glucose tolerance test and the response to insulin, *J. Clin. Invest.* **36**:504–514.

Simpson, N. E., 1962, The genetics of diabetes: A study of 233 families of juvenile diabetics, *Ann. Hum. Genet.* **26**:1–21.

Slack, J., 1974, Genetic differences in liability to atherosclerotic heart disease, *J. Roy. Coll. Phycns. Lond.* **8**:115–126.

Slack, J., and Evans, K. A., 1966, The increased risk of death from ischaemic heart disease in first degree relatives of 121 men and 96 women with ischaemic heart disease, *J. Med. Genet.* **3**:239–257.

Strehler, B., 1966, Code degeneracy and the aging process. A molecular-genetic theory of aging, *Proc. 7th Int. Congr. of Gerontology* **1**:177–185.

Svejgaard, A., Platz, P., Ryder, L. P., Staub-Nielsen, L., and Thomsen, M., 1975, HLA and disease associations—A survey, *Transplant Rev.* **22**:3–43.

Talamo, R. C., 1975, Basic and clinical aspects of the alpha$_1$-antitrypsin, *Pediat.* **56**:91–99.

Tattersall, R. B., 1974, Mild familial diabetes with dominant inheritance, *Quart. J. Med.* **43**:339–357.

Vladutiu, A. O., and Rose, N. R., 1971, Autoimmune murine thyroiditis: Relations to histocompatibility (H-2) type, *Science* **174**:1137–1139.

Walford, R. L., 1969, *The Immunologic Theory of Aging,* Munksgaard, Copenhagen.

Walford, R. L., 1970, Antibody diversity, histocompatibility systems, disease states, and aging, *Lancet* **2**:1226–1229.

Walford, R. L., 1974, Immunologic theory of aging: Current status, *Fed. Proc.* **33**:2020–2027.

Yunis, E. J., Fernandes, G., and Greenberg, L. J., 1975, Deficiency, autoimmunity and aging, *Birth Defects Original Series* **11**:185–192.

Yunis, E. J., and Greenberg, L. J., 1974, Immunopathology of aging, *Fed. Proc.* **33**:2017–2019.

8

Suppressor Cells in Aging

RICHARD K. GERSHON
and CHARLES M. METZLER

It is well known that after a certain optimal age the immune system declines in function. This is not particularly surprising since the lymphoid system is not unique in showing declining function with age. What strikes some people as paradoxical is that this decline is often accompanied by an increase in autoantibody production. However, with the general recognition in the past few years that there are subsets of T cells which act to suppress the immune response, a hypothesis linking declining T cell function with increasing autoantibody production has gained acceptance in some circles. The apparent paradox could be resolved by hypothesizing that the increase in autoantibody production is the result of a decrease in suppressor T cell function. Support for this thesis has been found in the observation that athymic nude mice have more autoantibodies than do their littermate controls which have a thymus (Morse *et al.,* 1974). Further support has been gleaned from studies on the NZB mouse, which have been interpreted to indicate that the autoantibody production that these mice are famous for is associated with a loss of suppressor T cell function (Steinberg *et al.,* 1975; Talal and Steinberg, 1974).

It is our opinion that the available evidence is insufficient to warrant the theory that suppressor T cell function is preferentially lost with age and, further, that this theory is probably incorrect. To substantiate this statement we will present a brief review of what is presently known about suppressor T cells and then speculate on why we think the theory is wrong. The review presented here will be brief, since a number of reviews on suppressor T cell activity have recently appeared (Gershon, 1974a; Gershon, 1974b, Gershon, 1974c, Gershon, 1975; Gershon *et al.,* 1974, Katz and Benacerraf, 1974; Möller, 1975; Pierce and Kapp, 1976). Readers interested in experimental details should refer to this list.

RICHARD K. GERSHON and CHARLES M. METZLER • Department of Pathology, Yale University School of Medicine, New Haven, Connecticut.

RICHARD K.
GERSHON AND
CHARLES M.
METZLER

1. Immunological Tolerance

In a number of diverse situations it has been shown that animals that are operationally tolerant (i.e., unable to make a specific immune response to an immunogenic form of the antigen following a previous encounter with that antigen) have cells which, if mixed with other normal cells, convey the specific immunological unresponsiveness to the normal population. This has been referred to as "infectious immunological tolerance." Such demonstrations have been shown with soluble and particulate antigens, with low-zone and high-zone tolerance, and with either cell-mediated or humoral immunity as the assay. Thus it has been suggested that these "suppressor" T cells may play a role in either the induction and/or the maintenance of the tolerant state. There are also numerous reports of an inability to show suppressor T cell activity in cases of immunological tolerance. It is not clear at this time whether this means there are multiple mechanisms for tolerance induction, or whether these are simply examples of technical failures.

2. Antigen Competition

In addition to the specific suppressive effects produced by T cells there are also a number of experiments which show that T cells also produce nonspecific suppressive effects. For instance, it is well known that supernatants of mixed lymphocyte cultures contain helper activity to unrelated antigens. Therefore it is not surprising that there should be some counter-balancing suppressor activity of a nonspecific nature. This notion has been referred to as the "Second Law of Thymodynamics," that is, for every helper T cell effect there is an equal and opposite suppressor effect (Gershon, 1974a). In several instances it has been shown that antigen competition, a temporary period of anergy to one antigen produced by stimulation of the animal with another antigen, is mediated at least in part by suppressor T cells. The mechanisms by which they do so is not clear. However, after stimulation with antigen there is a suppressor influence present which is radiation-resistant. Thus animals stimulated with antigen, then lethally irradiated and reconstituted with normal T cells, are as anergic as mice which are immunized but not irradiated.

3. Effects of Mitogens

This phenomenon may or may not be related to antigen competition. Under appropriate circumstances it has been shown that mitogen stimulated T cells can perform suppressor T cell functions. However, it is not known whether this is a nonspecific effect or a polyspecific effect (i.e., whether the mitogen stimulates all potential clones, and the effect is indeed specific while appearing nonspecific). The mechanism through which mitogen-stimulated T cells suppress their target is not known, although theories abound. Nor is it known whether there is a fully differentiated T cell that will, no matter how stimulated, produce a suppressive effect or whether there are subpopulations of T cells that will, depending upon the signals they receive, help or suppress.

4. Response to "Thymus Independent Antigens"

We would like to comment briefly on studies which have shown that the immune response to what were once thought to be thymus-independent antigens can be augmented by the removal of T cells. The classical work in this area was done by Phil Baker and his colleagues using pneumococcal polysaccharide antigen SIII (Baker, 1975). They have shown that removal of some, but not all, host T cells can cause a marked increase in the immune response to SIII. Removal of all T cells fails to lead to an augmented response. We would interpret these results to indicate that there are some antigens (none of which are protein antigens, incidentally) which, for unknown reasons, have a preferential affinity for activating suppressor T cells and preventing helper T cell activity. When the interaction effects are changed by removing some of the T cells, helper activity can be seen. This is why the response is augmented only when some T cells are removed and is not augmented when all T cells are removed. These results suggest that, at least in some situations, the helper T cell is the target of the suppressor T cell activity.

5. Delayed Type Hypersensitivity

Direct proof that a T cell can be the target of the suppressor cell was obtained in studies of delayed type hypersensitivity. Here the effector cell of the delayed response is clearly a T cell, and T cell suppression of this response, therefore, clearly involves a T–T interaction.

6. Esoteria

In addition to suppressor T cell activity in immune responses to specific antigens, suppressor T cells have been implicated in other areas as well. For example, it has been shown that suppressor T cell activity can be responsible for chronic allotype suppression (Herzenberg and Herzenberg, 1974; Herzenberg *et al.*, 1975), for idiotype-specific suppression (Eichmann, 1975), and even for poly-specific suppression of immunoglobulin production (Waldmann *et al.*, 1975). In addition, not only have suppressor T cells been implicated in IR gene control, an IR suppressor gene(s) has been mapped to the mouse major histocompatibility complex (Debré *et al.*, 1975).

7. Immunoregulation

Interestingly, specific suppressor T cells can be demonstrated in immune animals as well as in tolerant animals. The presence of suppressor cells in both circumstances suggests that these cells play an important role in immunoregulation: in tolerant animals suppressor cells are dominant, and in immune animals helper T cells are dominant. Demonstrating the presence of suppressor T cells in hyperim-mune animals, however, requires an appropriate assay. This point is emphasized by the studies of Eardley and Gershon (1975) who showed that immunized cells transferred to normal mice suppressed the response of the normal mice; however, the same immune cells transferred into irradiated mice produced considerable helper activity. The key cell in the normal mouse, which is responsible for the activation of the suppression and which is killed by irradiation, is a T cell. It has been clearly ruled out that this cell acts to suppress the response by merely occupying space and thus preventing the added helper cells from working. The interactions involved are more complex. Several laboratories are trying to solve this byzantine series of interactions which result in either a net effect of suppression or help, and there is considerable hope that this problem may soon be solved.

One point that is really quite important in trying to determine whether or not a specific immunologic deficit is due to an abnormality of suppressor T cell function, however, is understanding that functional suppressor T cell activity is dependent upon the activity of other cells. For example, it is quite clear that the level of B cell activity in an antibody response can determine whether or not suppressor T cells are activated (Gershon *et al.*, 1974). In addition, there is a large body of evidence which indicates that T cells with the attributes of cells that have been referred to as T1 by Raff and Cantor (1971) act as suppressor cells, in that their removal often augments immune responsiveness. However, in most of these situations, when very carefully examined, it was found that removal of that particular T cell population can also lead to a lack of helper activity. One of the key factors that determines how this particular cell class works seems to be the degree of intensity of antigen stimulation. We will return to the potential role of this particular class of T cells below.

Since suppressor T cell activities are thus dependent upon the activity of the cell that the suppressor T cell is regulating (the regulatee), the interpretation of many experiments is often difficult. One cannot be sure whether the abnormality one finds is due to an inherent defect in the suppressor T cell or to an inherent defect in the cell which is responsible for suppressor cell activation. Lack of a response in a given animal may be due to excess suppressor activity or poor helper activity; or conversely, too much activity may be due to excess helper activity or to a paucity of suppressor activity. This particular point, which we find so important, is usually not considered when interpreting experimental results.

8. The NZB Paradox

Perhaps one of the main reasons for thinking that a deficit in suppressor T cell activity is causally associated with the appearance of autoantibodies stems from studies done on NZB mice. These mice exhibit classical autoimmune disease that is very similar to the human disease systemic lupus erythematosis. A number of years ago it was shown that it was quite difficult to induce tolerance in NZB mice and that the difficulty increased with age. With the suggestion that tolerance might be mediated by suppressor T cells, a number of workers have used several assays to show that suppressor T cell activity declines with age in NZB and related mice. The two standard assays used have been variations of the regulation of graft versus host responses. In one of the assays, it was shown that young T cells from NZB mice could suppress the GVH response produced by more aged T cells (Steinberg *et al.*, 1975). In the other, it was shown that there was an abnormality in the kinetics of the DNA synthetic response of older NZB T cells compared with the response of younger T cells (Dauphinee and Talal, 1973). Both studies suggested to the authors that NZB mouse disease could be explained by a breakdown in suppressor T cell activity with age. The most striking experiments confirming this notion were those which showed that continual injection of young NZB thymocytes into mice, as they aged, prevented the development of the disease (Steinberg *et al.*, 1975).

These then are the experiments which have suggested that the autoimmune disease of NZB mice is produced by a breakdown of suppressor T cell activity and that aging is a contributory factor. There is, however, a great deal of difficulty in extrapolating from these results (and the interpretations derived therefrom) to a general statement that a breakdown in suppressor T cell activity occurs with age. One difficulty is in extrapolating anything from NZB mice in which other work has shown that C type virus infection plays an important role in disease causation (Yoshiki *et al.*, 1974). Thus in these mice one never knows which is the cart and which is the horse. Is a viral infection responsible for the breakdown in T cell regulation, are the two events independent, or is the deficient regulation which occurs with age in these mice responsible for their viral infection? Despite these questions, there is a more fundamental problem with interpreting the above results. This problem stems from the material we just presented which showed that the assay used for study was a key factor in demonstrating suppressor T cell activity. Thus one of the assays used in demonstrating a lack of suppressor T cell activity in NZB mice was the same assay originally used to demonstrate helper interactions between subpopulations of T cells, and indeed formed the basis on which the T1–T2 helper phenomenon was founded (Cantor *et al.*, 1970). It turns out that, by appropriately manipulating the number of each cell type used in the assay, one can use this assay to demonstrate either helper or suppressor activity depending on one's interest, point of view, or other factors. Thus the original studies show that the aged NZB mice were deficient in helper cells, whereas the same assay has been used more recently to show that they are deficient in suppressor cells. Which is true? As we will suggest, we think both are.

The other assay involves a measurement of DNA synthesis of injected cells in a GVH situation (Gershon and Liebhaber, 1972). It has been found that NZB thymic T cells, localizing in spleens of lethally irradiated histo-incompatable recipients, synthesize excess DNA. The excess DNA increases as the animals age (Dauphinee and Talal, 1973). In other strains the T cells reach an earlier peak in DNA synthesis and then shut themselves off. This again has been attributed to a deficit in suppressor T cell activity of the spleen-localizing cells, which many workers think are the suppressor T cells. However, in those studies, while it has been noted that the cells that localize in the spleen behave peculiarly with this excess of DNA synthetic activity, the cells that localize in the lymph nodes do not. In fact, the lymph-node-localizing cells respond much more poorly than do the cells of other strains of mice (Gershon and Kondo, Unpublished). This deficit also increases with age. This might be interpreted to indicate that NZB mice do not lose suppressor cell activity with age, but rather that there is a tendency for excess suppressor activity in one place and a compensatory deficit elsewhere. This situation may be likened to those situations where suppressor T cells have been shown to inactivate antibody production but not delayed type hypersensitivity (DTH), and vice versa. Perhaps it is the lymph-node-seeking cells involved in delayed type hypersensitivity that are being excessively suppressed; and as a consequence, there is excess or deficient regulation of those T cells involved in antibody responses. One must recall that the defect in NZB mice is one of excess autoantibody production and defective immunological tolerance when assayed by antibody production.

NZB mice clearly do not have excessive DTH responses, nor is it difficult to produce homograft tolerance in them. Therefore we would argue that it is more likely that NZB mice have a defect in regulatory interactions between their T cells rather than having an intrinsic defect in suppressor T cell activity. This interpretation is supported by studies that used a different assay than the ones discussed above and these studies conclude that NZB mice have excess, rather than defective, suppressor T cell activity (Roder *et al.,* 1975). This whole story may seem a bit arcane, but the recent elegant, and we would say breakthrough, work of Cantor and Boyse (1975a,b) allows a rational speculation as to what may be occurring with age in T cell regulation.

9. Defining T Cell Subsets Using Antisera Directed Against Ly Differentiation Antigens

Cantor and Boyse have defined three T cell subsets by the use of antisera directed against allelic determinants that are expressed only on T cells. One subset represents approximately 30% of the T cell pool of young adult mice (8 weeks). This subset (Ly1) has the Ly1 antigen on it and does not express the other two. Another subset (Ly2,3) has both the Ly2 antigen and Ly3 antigen on it, and does not express the Ly1 antigen. This subset represents somewhere between 5–10% of the peripheral T cell population of young adult mice. The third subset (Ly1,2,3) expresses all three of the Ly antigens and represents about 50% of the peripheral T cell pool of young adult mice. Interestingly, essentially all the T cells in the cortex of the thymus also express all the Ly1,2,3 antigens, but, in addition, they express the TL antigen that peripheral Ly1,2,3 cells do not. Thus there are at least four subsets of the T cells: Ly1,2,3 TL$^+$, Ly1,2,3 TL$^-$, Ly1, and Ly2,3. Because of the difficulty in positively selecting cells, the precise role of the cells bearing all three of the Ly antigens is not yet known. However, using negative selection experiments, Cantor, together with a series of collaborators, has worked out the functions of the Ly1 and the Ly2,3 cells. Much of this work is unpublished at the time of this writing, but it can be essentially summed up as follows.

The Ly1 cell is responsible for all helper effects that have yet been described or ascribed to T cells. The Ly2,3 cell is responsible for all the suppressor effects. In addition, the Ly2,3 cell is the cell responsible for cell-mediated lympholysis, which is why this particular T cell subset has been called the killer cell. Lastly, the Ly1 cell is both necessary and sufficient to mediate delayed-type hypersensitivity reactions, while the Ly2,3 cell again is able to suppress DTH reactions. Thus, by the use of negative selection experiments, Cantor and his colleagues have mapped out most known T cell functions and they fall into either the Ly1 or the Ly2,3 class of T cells. It should be emphasized that these two markers (i.e., Ly1 and Ly2,3) seem to be quite stable. Although Cantor and his colleagues have looked extensively, they have never found that the Ly1 cell can express the Ly2,3 antigen nor can the Ly2,3 cell ever express the Ly1 antigen.

This leaves us with the conundrum of what is the role of the Ly1,2,3 TL$^-$ cell, which represents at least half of the peripheral T cells of mature mice. There is no defined T cell function left to assign to this class. There is some suggestive evidence, however. Cantor has found that there is a preferential decrease in Ly1,2,3 cells after adult thymectomy. Adult thymectomy, it should be remembered, has been used to preferentially remove cells previously called T1. Thus it is likely that many functions previously described to T1 type cells will fall into the Ly1,2,3 class. Our guess is that it is this class of T cells which has bi-directional regulatory capacity; i.e., it is this cell which is responsible for recognizing the activity of other cells and regulating them on that basis. The Ly1,2,3 cell could perform this regulatory function in one of two ways: (a) it could, depending upon the signal it receives, differentiate into an Ly1 cell and therefore add to helper activity, or conversely differentiate into an Ly2,3 cell and therefore add to suppressor activity; (b) it could be a stable line in itself and could regulate the Ly1 and the Ly2,3 cells directly without itself differentiating into one of those other two types of cells.

The stability of the markers (that is Ly2,3 being suppressor, Ly1 being helper) is best illustrated by studies using Con A to activate these cells. In these studies, it was shown quite dramatically that the Ly1 cell activated by Con A was a helper cell and the Ly2,3 cell activated by Con A was a suppressor cell. The most reasonable interpretation of these experiments is to say that these cells have differentiated to have specific function and the activity that they exhibit depends solely upon those factors which govern whether or not they are turned on. The amount of Ly1,2,3 activity might be one of those factors.

It is also likely that it is the Ly1,2,3 cell which (or whose activity) declines with age, because this is the cell that disappears most rapidly after adult thymectomy and is the cell with many of the characteristics of immature cells. Aged mice tend to have inactive thymuses and may indeed have had functional thymectomies and thus have deficits in this type of cell. With a lack of the Ly1,2,3, one could find anything one wanted to, depending upon the assay. That is, one could say there was either too much or too little suppressor T cell activity, too much or too little helper T cell activity, because the lack of this cell is the cause of the aberrant expression of the more differentiated functional cells (Ly1 and Ly2,3). Whether this speculation will turn out to have any truth in it will probably be known in the near future, as the technology is now available for these questions to be answered.

10. Conclusion

It is too early in the game to say with any certainty what the basis for the immunological regulatory defect is in T cells of aged mice. Speculations may abound, but the prediction is that answers will be forthcoming within the next few years. We offer one further gratuitous prediction: With age there will be as much specificity in the decline of T cell functions as there is in the decline of another organ that expresses theta antigen and has complex interactions among component cells, the brain.

ACKNOWLEDGMENTS

The authors' research was supported by U.S.P.H.S. grants CA-08593, AI-10497 and CA-14216.

References

Baker, P. J., 1975, Homeostatic control of antibody responses: A model based on the recognition of cell-association antibody by regulatory T cells, *Transpl. Rev.* **26**:3–20,

Cantor, H., and Boyse, E. A. 1975a, Functional subclasses of T lymphocytes bearing different Ly antigens. I. The generation of functionally distinct T-cell subclasses is a differentiative process independent of antigen, *J. Exp. Med.* **141**:1376–1389.

Cantor, H., and Boyse, E. A. 1975b, Functional subclasses of T lymphocytes bearing different Ly antigens. II. Cooperation between subclasses of Ly+ cells in the generation of killer activity, *J. Exp. Med.* **141**:1390–1399.

Cantor, H., Asofsky, R., and Talal N., 1970, Synergy among lymphoid cells mediating the graft-versus-host response. I. Synergy in graft-versus-host reactions produced by cells from NZB/B1 mice, *J. Exp. Med.* **131:**223–234.

Dauphinee, M. J., and Talal N., 1973, Alteration in DNA synthetic response of thymocytes from NZB mice of different ages, *Proc. Nat. Acad. Sci. U.S.A.* **70:**3769–3772.

Debré, P., Kapp, J. A., Dorf, M. E., and Benacerraf, B., 1975, Genetic control of specific immune suppression. I. Experimental conditions for the stimulation of suppressor cells by the copolymer L-glutamic acid^{50}-L-tyrosine^{50} (GT) in nonresponder BALB/C mice, *J. Exp. Med.* **142:**1447–1454.

Eardley, D. D., and Gershon, R. K., 1975, Feedback induction of suppressor T-cell activity, *J. Exp. Med.* **142:**524–529.

Eichmann, K., 1975, Idiotype suppression. II. Amplification of a suppressor T cell with anti-idiotypic activity, *Europ. J. Immunol.* **5:**511–517.

Gershon, R. K., 1974a, T Cell Regulation: The "Second Law of Thymodynamics," in: *The Immune System, Genes, Receptors, Signals* (E. E. Sercarz, A. R. Williamson, and C. F. Fox eds.), pp. 471–484, Academic Press, New York.

Gershon, R. K., 1974b, Immunoregulation by T Cells, in: *Molecular Approaches to Immunology* (E. E. Smith and D. W. Ribbons, eds.), pp. 267–288, Academic Press, New York.

Gershon, R. K., 1974c, T cell control of antibody production, *Contemporary Topics in Immunobiology,* Vol. 3, pp. 1–40, Plenum, New York.

Gershon, R. K., 1975, A disquisition on suppressor T cells, *Transpl. Rev.* **26:**170–185.

Gershon, R. K., and Liebhaber, S. A., 1972, The response of T cells to histocompatibility-2 antigens. Dose response kinetics, *J. Exp. Med.* **136:**112–127.

Gershon, R. K., Orbach-Arbouys, S., and Calkins, C., 1974, B cell signals which activate suppressor T cells, *Prog. Immunol. II* **2:**123–133.

Herzenberg, L. A., and Herzenberg, L. A., 1974, Short-term and chronic allotype suppression in mice, *Contemporary Topics in Immunobiology,* Vol. 3, Plenum, New York, pp. 41–75.

Herzenberg, L. A., Okumura, K., and Herzenberg, L. A., 1975, in: *Suppressor Cells in Immunity,* S. K. Singhal and N. R. St. C. Sinclair, eds., pp. 42–49, The Univ. of Western Ontario Press, London, Ontario.

Kapp, J. A., Pierce, C. W., and Benacerraf, B., 1975, Role of suppressor T cells in an IR gene controlled immune response, in: *Suppressor Cells in Immunity* (S. K. Singhal and N. R. St. C. Sinclair, eds.), pp. 84–92, The Univ. of Western Ontario Press, London, Ontario.

Katz, D. H., and Benacerraf, B., 1974, *Immunological Tolerance, Mechanisms and Potential Therapeutic Applications,* pp. 1–645, Academic Press, New York.

Möller, G., ed., 1975, Suppressor T Lymphocytes, *Transpl. Rev.* **26:**1–205.

Morse, H. C., III, Steinberg, A. D., Vchur, P. H., and Reed, N. D., 1974, Spontaneous "Autoimmune Disease" in nude mice, *J. Immunol.* **113:**688–697.

Pierce, C. W., and Kapp, J. A., 1976, Regulation of the immune response by suppressor T cells, in: *Contemporary Topics in Immunobiology,* Vol. 5, Plenum, New York.

Raff, M., and Cantor, H., 1971, Subpopulations of thymus cells and thymus-derived lymphocytes, *Prog. in Immunol. I.* **83:**106.

Roder, J. C., Bell, D. A., and Singhal, S. K., 1975, Suppressor cells in New Zealand mice: Possible role in the generation of autoimmunity, in: *Suppressor Cells in Immunity* (S. K. Singhal and N. R. St. C. Sinclair, eds.), pp. 164–173, The Univ. of Western Ontario Press, London, Ontario.

Steinberg, A. D., Gerberg, N. L., Gershwin, M. E., Morton, R., Goodman, D., Chused, T. M., Hardin, J. A., and Barthold, D. R., 1975, Loss of suppressor T cells in the pathogenesis of autoimmunity, in: *Suppressor Cells in Immunity,* (S. K. Singhal and N. R. St. C. Sinclair, eds.), pp. 174–181, The Univ. of Western Ontario Press, London, Ontario.

Talal, N., and Steinberg, A., 1974, The pathogenesis of autoimmunity in New Zealand black mice. Current Topics, in: *Microbiol. and Immunol.* **64:**79–103.

Waldmann, T. A., Broder, S., Krakauer, R., Durm, M., Goldman, C., and Meade, B., 1975, The role of Suppressor T cells in immunodeficiency, in: *Suppressor Cells in Immunity* (S. K. Singhal and N. R. St. C. Sinclair, eds.), pp. 182–187, The Univ. of Western Ontario Press, London, Ontario.

Yoshiki, T., Mellors, R. C., Strand, M., and August, J. T., 1974, The viral envelope glycoprotein of murine leukemia virus and the pathogenesis of immune complex glomerulonephritis of New Zealand mice, *J. Exp. Med.* **140:**1011–1027.

9

Attempts to Correct Age-Related Immunodeficiency and Autoimmunity by Cellular and Dietary Manipulation in Inbred Mice

GABRIEL FERNANDES, ROBERT A. GOOD, and
EDMOND J. YUNIS

1. Introduction

The association of immunologic malfunction with aging has been viewed in several ways. The immunologic theory of aging, first clearly stated by Walford (1969), has been extensively promulgated by Burnet (1970b). This theory states that the immune system is essential to maintenance of health and that, to a major extent, the integrity of the immune system determines survival. Further, Walford has maintained that the immune system is involved in the pathogenesis of many of the diseases that occur in aging man and animals and may actually be involved in the pathogenesis of the aging process itself.

In our studies, the decline of effective immunologic function in man and mouse during the aging process has been associated with the same diseases and immuno-

GABRIEL FERNANDES and EDMOND J. YUNIS • Department of Laboratory Medicine and Pathology, University of Minnesota, Minneapolis, Minnesota 55455, and **ROBERT A. GOOD** • Sloan-Kettering Institute for Cancer Research, New York, New York. Present address of E. J. Y. is Sidney Farber Cancer Institute, Harvard Medical School, Boston Massachusetts.

GABRIEL
FERNANDES, ROBERT
A. GOOD, AND
EDMOND J. YUNIS

logic perturbations that plague man and other animals lacking a normal T cell immunity system (Good and Yunis, 1974). Observations consistent with the clonal selection theory of immunity function have provoked Burnet (1958) to maintain that clones of cells, ordinarily forbidden expression by an intact immunity system, appear by somatic mutation and persist when immunity functions are defective. This, he feels, accounts for the frequent autoimmunity observed in aging and immunodeficient man and animals (Burnet 1970a).

On the other hand, Good and Yunis (1974) have interpreted the association of autoimmunity with immune deficiency states, as seen in aging and following neonatal thymectomy, to be consistent with a forbidden antigen theory of autoimmunity. We have argued that under several circumstances of immunodeficiency, antigens which otherwise would have been prohibited from entering the body, or else promptly eliminated from it, are permitted to enter or persist as infectious agents or antigens that can generate cross-reacting antibodies as part of an ineffective immune response (Yunis *et al.*, 1969; Teague *et al.*, 1970; Yunis *et al.*, 1972; Good and Yunis, 1974).

From either perspective, autoimmunity phenomena, autoimmune disease, and immunologic injury might be expected to occur with great frequency in aging and to produce the serious diseases associated with aging. Gatti and Good (1970) and Greenberg and Yunis (1972) have reviewed the relationship between the various components of the aging process and the functional state of the immunity system. They have classified aging according to its primary and secondary events and proposed that the primary component be considered separately from the secondary ones. They have argued that the primary components of immunologic aging are embodied in a chronological process which is genetically programmed to result in a decline in effective function and control of immunity. Indeed, Good and Finstad (1968) have argued that survival advantage for the species might be found in such a programmed decline of immunological function, which could be intrinsic to all body cells or, perhaps, be centered in the central nervous system–endocrine function.

According to this view, the genetically programmed clock operates at a rate consistent with the median life span of the species and adheres to limits imposed by the Hayflick (1965) formulation, for example. To conform to this limitation, it is probable that the thymic process of spawning T lymphocytes ceases either through CNS–endocrine control or because of its intrinsic temporal limitations, which bring about a progressive decline of thymic function. An involuted thymus would thus impose an essential limit on the immunologic vigor of the T cell system. We would add, of course, a programmed involution with aging of the site for generation and differentiation of B lymphocytes, which is located in the bursa of Fabricius of birds, a central lymphoid organ. The involution of either or both of these central lymphoid organs and loss of their generating and supporting functions with age impose a restriction on immunological vigor that is determined by the limited programmed potentiality for replication of the B and T lymphoid elements found in the peripheral systems.

All the remaining immunological components of aging can therefore be viewed as events secondary to this essential feature of the aging process. These secondary immunologic components of aging encompass disease processes and pathology commonly associated with aging, but not directly functions of the aging process *per se*. In recounting such processes and diseases associated with aging of both mice

113

ATTEMPTS TO
CORRECT
AGE-RELATED
IMMUNODEFICIENCY
AND
AUTOIMMUNITY BY
CELLULAR AND
DIETARY
MANIPULATION IN
INBRED MICE

and men, one must focus on the high frequency of cancer, autoimmune phenomena, autoimmunity diseases, arthritis, amyloidosis, hyalinization of blood vessels and other tissues, hyalinization and sclerosis of the renal glomeruli, increased frequency of serious infections due to pathogens of low grade virulence (for members of the species who have vigorous immunity function), and varying degrees of immunodeficiencies that involve both the T and B cell functions (Good, 1975a; Hansen and Good, 1974; Yunis *et al.*, 1975).

Several biologists have advanced theories of aging, none of which is entirely satisfactory. These include:

1. The free radical theory, which suggests the occurrence of age-associated interference with oxidative processes of proteins, which leads to molecular malfunction, misinformation, or mutations (Harman, 1968).
2. The somatic mutation theory, which postulates that mutations in somatic cell DNA result in physiologic dysfunctions and deficiencies, ultimately leading to death (Curtis, 1971).
3. The accumulation of errors theory of aging, which states that age-associated progressive accumulation of errors of transcription and/or translation results in accumulation of abnormalities of cellular information and deterioration of nuclear cytoplasmic functional controls (Price and Makinodan, 1973).
4. The cross-linkage theory of aging, which postulates that aging is caused by the progressive cross-linkage of informational molecules and other molecules essential to life, which include nucleic acids, nucleoproteins, enzymes, and structural proteins, e.g., collagen (Bjorksten, 1958; Alexander, 1967).
5. The chalone theory of aging, which proposes that aging is related to the appearance of specific molecules or chalones that inhibit essential processes of CNS and other organs (Bullough, 1971).
6. The CNS-hormonal theory of aging, which states that age-related changes are central nervous system based, hormonally controlled and programmed, and result in progressive decline of mechanisms governing the rate of vital processes and corrective adjustments following cellular and environmental perturbation (Bellamy, 1967; Makinodan, 1973).

In addition, other theories of aging have been proposed, including the stress theory of Selye and Prioreschi (1960), the molecular vs. systemic theory of Sacher (1968), and the integrated theory of Hart and Carpenter (1971). Although the decline of the immune system could have at its origin any of the processes considered in these generalizations and could be entirely secondary to a fundamental aging process, we view the nature and substance of this immunologic decline as a particularly appropriate focus for our attention. This is because engineering to correct the immunodeficiencies and immunologic disturbances associated with aging by reconstructive cellular or molecular manipulations is possible. Such engineering practices could have great potential for correcting some of the diseases that represent the awful consequences of aging itself, such as arthritis and other autoimmunity diseases, infectious vascular insufficiency, renal and central nervous system malfunctions, and cancer.

In this chapter, we focus our attention on efforts to analyze, manipulate, and correct age-associated immunological disorders in mice and on efforts to signifi-

GABRIEL
FERNANDES, ROBERT
A. GOOD, AND
EDMOND J. YUNIS

cantly alter the life-span of animals adversely affected by several immunologically based diseases that are both age-associated and genetically determined.

Specific thymic alterations related to aging have been described and extensively discussed by Hammar (1926) and reviewed by many others in *The Thymus in Immunobiology* (Good and Gabrielsen, 1964). It has been known for many years that, beginning at the time of sexual maturation, there begins in the central lymphoid organs a process of apparently programmed involution, which is succeeded by a period of gradual involution of the peripheral lymphoid apparatus and declining vigor of immunologic function. In both mice and man, the rate of this immunologic involution is highly variable. The variability and thus the rate of immunologic decline clearly implicates genetic determinants described later, but proceeds, as with other aging processes, according to a schedule that, in a broad framework, is characteristic of the species.

Among inbred strains of mice, the rates of aging in general, and immunologic aging in particular, have clearly defined time constraints. CBA/H mice tend to be very long-lived and to maintain immunologic function longer than other strains when measured by several standards. By contrast, NZB and (NZB × NZW)F$_1$ mice are both short-lived and develop immunodeficiencies and immunologic abnormalities early in life (Teague *et al.,* 1970; Rodey *et al.,* 1971). It is important to note that we are here primarily discussing age-related changes within the species, without attempting to explain the possible evolutionary processes determining the life span of each species (see Chapter 7 in this volume). For instance, both survival and maintenance of immunologic function seem very short when CBA/H mice are compared to man, yet survival and the temporal state of immunologic function of NZB mice may seem long by standards that could be applied to the Snell-Bagg or Ames dwarf mice (Duquesnoy, 1975).

Thus aging, diseases of aging, and thymic and immunologic involution may occur early in certain inbred strains of mice and much later in others; but in all strains studied, even the very long-lived strains, evidence of immunologic involution may be found. In humans, involution of the thymus and the subsequent loss of immunologic vigor also occurs commonly, but with considerable individual variation. It remains to be determined whether or not the decline of immunologic vigor, which seems to be centrally and genetically determined, is directly or indirectly controlled by the major histocompatibility complex (HLA) linkage group of chromosome 6 of man and chromosome 17 of mouse. This linkage group could be considered as a "supergene," since it may well control individuality, cell surface antigenicity, complement function, capacity to initiate and vigorously produce antibody, recognition of foreign matter (as in mixed leukocyte responses), and immunologic capacity to reject foreign cells. It is also a major determinant of susceptibility or resistance to diseases that are commonly linked to aging, e.g., arthritis, diabetes, demyelinating disease of the central nervous system, and malignancies. Thus it is provocative to think that it must also be associated with aging. To date, this has not been established.

Walford (1974a) proposed that conditions which prolong life must be based on conditions which influence either endocrine function or the immunity system. He showed that the life-span of fish whose body temperature had been lowered to 15°C was markedly prolonged as compared to that of controls kept at 20°C. He argued that this finding may be a function of the well-known temperature depressing influence on immunity functions seen in the poikilotherms (Hildemann, 1963). Even

115

ATTEMPTS TO
CORRECT
AGE-RELATED
IMMUNODEFICIENCY
AND
AUTOIMMUNITY BY
CELLULAR AND
DIETARY
MANIPULATION IN
INBRED MICE

though the prolongation of life by temperature depression was accompanied by measurable changes in collagen, reflecting a deceleration of the aging process, Walford argues that the important influence on life span could be preeminently an immunological one.

In a similar fashion, Walford *et al.* (1974b), showed that calorie restriction, which decreases both cellular and humoral immune functions early in life, also results in preservation of immunological function late in life. By contrast, well-fed mice which showed vigorous immunological function early in life were characterized as well by early decline of immunologic functions and earlier death. Makinodan *et al.* (1971) and Nordin and Makinodan (1974) showed clearly the decline of B cell functions with aging.

Our own investigations over the past 20 years (Good, 1954; Good *et al.*, 1962; Good, 1973a,b; Good and Yunis, 1974) have been especially concerned with the consequences of deficiency and decline of the T-cell-immunity system. The T cell component of the immunity system underlies not only delayed allergic responses and allograft rejection but is also responsible for the vital defense of the body against facultative intracellular bacterial pathogens, fungi, and many viruses. It is essential as well for initiating humoral immunologic responses to many antigens by its helper cells. It probably applies the damper to ongoing immunologic processes with its suppressor cells, and inhibits accumulation of foreign organisms and, perhaps, malignant cells with its killer cells. Thus it is among the most vital and powerful components of the bodily defense. It can talk to macrophages, eosinophils, and granulocytes through products generated and released by its stimulated T cells which can act either directly or indirectly in the bodily defense.

Shortly after we (Archer and Pierce, 1961; Archer *et al.*, 1962; Martinez *et al.*, 1962; Good *et al.*, 1962) and Miller independently (1961) discovered the essential role of the thymus in development and maintenance of the immunologic functions, we encountered evidence that autoimmune phenomena, autoimmune disease, amyloidosis, wasting disease, hyalinization of vessels, and cardiovascular–renal diseases regularly accompany T cell deficiency. We discovered that neonatally thymectomized rabbits, irradiated thymectomized rabbits, and neonatally thymectomized mice (Papermaster and Good, 1962; Kellum *et al.*, 1965; Cooper *et al.*, 1966; Yunis *et al.*, 1965), like aging mice of certain strains (Teague *et al.*, 1970) and immunodeficient man (Good, 1973a,b; Hallgren *et al.*, 1973) develop not only many infections, but autoantibodies, autoimmunity disease, amyloidosis, and immunologically based kidney disease as well as a consequence of the immunological perturbations associated with their T cell immunodeficiency (Good and Yunis, 1974). Furthermore, we found that when we corrected with thymus cells, thymus grafts, or fully differentiated T cells (Yunis *et al.*, 1965, 1966) the immunodeficiencies imposed by neonatal thymectomy, and in several strains of mice by aging, we could prevent immunologic diseases or even reverse immunological and autoimmune disorders (Yunis *et al.*, 1972).

We have been concerned from the earliest days not only with the association of immunodeficiency with aging, but with the similar manifestations of aging occurring in animals made immunodeficient by thymectomy early in life (Good *et al.*, 1962; Good and Yunis, 1974). We have also been interested in the possibilities of correcting both kinds of immunological abnormalities by cellular and macromolecular engineering (Yunis *et al.*, 1965; Stutman *et al.*, 1967; Gatti *et al.*, 1968; Good *et al.*, 1969; Good, 1973a, 1975b). Field studies underscored the association of nutri-

GABRIEL
FERNANDES, ROBERT
A. GOOD, AND
EDMOND J. YUNIS

tional deficiency with immunodeficiency (Good *et al.*, 1972). Furthermore, the association of nutritional deficiency and failure of growth and reproduction in chickens (Fernandes, 1960; Fernandes and Ranadive, 1962) persuaded us to make extensive investigations of the influence of nutrition on immunity, using rats, mice, and guinea pigs in a controlled laboratory situation (Good and Jose, 1975c; Jose and Good, 1971; Jose *et al.*, 1973; Cooper *et al.*, 1974; Fernandes *et al.*, 1972, 1973a). In the course of these investigations we found that the immunodeficiencies and immunological perturbations associated with aging in certain inbred strains of mice can be manipulated by dietary restriction (Fernandes *et al.*, 1976a,b).

It is our intent here to briefly summarize information about the immunodeficiencies and immunological perturbations that occur with aging, as well as those produced by neonatal thymectomy in certain strains of mice. We will then delineate possibilities for correction of these deficiencies by cellular engineering. In addition, we will describe nutritional manipulation of the immunologic system and of the abnormalities associated with aging in certain strains of mice. By careful control of diet, it has already been possible to prolong life in several strains of mice. Perhaps our most dramatic experiments show that calorie restriction promoted the doubling of the life span of (NZB × NZW)F_1. This was the case when life span was viewed as mean or median interval of survival, 20% longest survival, or the longest surviving individual of the strain. Finally, we have been able to show that immunodeficiency and longevity in inbred mice can also be manipulated genetically in a dramatic fashion. Representative analyses and experimental manipulations will be presented. The experimental basis for these analyses is the observation of similarities in the immunodeficiency state of neonatally thymectomized and aging mice of the autoimmunity susceptible NZB, (NZB × NZW)F_1, C57BL/Ks, and A strains, which are summarized in Table 1. The table shows that the perturbations that occur with aging in the autoimmune susceptible mice occur sooner after neonatal thymectomy than in untreated mice. However, they also often appear following neonatal thymectomy in strains of mice which, without neonatal thymectomy, rarely develop autoimmune phenomena until very late in life.

2. Histopathology of Autoimmunity Susceptible Mice and Neonatally Thymectomized Mice and Rabbits

In autoimmunity susceptible strains of mice there is an extraordinary age-associated histiocytosis, plasmacytosis, and immunoblastosis (Yunis *et al.*, 1972). Similar lesions were observed in neonatally thymectomized rabbits and mice (Good and Yunis, 1974). Renal lesions reflecting immunological assault are seen in both the autoimmunity susceptible mice and the neonatally thymectomized mice, as well as in the autoimmunity resistant strains. Amyloidosis was also a common feature after thymectomy and in aging mice. Figure 1 illustrates the wasting syndrome seen in neonatally thymectomized mice.

3. Cellular Engineering to Correct Immunodeficiency, Wasting Disease, and Autoimmunity in Neonatally Thymectomized Mice

In extensive studies with thymectomized C3Hf, Af, and CBA/H mice, it has been possible to routinely prevent runting and wasting disease, the development of

Autoimmune susceptible mice	Neonatally thymectomized autoimmune susceptible and autoimmune resistant mice
1. Relative decrease in number of T lymphocytes after early maturation.	1. Decreased numbers or absence of 0^+ T lymphocytes.
2. Loss of helper function to produce antibodies to SRBC.	2. Inability to produce antibody to SRBC; absence of helper function.
3. Loss of T lymphocytes to exert suppressor function.	3. Absence of suppressor T cells.
4. Inability to develop killer cells against allogeneic tumor cells (DBA/2 mastocytoma, EL-4 lymphoma, etc.).	4. Inability to develop T killer cells against allogeneic tumor cells (DBA/2 mastocytoma, EL-4 lymphoma).
5. Prolonged survival of skin allografts.	5. Failure of skin allograft rejection.
6. Loss of ability to initiate graft-versus-host reactions.	6. Inability to initiate graft-vs.-host.
7. Loss of cells that proliferate with stimulation by PHA and Con A lectins.	7. Absence of cells that proliferate with PHA and Con A.
8. Progressive wasting disease.	8. Rapidly progressive wasting disease.
9. Autoantibody vs. T lymphocytes, Coombs positive hemolytic anemia, anti-DNP, anti-DNA increase with time.	9. Coombs positive hemolytic anemia, anti-nuclear antibodies (anti-DNP), anti-DNA antibody.
10. Immune complex renal and vascular disease.	10. Immune complex renal and vascular disease.
11. Histopathology of spleen, kidneys, marrow show extensive proliferation of histocytes, immunocytes, immunoblasts, and plasma cells.	11. Histopathology of spleen, lymph nodes, and marrow show extensive proliferation of histiocytes, immunocytes, immunoblasts, and plasma cells.
12. Hypergammaglobulinemia, amyloidosis-secondary type.	12. Hypergammaglobulinemia, amyloidosis-secondary type.
13. Early death in NZB (NZB × NZW)F$_1$, A/J, A/Umc, and C57BL/Ks strains.	13. Early death from autoimmune disease and infection.

[a]Autoimmune susceptible mice thymectomized at birth (A/J and A/Umc) develop autoimmune phenomena and disease much earlier than newborn thymectomized autoimmune resistant mice (C3H, DBA/2, etc.).

autoimmune phenomena, and immunologic injury to kidneys and other organs by treating the mice either with thymus transplants from syngeneic or allogeneic donors, or with spleen cells from syngeneic donors (Yunis *et al.*, 1972). Thymectomized mice reconstituted immunologically by such manipulations failed to develop immunologically based diseases and autoimmune diseases, while control thymectomized mice showed these phenomena in high frequency (Tables 2, 3, and 4). It can be seen from Table 2 that spleen cells from young autoimmune susceptible Af mice could immunologically reconstitute neonatally thymectomized autoimmunity susceptible Af mice. By contrast, spleen cells from older mice of the same strain failed to reconstitute the immunologic functions of these thymectomized mice and thus did not promote avoidance of infection, autoimmunity, and immunologic injury, nor did they improve their survival. On the other hand, spleen cells of 2-month-old CBA/H mice and, to a slightly lesser degree, spleen cells from 23-month-old CBA/H mice corrected the immunodeficiency when given intraperitoneally to the neonatally thymectomized CBA/H mice.

4. Prevention of Immunodeficiency by Thymus Transplants

In studies of the ability of thymus transplants to reconstitute immunological functions of thymectomized mice, it was shown that syngeneic thymus transplants from both A or allogeneic CBA/H mice corrected quite well the immunologic defect of neonatally thymectomized mice. Thymus grafts from older 22- or 23-month-old donors, however, regularly failed to correct the immunodeficiency or to prevent immunological diseases. These observations are summarized in Table 3.

5. Reversal of Autoimmunity Disease by Cellular Engineering

Of greater potential interest are the possibilities of reversing already existing autoimmunity manifestations by cellular engineering when the autoimmunity phenomena had (a) appeared spontaneously, (b) been accelerated in autoimmunity susceptible strains of mice, or (c) been induced in autoimmunity resistant strains of

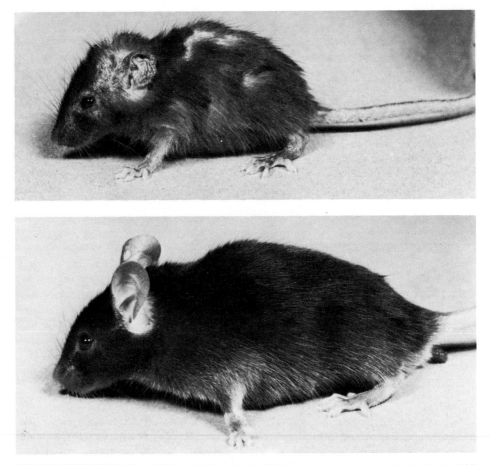

Figure 1. A comparison between a three-month-old C57BL/Ks mouse (top) thymectomized at birth, which shows acute wasting disease, and a normal sham-operated littermate mouse shown at the bottom.

Strain	Treatment	Six-month survivors	Allogeneic skin rejection, mean + SD (days)
Af	100×10^6 2-month Af	21/22 (95%)	13 ± 1.2 (8)
	100×10^6 12-month Af	15/19 (79%)	16.7 ± 2.4 (15)
	100×10^6 22-month Af	0/8	—
	untreated	0/8	—
CBA/H	100×10^6 2-month CBA/H	9/9 (100%)	16 ± 2.8 (9)
	100×10^6 23-month CBA/H	5/8 (62%)	15.6 ± 3.7 (3)
	untreated	0/9	—

mice by neonatal thymectomy. Teague and Friou (1964) injected A/J mice, which had developed antinuclear antibodies during aging, with syngeneic thymus cells obtained from young animals that were antinuclear antibody negative. After such treatment, the anti-DNP antibody titers decreased and actually disappeared (Teague and Friou, 1964). In additional experiments where spleen cells of young A/J mice were injected into older A/J mice prior to development of the regularly occurring autoimmunity, the autoantibodies to nucleoprotein were prevented from appearing (Teague and Friou, 1969).

Table 4 summarizes some of our efforts to reverse postthymectomy wasting and autoimmunity by injection of spleen cells from young syngeneic donors. It can be seen that immunologic reconstitution by spleen cells, even after the autoimmunity had developed, could rather strikingly reverse the autoimmune disease. Similarly, treatment using multiple thymus transplants, and even allogeneic thymus cells when the histocompatibility barrier was not too great, permitted reversal of postthymectomy autoimmune disease in mice (Yunis et al., 1965; Stutman et al., 1967).

In experiments with other strains that spontaneously developed autoimmune disease and profound immunodeficiency (Steinberg et al., 1970), injection of (NZB × NZW)F$_1$ hybrid mice with thymus cells from very young donors inhibited the development of anti-DNA antibodies in these animals. Gelfand and Steinberg (1973)

TABLE 3. Age of Donor of Thymus and Reconstitution of Thymectomized Mice[a]

Strain	Treatment	Six-month survivors	Allogeneic skin rejection, mean + SD (days)
Af	2-month Af	10/22 (45%)	15.1 ± 2.6 (10)
	12-month Af	7/14 (50%)	16.6 ± 1.9 (8)
	22-month Af	1/9 (11%)	15 days
CBA/H	2-month CBA/H	7/10 (70%)	15 ± 2.8 (6)
	23-month CBA/H	1/10 (10%)	30

[a]Treatment intraperitoneally at 2 weeks of age.

GABRIEL
FERNANDES, ROBERT
A. GOOD, AND
EDMOND J. YUNIS

TABLE 4. Reversal of Postthymectomy Wasting and Conversion of Coombs Positive to Coombs Negative by Spleen Cell Injection

Strain		Pretreatment 45–60 days of age		Posttreatment 45–60 days		Posttreatment 120 days	
		Number	Percent Coombs	Percent survival	Percent Coombs	Percent survival	Percent Coombs
Af	Treated	14	78 (11/14)	85 (12/14)	25 (3/12)	57 (8/14)	0
	Control	14	71 (10/14)	36 (5/14)	60 (3/5)	0	
(C3Hf × Af)F$_1$	Treated	6	33 (2/6)	100 (6/6)	17 (1/6)	66 (4/6)	0
	Control	6	50 (3/6)	17 (1/6)	Pos. (1/1)	0	
C3Hf	Treated	8	0	75 (6/8)	0	75 (6/8)	0
	Control	7	0	14	0	0	

reconstituted immunologic functions of (NZB × NZW)F$_1$ mice, which had already developed autoimmunity and immunodeficiency, by intravenous injection of spleen or lymph node cells from young donors. In the aggregate, these findings indicate that both immunodeficiency and autoimmunity, which develop spontaneously in certain strains of mice and which can be produced experimentally by neonatal thymectomy, can be both prevented and reversed by administration of appropriate cells. These findings encourage further efforts to develop cellular engineering designed to forestall certain immunologic and autoimmunity events that occur with aging. Such engineering may ultimately prove to be a valuable clinical tool.

The possibility of developing a clinically useful cellular engineering to address problems of immunodeficiency and immunologic abnormality of aging was first raised by the work of Yunis et al. (1964). In these experiments we showed that immunologic function, growth, and longevity of neonatally thymectomized mice was restored by intraperitoneal administration of 100-to-400 million syngeneic, hemiallogeneic, or allogeneic cells from adult donors. Similarly, neonatally thymectomized mice were restored with allogeneic adult spleen cells. Postthymectomy wasting disease and autoimmunity were reversed by injection of 200 million hemiallogeneic or allogeneic spleen cells.

In the experiments using the allogeneic cells, the single most important factor in preventing graft-vs.-host reactions was to have the allogeneic cells matched with the recipient at the entire H-2 major histocompatibility barrier. When this was done with mice, the wasting disease and immunologic disturbance produced by neonatal thymectomy could be completely corrected with allogeneic cells. Now it is known that graft-vs.-host reaction can be completely avoided, even though donor and recipient are mismatched at the major histocompatibility barrier if postthymic allogeneic cells can be eliminated from the hematopoietic preparations (Yunis et al., 1974; Tulunay et al., 1975; Yunis et al., 1976).

6. Prevention or Delay of Age-Associated Autoimmunity by Genetic Manipulation

It is known that certain strains of mice are susceptible to development of autoimmune disease—NZB, (NZB × NZW)F$_1$, C57BL/Ks, A/J, and Af, for example.

Autoimmunity resistant strains include C3Hf, CBA/H, C57BL/6, and Balb/C. We mean by "autoimmunity susceptible" that the mice will develop, relatively early in life, autoimmune phenomena and immunodeficiency disease. By contrast, the autoimmunity resistant strains of mice do not develop evidence of autoimmunity and immunodeficiency until very late in life, if at all. Even autoimmunity resistant mice can often be made to develop both immunodeficiency and autoimmunity if they are thymectomized in the neonatal period.

Because of the apparent resistance of certain strains of mice to immunodeficiency and autoimmunity with aging, we thought it would be of interest to determine whether heterozygosity would influence the expression of these immunological phenomena with aging. To test this postulate, hybrids were prepared and the influence of the breeding on longevity, autoimmunity, and immunologic function was evaluated. Results of the influence of heterozygosity on survival are summarized in Table 5.

It can be seen that although NZB mice are short-lived and NZW mice somewhat longer-lived, (NZB × NZW)F_1 had the shortest life span of all. (NZW × NZB)F_1 were equally short-lived. By contrast, when (NZB × CBA)F_1 hybrids were prepared, the hybrids approached the longevity of the longer-lived CBA parents. Similarly, the F_1 hybrids of NZB mice prepared with C3H, or even the autoimmunity susceptible Af, showed longer life span in each instance than the NZB. Perhaps the most interesting observation was that (NZB × Af)F_1 hybrids even showed what might be termed hybrid vigor, because the hybrids survived longer than members of either parent strain. This same hybrid vigor was also observed when (C3H × NZB)F_1 hybrids were prepared. In this instance, 34% of the F_1 animals lived beyond 30 months, whereas none of the $C3H_f$ mice reached 30 months of age, and none of the NZB mice reached 24 months of age. This genetic influence not only affected longevity but also the decline of immunologic vigor and development of autoimmunity that is regularly expressed in NZB mice (Yunis *et al.*, 1975; Fernandes *et al.*, 1976c).

Talal and Steinberg (1974) have reviewed others' findings of similar genetic

TABLE 5. Hybrid Vigor and Aging

Parent strain and hybrids	Number[a]	Percent survivors				
		12 mo.	18 mo.	24 mo.	30 mo.	36 mo.
NZB	30	50	5	0	0	0
NZW	30	100	70	10	0	0
C₃Hf	30	78	45	5	0	0
Af	50	86	69	24	0	0
CBA/H	30	100	92	75	36	12
(NZB × NZW)F1	30	30	0	0	0	0
NZB × C₃Hf	30	100	93	70	27	0
C₃Hf × NZB	30	97	83	58	34	0
NZB × C₃H	60	100	93	78	26	0
C₃H × NZB	30	93	72	41	14	0
NZB × CBA/H	20	100	95	60	30	10
CBA/H × NZB	40	100	100	90	40	0
NZB × A	20	89	74	44	19	0

[a]Equal numbers of males and females.

influences on immunologic function and expression of autoimmunity in hybrids prepared with NZB mice. Their studies, which also involve cross analyses, are compatible with the view that the susceptibility is not inherited from either parent as a transmissible agent and suggest that more than one gene is involved.

7. The Decline of Immunologic Vigor with Aging in NZB Mice

Early in life, NZB and (NZB × NZW)F_1 mice have vigorous immunologic capacity. Even in the newborn period, e.g., at 10 days of age, the spleens of NZB mice have much greater capacity to induce graft-vs.-host reaction than does the spleen of very long-lived CBA mice and longer-lived NZW mice. Indeed, the thymus cells of NZB mice, quite in contradiction to those of CBA and NZW, which for the most part lack cells having capacity to induce graft-vs.-host reaction, show ability to induce splenomegaly when injected into (NZB × NZW)F_1 hybrids or (NZB × CBA)F_1 hybrids. Data documenting the very early development of this form of cell-mediated immunity are presented in Table 6. The table shows that capacity to induce graft-vs.-host reactions develops early in NZB mice and undergoes an earlier decline with aging than is the case with NZW or CBA mice.

Similarly, the response to the plant lectins PHA and Con A develops early during growth and declines chronologically earlier with aging in NZB and (NZB × NZW)F_1 than in other strains of mice. Further, the capacity to reject allografts of skin and to respond to immunization with allogeneic tumor cells, such as DBA/2 mastocytoma, EL-4 lymphoma cells of methyl cholanthrene-induced sarcoma cells, and spontaneous mammary adenocarcinoma are vigorous early and decline early during adult life (Fernandes *et al.*, 1976c). All these forms of cell-mediated

TABLE 6. Variations in the Graft-vs.-Host Response of Thymus, Spleen, and Lymph Node Cells from NZB, NZW, and CBA/H Mice[a]

Strain	Age	Cells	Positive/tested
NZB	10 day	Thymus (20 × 10⁶)	8/8
NZW	10 day	Thymus (20 × 10⁶)	0/9
CBA/H	10 day	Thymus (20 × 10⁶)	4/9
NZB	10 day	Spleen (10 × 10⁶)	8/8
NZW	10 day	Spleen (10 × 10⁶)	4/8
CBA/H	10 day	Spleen (10 × 10⁶)	5/9
NZB	2 mo.	Spleen (10 × 10⁶)	9/9
		L. node (5 × 10⁶)	6/6
NZW	2 mo.	Spleen (10 × 10⁶)	8/8
		L. node (5 × 10⁶)	7/7
CBA/H	2 mo.	Spleen (10 × 10⁶)	12/12
		L. node (5 × 10⁶)	5/5
NZB	12 mo.	Spleen (10 × 10⁶)	2/11
		L. node (5 × 10⁶)	6/6
NZW	12 mo.	Spleen (10 × 10⁶)	8/8
		L. node (5 × 10⁶)	6/6
CBA/H	14 mo.	Spleen (10 × 10⁶)	11/11
		L. node (5 × 10⁶)	8/8

[a] (NZB × NZW)F_1, (NZB × CBA/H)F_1. eight-day-old mice were injected I.P. and eight days later the animals were killed to determine the positive spleen index 1.30.

ATTEMPTS TO
CORRECT
AGE-RELATED
IMMUNODEFICIENCY
AND
AUTOIMMUNITY BY
CELLULAR AND
DIETARY
MANIPULATION IN
INBRED MICE

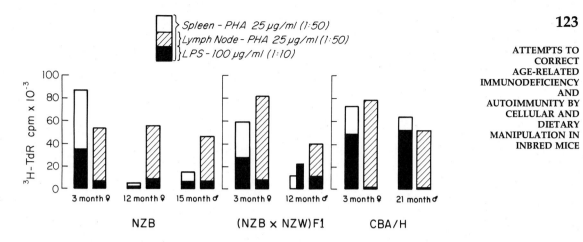

Figure 2. Effect of age on the *in vitro* response to phytohemagglutinin (PHA) and lipopolysaccharide (LPS) of spleen and lymph node cells in three different strains of mice. Cultures (2% FCS) were incubated with or without serially diluted mitogen concentration for 48 hr and for an additional 16 hr with [³H]thymidine (³H-TdR) in microtiter plates. Data presented here are the mean of two experiments carried out in identical *in vitro* conditions.

immunity in NZB mice are well developed very early in life but decline in the latter half of the first year to extremely low levels, as noted in studies focusing on spleen cells. We have found, however, that the decline of lymphoid cell function is not uniform for all lymphoid organs and that some of these functions decline to a lesser degree or not at all in aging cervical and axillary lymph nodes. Thus, in the NZB mice, there occurs with aging not only a decline of immunologic vigor but also a form of ecotaxopathy. Observations reflecting these changes are presented in Figure 2.

Some of the changes of immunologic function occurring with ontogeny in NZB mice have been analyzed and at least partly explained in terms of the shifts of the so-called suppressor lymphocyte subpopulation. Very early in life, suppressor cells are readily demonstrable in the spleen of NZB and (NZB × NZW)F₁ mice. These cells decrease in number or in vigor of expression by 2 months of age and decrease further in number or expression during the latter half of the first year. The disappearance or decline in suppressor T cell function has been linked by Dauphinee and Talal (1975) and Barthold *et al.* (1974) to the susceptibility of NZB mice to development of autoimmune disease. Stutman (1972) and we (Fernandes *et al.*, 1976c) have also noted the apparent decline of θ^+ cells in the lymphoid organs of NZB mice. In our analyses, however, this decline in number of θ^+ cells in spleens of both NZB and (NZB × NZW)F₁ mice seems to be relative rather than absolute. Because of the marked enlargement of the spleens in aging NZB mice and their lesser enlargement in (NZB × NZW)F₁ mice, the absolute number of positive cells is actually increased, while the relative number of these cells in the spleen is significantly decreased.

The basis for the rather extreme decrease in immunologic vigor of NZB and (NZB × NZW)F₁ mice, as reflected in (a) spleen cell responses to mitogens, (b) results of mixed leukocyte cultures using spleen cells, (c) spleen capacity to induce GVH reactions and (d) to form antibody to SRBC, (e) capacity of the spleen to

GABRIEL
FERNANDES, ROBERT
A. GOOD, AND
EDMOND J. YUNIS

develop plaque-forming cells to SRBC stimulation, (f) prolongation of skin allograft rejection, and finally, (g) capacity to generate killer lymphocytes, still remains somewhat obscure (Talal and Steinberg, 1974). Until recently, no experiments had been reported that demonstrated the presence of a suppressor cell population in aging mice of these strains. Recently, however, Roder *et al.* (1975) presented evidence for a suppressor cell population in the (NZB $\times$ NZW)F_1 mice, which may account in part for the decline of immunologic vigor with aging.

Antibodies directed at T lymphocytes have been described in mice of these strains (Shirai and Mellors, 1972). Such autoantibodies could also play an important role in the decline. It has also been suggested that deficiency of thymosin could account for the loss of immunologic vigor (Goldstein *et al.*, 1970). Indeed, evidence of restoration of cell numbers and T cell functions by thymopoietin treatment has been presented (Gershwin *et al.*, 1974). However, our observations of a very different distribution of cellular and immunologic function in different lymphoid organs, e.g., spleen and lymph nodes, must be taken into account, and unless the suppressor cells, the anti-T-cell autoantibodies, or the thymic factors are differently distributed in the spleen and lymph nodes, difficulties in complete explanation for the immunodeficiency of NZB and (NZB $\times$ NZW)F_1 mice will still be with us. Similar detailed studies focusing on the number of lymphocytes and the number of subsets of the lymphocyte subpopulation, as well as the functional capacity of both T and B cells, need to be done in other short-lived and autoimmunity susceptible strains of mice, as well as for the very aged members of long-lived mouse populations. Already, data from our own studies indicate both parallels and significant differences in the decline of T cell immunologic vigor with aging in these strains, and much more study is needed for a full understanding of the nature and pathogenesis of immunodeficiency in aging mice.

8. Analysis of Age-Related Immunodeficiencies by Cell Transfer to Irradiated Hosts

Makinodan *et al.* (1971) have used supralethally irradiated recipient mice to incisively analyze the decline of B cell function with age in long-lived strains of mice. We have also been using this approach to analyze T-cell-dependent antibody (B cell) responses of our short-lived strains. From these studies we have learned that such responses decline with aging in mice of the NZB strain. In Table 7 we summarize data in which young CBA/H, NZB, or (NZB $\times$ NZW)F_1 lethally irradiated 3-month-old mice were reconstituted by young, middle-aged, or old syngeneic donors and challenged intravenously by SRBC. Four days later the spleen cells were assayed in their capacity to respond *in vitro* to SRBC by developing plaque-forming cells. It can be seen from the table that spleen cells from CBA/H mice have poorly developed capacity to produce plaque-forming cells after injection into young irradiated recipients at 2 months of age. They develop this capacity to a high peak during midlife and then show a slight decline of this function late in life. NZB mice, on the other hand, have very vigorous plaque-forming capacity very early in life but lose this ability almost completely by 12 months of age. (NZB $\times$ NZW)F_1 hybrids demonstrate a relatively feeble response early and late in life. Considerable

125

ATTEMPTS TO
CORRECT
AGE-RELATED
IMMUNODEFICIENCY
AND
AUTOIMMUNITY BY
CELLULAR AND
DIETARY
MANIPULATION IN
INBRED MICE

TABLE 7. Response to SRBC in Lethally X-Irradiated Mice Injected with Spleen Cells from Young or Old Mice to Develop PFC

Strain	Host (950R)	Donor cells (40×10^6)	PFC response
CBA/H	Young	Young (2 mo.)	++
CBA/H	Young	Middle (12 mo.)	++++
CBA/H	Young	Old (24 mo.)	+++
NZB	Young	Young (2 mo.)	++++
NZB	Young	Old (12 mo.)	+
(NZB × NZW)F$_1$	Young	Young (2 mo.)	++
(NZB × NZW)F$_1$	Young	Old (12 mo.)	++

variation in ability to develop plaque-forming cells was observed at 10 months of age. In general, capacity to produce IgM and IgG direct and indirect plaque-forming cells after SRBC was parallel in all three strains.

9. Host Environmental Factors and Aging

In another analysis we have attempted to dissect the influences of the age of the cells and the adequacy of the environment in evaluating antibody production responses to SRBC in two autoimmunity susceptible strains of mice. A summary of the findings of these experiments is presented in Table 8. It can be seen from the table that spleen cells from both A/Umc strain and NZB young donor mice form antibody producing cells well in a young recipient, but spleen cells from an old donor in a young irradiated recipient, or spleen cells from a young donor given to an old irradiated recipient do not generate plaque-forming cells very well. However, it

TABLE 8. Immune Response to SRBC in Young and Old Lethally X-Irradiated Host Mice Injected with Spleen Cells from Young or Old Mice

Strain	Donor	Host (950R)	PFC response
	(50×10^6)		
A/Umc	Young[a]	Young	+++
	Old[b]	Young	+
	Young	Old	+
	Old	Old	+
NZB	Young	Young	++++
	Young	Old	+
	Old[c]	Young	++
	—	Young (no X ray)	++++
	—	Old (no X ray)	+

[a]3-month-old.
[b]20-month-old.
[c]12-month-old.

GABRIEL
FERNANDES, ROBERT
A. GOOD, AND
EDMOND J. YUNIS

would appear that with NZB mice, spleen cells from an old donor given to the young irradiated recipient manifest a greater response to SRBC than do those from a young donor given to an aging recipient. These findings are consistent with the view that the immunodeficiency of aging in a short-lived strain or autoimmunity susceptible strain involves both the lymphoid cells themselves and the environment in which they must function. These findings are similar to those described for long-lived strains (Makinodan, 1972; Mathies *et al.*, 1973).

10. Ecotaxopathy with Aging

To determine whether an abnormality of distribution of lymphoid cells occurs with aging in autoimmune susceptible and autoimmune resistant mice, experiments were carried out to trace ^{51}Cr-labeled lymphoid cells. In these experiments we were able to show that in both old and young NZB mice, lymphocytes from old donors were distributed in abnormally large numbers in the liver and in abnormally small numbers in the spleen and lymph node, as compared to the distribution found for labeled cells of young donors given to young recipients. The cells from old donors did not home to bone marrow of old mice but homed better to bone marrow of young mice. Cells from young animals given to old animals with significant autoimmunity disease also were deployed excessively to the liver and poorly to spleen and marrow, as compared to tagged cells of young animals injected intravenously into old animals.

These findings, which are summarized in Table 9, indicate that in NZB mice there is a significant age-related pathology of the normal ecotaxis, which has both cellular- and organ-determined components. One of the most interesting findings was that spleen cells from young NZB donors homed well to lymph nodes of both young and old recipients, but spleen cells from old donors homed very poorly to lymph nodes of either young or old recipients. This is in contrast to findings in young and old CBA/H mice, which are long-lived and autoimmunity resistant because old donor cells were here able to home to lymph nodes very well. However, to some

TABLE 9. Ability of ^{51}Cr-Labeled Spleen Cells from NZB Mice to Migrate into the Lymphoid Organs[a]

	Migration of cells			
Organ	Young donor, young host	Young donor, old host	Old donor, young host	Old donor, old host
Spleen	+++	++	++	++
Liver	++++	++++	++++	++++
Kidney	++	++	+	+
L. nodes	++	++	+ −	+ −
Bone marrow	++	+ −	+	+ −

[a]^{51}Cr-labeled spleen cells were injected I.V. and after 24 hours each organ was removed and was counted in a Gamma counter. Young donors' age was 2–3 months and old animals were 10–12 months old.

degree ecotaxopathy existed in this case also, for old cells were observed distributing themselves excessively in the liver of young animals.

11. Influence of Nutrition on Decline of Immunity with Aging in NZB Mice

127

ATTEMPTS TO
CORRECT
AGE-RELATED
IMMUNODEFICIENCY
AND
AUTOIMMUNITY BY
CELLULAR AND
DIETARY
MANIPULATION IN
INBRED MICE

Our studies of the association of nutritional deprivation and immunity began with field observations (Good and Jose, 1975c). It soon became clear to us, however, that an incisive study of the relation of nutrition to immunological function could not be made in field studies. This was true because the complexity of the influence of concomitants of nutritional deficiency, which may exist simultaneously in children with vigorous nutritional deficiencies, precluded analysis of the variables involved. These concomitants included bacterial and viral infections, simultaneous deficiency of multiple dietary components, e.g., vitamins, minerals, proteins, calories, fat, and other environmental factors. Consequently, we have embarked on a comprehensive analysis of the influence of well-defined dietary restriction under as well-controlled laboratory conditions as possible.

From these studies with inbred mice, rats, and guinea pigs, we have been able to evaluate the influence of acute and chronic protein and protein-calorie malnutrition on different components of the immune response. We have studied the influence of moderate and severe chronic protein deprivation in mice, rats, and guinea pigs on antibody production, plaque-formation to SRBC, various parameters of T cell responses to lectins, allogeneic cells and defined antigens, skin allograft rejection, ability to initiate graft-vs.-host reactions, ability to resist infections with virus or bacteria, and ability to develop cellular and humoral immunity and blocking antibody (or antigen–antibody complex) against allogeneic and syngeneic tumor cells (Cooper et al., 1975; Good and Jose, 1975c). In addition, nutritional deprivation in guinea pigs was induced, with an eye on production of enhanced delayed allergy and production of lymphokines by lymphoid cells (Kramer and Good, 1975).

Our initial studies in the laboratory were rather fortuitous. We were concerned with the influence of diet on reproduction of NZB mice (Fernandes et al., 1973b). It was observed that two commercial diets (Purina) which had different protein and fat compositions had strikingly different effects on NZB mice. The diet high in fat and low in protein, which favored effective reproduction of NZB mice, also significantly shortened the life span and fostered the development of autoimmunity (Fernandes et al., 1972, 1973b). By contrast, the diet relatively high in protein and low in fat prolonged life significantly and decreased autoimmunity phenomena significantly, while being less favorable for reproduction. Because the two diets used were not the sort of defined diet one would like to use for a precise analysis of the influence of dietary constituents on physiology or pathology, we used better-defined diets in studies of immune responses and longevity in several mouse strains, including NZB, (NZB × NZW)F_1, DBA/2, and C3H.

Although these studies are still incomplete, it is clear from our findings to date that by regulating dietary components, we can dramatically influence the age-related immunological decay of NZB mice (Fernandes et al., 1976a). Further, with other dietary manipulations we have been able to produce a truly amazing increase in longevity of (NZB × NZW)F_1 mice (Fernandes et al., 1976b). Chronic, moderate

GABRIEL
FERNANDES, ROBERT
A. GOOD, AND
EDMOND J. YUNIS

protein restriction for NZB mice, achieved by reduction of dietary protein intake from the time of weaning to a level of approximately ¼ to ⅓ that of the standard diet, produced some interesting findings. The low protein intake was associated with decreased weight gain in both male and female NZB mice. Mice fed the low-protein diet did not develop splenomegaly, which generally occurs by 7 to 10 months of age in NZB mice fed a normal amount of protein. Further, 7- to 10-month-old NZB mice fed the low protein (6%) diet maintained (1) more vigorous antibody production to sheep red blood cells, (2) greater capacity to produce graft-vs.-host reactions, and (3) more vigorous cell-mediated "killer" cell immunity after immunization against DBA/2 mastocytoma cells than did NZB mice on a normal (22%) protein diet. The decrease of PHA and Con A response, which normally occurs with aging in NZB mice, was abrogated to some degree by protein restriction. However, response to LPS, which also declines with age in NZB mice, did not appear to be influenced by diet. The low protein diet inhibited the rise of IgG1 levels, prevented the increase of IgM levels and the fall of IgA levels that usually occurs with aging in NZB mice. The low protein diet, although delaying the onset of hemolytic anemia, did not prevent the development of this autoimmune disease and did not significantly prolong life span.

These studies indicate that the immunodeficiency associated with aging in NZB mice can be dramatically altered by diet. This is contradictory to studies of chronic—moderate protein deprivation in mice of other strains not prone to development of immunodeficiency and autoimmunity, in which cases, instead of being preserved, the antibody production against SRBC and formation of plaque-forming cells to SRBC is depressed by the chronic protein deprivation.

12. Increased Longevity of (NZB × NZW)F$_1$ Mice with Calorie Restriction

The striking influence of protein restriction on immunity functions in NZB mice, Walford's evidence in C57BL/6 mice (this volume), and an extensive literature indicating that the longevity of long-lived strains of mice and rats can be increased by calorie restriction (McCay *et al.*, 1939; Ross, 1969; Comfort, 1974) encouraged us to study the influence of calorie, protein, and fat manipulation on the autoimmunity susceptible, short-lived strains of mice (Dubois and Strain, 1973).

At this time, these studies have only begun, and our analysis of this issue remains incomplete. However, certain observations can be reported which are most provocative. Our study of the influence of diet on longevity of mice of (NZB × NZW)F$_1$(B/W) and DBA/2 strains showed that the life span of both male and female B/W mice is dramatically prolonged by dietary restriction. Indeed, the median and mean survival of both male and female B/W mice was increased by more than ⅔. The 20% longest survival interval for both males and females was at least doubled, and the longest survival time was more than doubled simply by reducing caloric intake to ½. In DBA/2 mice, which are also susceptible to development of autoimmune disease but have an intermediate longevity, caloric restriction did not produce such an effect. However, in this strain, normal calorie and moderate protein restriction prolonged life significantly.

These observations and those of our earlier studies show that dietary manipulations can have a profound influence not only on immune functions, but also on the longevity of short-lived strains of mice. Figure 3 presents representative data concerning the prolongation of life of B/W mice fed a calorie restricted diet. Our initial efforts to study the influence of the low calorie intake are, in one sense, consonant with the earlier observations of Walford. They present, however, an interesting paradox that requires further analysis. After B/W mice had been on a calorie restricted diet for two months, their ability to produce plaque-forming cells after antigenic stimulation with SRBC was reduced to less than half of the plaque-forming cells that appeared in the spleens of mice fed a full calorie intake. Yet, when we studied the response of spleen cells from sensitized animals injected with sheep red blood cells in a lethally irradiated host, we observed—not a reduction—but a marked increase in ability to develop plaque-forming cells.

129

ATTEMPTS TO
CORRECT
AGE-RELATED
IMMUNODEFICIENCY
AND
AUTOIMMUNITY BY
CELLULAR AND
DIETARY
MANIPULATION IN
INBRED MICE

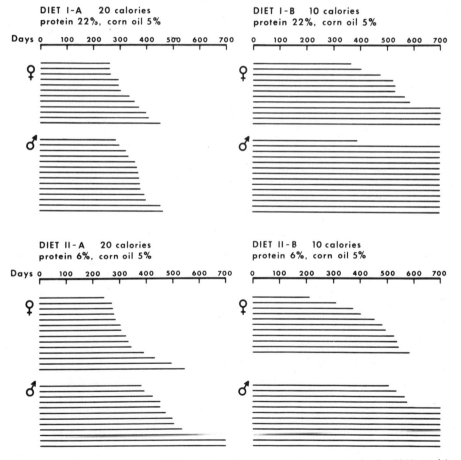

Figure 3. Survival of (NZB x NZW)F₁ (B/W) mice maintained on normal-protein (22% casein) and low-protein (6% casein) diets with daily feedings of either 10 or 20 calories per day. Each line represents life span of a single mouse.

GABRIEL
FERNANDES, ROBERT
A. GOOD, AND
EDMOND J. YUNIS

Taken together, these findings are most compatible with the view that restriction of calories in the diet of NZB mice puts a brake on their immunity system. This brake probably operates through the influence of a suppressor cell population, from which the immune response is uncoupled when the stimulated sensitized cells are introduced into the irradiated host. It is clear from these studies that much work is needed to fully understand the nature of these powerful influences.

ACKNOWLEDGMENTS

This work was aided by Public Health Service Research Grants CA-08748, CA-17404 and CA-11933 (NCI); AI-10153, AI-08145 and AI-11843 (NIAID); NS-11457 (NINCDS); HL-06314; the Department of Laboratory Medicine and Pathology, University of Minnesota, and the National Foundation–March of Dimes.

References

Alexander, P. 1967, The role of DNA lesions in processes leading to aging in mice, *Symp. Soc. Exp. Biol.* **21**:29–50.

Archer, O. K., and Pierce, J. C., 1961, Role of thymus in development of the immune response, *Fed. Proc.* **20**:26.

Archer, O. K., Pierce, J. C., Papermaster, B. W. and Good, R. A., 1962, Reduced antibody response in thymectomized rabbits, *Nature* **195**:191–192.

Barthold, D. R., Kysela, S., and Steinberg, A. D., 1974, Decline in suppressor T cell function with age in female NZB mice, *J. Immunol.* **112**:9–16.

Bellamy, D., 1967, Hormonal effects in relation to aging in mammals, *Symp. Soc. Exp. Biol.* **21**:427–450.

Bjorksten, J., 1958, A common molecular basis for the aging syndrome, *J. Am. Geriatr. Soc.* **6**:740–748.

Bullough, W. S., 1971, Ageing of mammals, *Nature* **229**:608–610.

Burnet, F. M., 1958, *The Clonal Selection Theory of Acquired Immunity,* Vanderbilt Univ. Press, Nashville, Tenn.

Burnet, F. M., 1970a, *Immunological Surveillance,* Pergamon Press, New York.

Burnet, F. M., 1970b, An immunologic approach to ageing, *Lancet* **2**:358–360.

Comfort, A., 1974, The position of aging studies, *Mech. Ageing Dev.* **3**:1–31.

Cooper, M. D., Peterson, R. D. A., South, M. A., and Good, R. A., 1966, The functions of the thymus system and the bursa system in the chicken, *J. Exp. Med.* **123**:75–102.

Cooper, W. C., Good, R. A., and Mariani, T., 1974, Effect of protein insufficiency on immune responsiveness. *Am. J. Clin. Nutr.* **27**:647–664.

Cooper, W. C., Mariani, T. N., and Good, R. A., 1975, The effects of protein deprivation on cell-mediated immunity, in: *Immunodeficiency in Man and Animals* (D. Bergsma, R. A. Good and J. Finstad, eds.), Sinauer Associates, Sunderland, Mass. pp. 223–228. (Birth Defects: Original Article Series, Vol. XI, No. 1, 1975)

Curtis, H. J., 1971, Genetic factors in aging, *Adv. Genet.* **16**:305.

Dauphinee, M. J., and Talal, N., 1975, Reversible restoration by thymosin of antigen-induced depression of spleen DNA synthesis in NZB mice. *J. Immunol.* **114**:1713–1716.

Dubois, E., and Strain, L., 1973, Effect of diet on survival and nephropathy of NZB × NZW hybrid mice, *Biochem. Med.* **7**:336–342.

Duquesnoy, R. J., 1975, The pituitary dwarf mouse. A model for study of endocrine immunodeficiency disease, in: *Immunodeficiency in Man and Animals* (D. Bergsma, R. A. Good and J. Finstad, eds.), pp. 536–543, (Birth Defects: Original Article Series, Vol. XI, No. 1, 1975), Sinauer Associates, Sunderland, Mass.

Fernandes, G., 1960, Value of penicillin mycelium residue and liver meal residue as a supplement to chick diet, *Indian J. Vet. Sci.* **30**:99–105.

Fernandes, G., and Ranadive, K. J., 1962, The value of pharmaceutical waste as a supplement to poultry ration, *Proc. 12th World's Poultry Congress,* Sydney, Australia, pp. 264–271.

Fernandes, G., Yunis, E. J., Smith, J. and Good, R. A., 1972, Dietary influence on breeding behavior, hemolytic anemia, and longevity in NZB mice, *Proc. Soc. Exp. Biol. Med.* **139**:1189–1196.

ATTEMPTS TO
CORRECT
AGE-RELATED
IMMUNODEFICIENCY
AND
AUTOIMMUNITY BY
CELLULAR AND
DIETARY
MANIPULATION IN
INBRED MICE

Fernandes, G., Yunis, E. J., Jose, D. G., and Good, R. A., 1973a, Dietary influence on antinuclear antibodies and cell-mediated immunity in NZB mice, *Int. Arch. Allergy Appl. Immunol.* **44**:770–782.

Fernandes, G., Yunis, E. J., and Good, R. A., 1973b, Reproductive deficiency of NZB male mice: possibility of a viral basis, *Lab. Invest.* **29**:278–281.

Fernandes, G., Yunis, E. J., and Good, R. A., 1976a, Influence of protein restriction on immune function in NZB mice, *J. Immunol.* **116**:782–790.

Fernandes, G., Yunis, E. J., and Good, R. A., 1976b, The influence of diet on survival of mice. *Proc. Natl. Acad. Sci.* **73**:1279–1283.

Fernandes, G., Yunis, E. J., and Good, R. A., 1976c, Age and genetic influence on immunity in NZB and autoimmunity resistant mice, *Clin. Immunol. Immunopathol.* (Sept. 1976).

Gatti, R. A., and Good, R. A., 1970, Aging, immunity and malignancy, *Geriatrics* **25**:158–168.

Gatti, R. A., Meuwissen, H. J., Allen, H. D., Hong, R., and Good, R. A., 1968, Immunologic reconstitution of sex-linked lymphopenic immunologic deficiency, *Lancet* **2**:1366–1369.

Gelfand, M. C. and Steinberg, A. D., 1973, Mechanism of allograft rejection in New Zealand mice. I. Cell synergy and its age-dependent loss, *J. Immunol.* **110**:1652–1662.

Gershwin, M. E., Ahmed, A., Steinberg, A. D., Thurman, G. B., and Goldstein, A. L., 1974, Correction of T cell function by thymosin in New Zealand mice, *J. Immunol.* **113**:1068–1071.

Goldstein, A. L., Asanuma, Y., Battisto, J. R., Hardy, M. A., Quint, J., and White, A., 1970, Influence of thymosin on cell-mediated and humoral immune responses in normal and in immunologically deficient mice, *J. Immunol.* **104**:359–366.

Good, R. A., 1954, Agammaglobulinemia—a provocative experiment of nature, *Bull. Univ. Minnesota Med. Found.* **26**:1.

Good, R. A., Dalmasso, A. P., Martinez, C., Archer, O. K., Pierce, J. C., and Papermaster, B. W., 1962, The role of the thymus in development of immunologic capacity in rabbits and mice, *J. Exp. Med.* **116**:773–796.

Good, R. A., and Gabrielsen, A. E., eds., 1964, *The Thymus in Immunobiology,* Hoeber-Harper, New York.

Good, R. A., and Finstad, J., 1968, The development and involution of the lymphoid system and immunologic capacity, *Trans. Am. Clin. Climatol. Assoc.* **79**:69–107.

Good, R. A., Gatti, R. A., Hong, R., and Meuwissen, H. J., 1969, Graft treatment of immunological deficiency, *Lancet* **1**:1162.

Good, R. A., 1973a, Immunodeficiency in developmental perspective, *Harvey Lectures, Series* **67**:1–107.

Good, R. A., 1973b, Overview of development, organization, function of lymphoid system and human disease, in: *Membranes and Viruses in Immunopathology* (S. B. Day and R. A. Good, eds.), pp. 425–436, Academic Press, New York.

Good, R. A., Jose, D. G., and Cooper, W. C., 1972, The relation between nutritional deprivation and immunity, in: *Microenvironmental Aspects of Immunity* (B. D. Jankovic and K. Isakovic, eds.), pp. 321–326, Plenum Press, New York.

Good, R. A., and Yunis, E. J., 1974, Association of autoimmunity, immunodeficiency and aging in man, rabbits and mice, *Fed. Proc.* **33**:2040–2050.

Good, R. A., 1975a, The primary immunodeficiency diseases, in: *Textbook of Medicine,* 14th Ed. (P. B. Beeson and W. McDermott, eds.), pp. 104–109, W. B. Saunders, Philadelphia.

Good, R. A., 1975b, Bone marrow transplantation: cellular engineering to correct primary immunodeficiency, aregenerative anemia and pancytopenia, in: *Immunodeficiency in Man and Animals* (D. Bergsma, R. A. Good and J. Finstad, eds.), pp. 377–379 (Birth Defects: Original Article Series, Vol. XI, No. 1, 1975), Sinauer Associates, Sunderland, Mass.

Good, R. A., and Jose, D., 1975c, Immunodeficiency secondary to nutritional deprivation: clinical and laboratory observations, in: *Immunodeficiency in Man and Animals* (D. Bergsma, R. A. Good and J. Finstad, eds.), pp. 219–222, (Birth Defects: Original Article Series, Vol. XI, No. 1, 1975), Sinauer Associates, Sunderland, Mass.

Greenberg, L. J., and Yunis, E. J., 1972, Immunologic control of aging: a possible primary event, *Gerontologia* **18**:247

Hallgren, H. M., Buckley, C. E., III, Gilbertsen, V. A., and Yunis, E. J., 1973, Lymphocyte phytohemagglutinin responsiveness, immunoglobulins and autoantibodies in aging humans, *J. Immunol.* **111**:1101–1107.

Hammar, J. A., 1926, Die Menschen-thymus in Gesundheit und Krankheit. I. Das normale Organ, *Z. Mikroskop.-Anat. Forsch.* **6**:1.

Hansen, J. A., and Good, R. A., 1974, Malignant disease of the lymphoid system in immunological perspective, *Hum. Pathol.* **5**:567–599.

Harman, D., 1968, Free radical theory of aging: effect of free radical reaction inhibitors on the mortality rate of male LAF_1 mice, *J. Gerontol.* **23**:476–482.

Hart, J. W., and Carpenter, D., 1971, Toward an integrated theory of aging, *Amer. Lab.* **3**:31–35.

Hayflick, L., 1965, The limited *in vitro* lifetime of human diploid cell strains, *Exp. Cell Res.* **37**:614–636.

Hildemann, W. H., and Cooper, E. L., 1963, Immunogenesis of homograft reaction in fishes and amphibians, *Fed. Proc.* **22**:1145–1151.

Jose, D. G., and Good, R. A., 1971, Absence of enhancing antibody in cell-mediated immunity to tumor heterografts in protein deficient rats, *Nature* **231**:323–325.

Jose, D. G., Stutman, O., and Good, R. A., 1973, Long-term effects on immune function of early nutritional deprivation, *Nature* **241**:57–58.

Kellum, M. J., Sutherland, D. E. R., Eckert, E., Peterson, R. D. A., and Good, R. A., 1965, Wasting disease, Coombs positivity and amyloidosis in rabbits subjected to central lymphoid tissue extirpation and irradiation, *Int. Arch. Allergy* **27**:6–26.

Kramer, T. and Good, R. A., 1975, Effects of protein insufficient diets on the ability of guinea pigs to produce antigen specific MIF, *Fed. Proc.* **34**:829, 3448A.

McCay, C. M., Maynard, L. A., Sperling, G., and Barnes, L. L., 1939, Retarded growth, life span, ultimate body size and age changes in the albino rat after feeding diets restricted in calories, *J. Nutr.* **18**:1–13.

Makinodan, T., Parkins, E. H., and Chen, M. G., 1971, Immunologic activity of the aged, *Adv. Gerontol. Res.* **3**:171–198.

Makinodan, T., 1972, Age-related changes in antibody forming capacity, in: *Tolerance, Autoimmunity and Aging* (M. Sigel and R. A. Good, eds.), pp. 3–17, Charles C Thomas, Springfield, Ill.

Makinodan, T., 1973, Cellular basis of immunosenescence, in: *Molecular and Cellular Mechanisms of Aging,* Vol. 27, *I.N.S.E.R.M.* pp. 153–166.

Martinez, C., Kersey, J., Papermaster, B. W., and Good, R. A., 1962, Skin homograft survival in thymectomized mice, *Proc. Soc. Exp. Biol. Med.* **109**:193–256.

Mathies, M., Lipps, L., Smith, G. S. and Walford, R. L., 1973, Age-related decline in response to phytohemagglutinin and pokeweed mitogen by spleen cells from hamsters and a long-lived mouse strain, *J. Gerontol.* **28**:425–430.

Miller, J. F. A. P., 1961, Immunological function of the thymus, *Lancet* **2**:748–749.

Nordin, A. A., and Makinodan, T., 1974, Humoral immunity in aging, *Fed. Proc.* **33**:2033–2035.

Papermaster, B. W., and Good, R. A., 1962, Relative contributions of the thymus and the bursa of Fabricius to the maturation of the lymphoreticular system and immunologic potential in the chicken, *Nature* **196**:838–840.

Price, G. B., and Makinodan, T., 1973, Aging: alteration of DNA protein information, *Gerontologia* **19**:58–70.

Roder, J. C., Bell, D. A., and Singhal, S. K., 1975, Suppressor cells in New Zealand mice: possible role in generation of autoimmunity, in: *Suppressor Cells in Immunity* (International Symposium) (S. K. Singhal and N. R. Sinclair, eds.), pp. 164–173, Univ. of Western Ontario, London, Canada.

Rodey, G. E., Good, R. A., and Yunis, E. J., 1971, Progressive loss *in vitro* of cellular immunity with aging in strains of mice susceptible to autoimmune disease, *Clin. Exp. Immunol.* **9**:305–311.

Ross, M. H., 1969, Aging, nutrition and hepatic enzyme activity patterns in the rat, *J. Nutr.* **97**:565–601.

Sacher, G. A., 1968, Molecular versus systemic theories on the genesis of ageing, *Exp. Gerontol.* **3**:265–271.

Selye, H., Prioreschi, P., 1960, Stress theory on aging, in: *Aging, Some Social and Biological Aspects,* p. 261, Am. Assoc. Adv. Sci., Washington, D.C.

Shirai, T., and Mellors, R. C., 1972, Natural cytotoxic autoantibody against thymocytes in NZB mice, *Clin. Exp. Immunol.* **12**:133–152.

Steinberg, A. D., Law, L. W., Talal, N., 1970, The role of the (NZB × NZW)F_1 thymus in experimental tolerance and auto-immunity, *Arthritis Rheum.* **13**:369–377.

Stutman, O., Yunis, E. J., Smith, J. M., Martinez, C., and Good, R. A., 1967, Reversal of post-thymectomy wasting disease in mice by multiple thymus grafts, *J. Immunol.* **98**:79–87.

Stutman, O., 1972, Lymphocyte subpopulation in NZB mice: deficit of thymus-dependent lymphocytes, *J. Immunol.* **109**:1204–1207.

Talal, N., and Steinberg, A. D., 1974, The pathogenesis of autoimmunity in New Zealand black mice, *Curr. Top. Microbiol. Immunol.* **64**:79–103.

133

ATTEMPTS TO
CORRECT
AGE-RELATED
IMMUNODEFICIENCY
AND
AUTOIMMUNITY BY
CELLULAR AND
DIETARY
MANIPULATION IN
INBRED MICE

Teague, P. O., and Friou, G. J., 1964, Inhibition of autoimmunity in A/J mice by transfer of isogenic thymic or spleen cells from young animals, *Arthritis Rheum.* **8**:474.

Teague, P. O., and Friou, G., 1969, Antinuclear antibodies in mice. II. Transformation with spleen cells, inhibition or prevention with thymus or spleen cells, *Immunology* **17**:665–675.

Teague, P. O., Yunis, E. J., Rodey, G., Fish, A. J., Stutman, O., and Good, R. A., 1970, Autoimmune phenomena and renal disease in mice: role of thymectomy, aging, and involution of immunologic capacity, *Lab. Invest.* **22**:121–130.

Tulunay, O., Good, R. A., and Yunis, E. J., 1975, Protection of lethally irradiated mice with allogeneic fetal liver cells: influence of irradiation dose on immunologic reconstitution, *Proc. Natl. Acad. Sci. USA* **72**:4100–4104.

Walford, R. L., 1969, *The Immunologic Theory of Aging,* Munksgaard, Copenhagen.

Walford, R. L., 1974a, Immunologic theory of aging: current status, *Fed. Proc.* **33**:2020–2027.

Walford, R. L., Liu, R. K., Gerbase-Delima, M., Mathies, M., and Smith, G. S., 1974b, Longterm dietary restriction and immune function in mice: response to sheep red blood cells and to mitogenic agents, *Mech. Ageing Dev.* **2**:447–454.

Yunis, E. J., Hilgard, H., Sjodin, K., Martinez, C., and Good, R. A., 1964, Immunologic reconstitution of thymectomized mice by injections of isolated thymocytes, *Nature* **201**:784–786.

Yunis, E. J., Hilgard, H., Martinez, C., and Good, R. A., 1965, Studies of immunologic reconstitution of thymectomized mice, *J. Exp. Med.* **121**:607–632.

Yunis, E. J., Martinez, C., Sjodin, K., and Good, R. A., 1966, Allograft tolerance in thymectomized mice injected with small doses of spleen cells, *Transplantation* **4**:582–586.

Yunis, E. J., Teague, P. O., Stutman, O., and Good, R. A., 1969, Post-thymectomy autoimmune phenomena in mice. II. Morphologic observations, *Lab. Invest.* **20**:46–61.

Yunis, E. J., Fernandes, G., and Stutman, O., 1971, Susceptibility to involution of the thymus dependent lymphoid system and autoimmunity, *Am. J. Clin. Pathol.* **56**:280–292.

Yunis, E. J., Fernandes, G., Teague, P. O., Stutman, O., and Good, R. A., 1972, The thymus, autoimmunity and the involution of the lymphoid system, in: *Tolerance, Autoimmunity and Aging* (M. Sigel and R. A. Good, eds.), pp. 62–120, Charles C Thomas, Springfield, Ill.

Yunis, E. J., Fernandes, G., Smith, J., Stutman, O., and Good, R. A., 1973, Involution of the thymus dependent lymphoid system, in: *Microenvironmental Aspects of Immunity* (B. D. Jankovic and K. Isakovic, eds.), pp. 301–306, Plenum Press, New York.

Yunis, E. J., Good, R. A., Smith, J., and Stutman, O., 1974, Protection of lethally irradiated mice by spleen cells from neonatally thymectomized mice, *Proc. Natl. Acad. Sci. U.S.* **71**:2544–2548.

Yunis, E. J., Fernandes, G., and Greenberg, L. J., 1975, Immune deficiency, autoimmunity and aging, in: *Immunodeficiency in Man and Animals* (D. Bergsma, R. A. Good and J. Finstad, eds.), pp. 185–192, (Birth Defects: Original Article Series, Vol. XI, No. 1, 1975), Sinauer Associates, Sunderland, Mass.

Yunis, E. J., Fernandes, G., Smith, J., and Good, R. A., 1976, Long survival and immunological reconstitution following transplantation with syngeneic or allogeneic fetal liver and neonatal spleen cells, *Transplant. Proc.* (March 1976).

10

High-Resolution Scanning Electron Microscopy and Its Application to Research on Immunity and Aging

MARGUERITE M. B. KAY

1. Introduction

The importance of membrane molecules that function as receptors and antigens in aging is attested to by the fact that such molecules emerging late in life can evoke a response from the immune system that can lead to the destruction of cells possessing those specificities. Examples include encephalopathies of autoimmune etiology in which viral antigens appear on neurons and acquired late-adulthood anemias in which immunoglobulins (Ig) M or G are present on erythrocyte membranes.

Until recently, any direct demonstration of a cell surface molecule required the use of transmission electron microscopy (TEM). The disadvantages of TEM for studies of cell membrane receptors and topology include the following: (a) The standard postfixative, osmium tetroxide, solubilizes membrane proteins and reduces the width of membranes by 5–7 nm (McMillan and Luftig, 1973). (b) Only a relatively small number of cells can be examined in any preparation. (c) The proportion of the total cell periphery that can be seen in any one section is extremely small (approximately 0.01%). Thus aggregates of membrane-bound molecules such as a cell "cap" which covers one-third to one-half the cell surface area can be easily missed. It is even easier to miss "patches" or individual molecules. (d)

MARGUERITE M. B. KAY • Laboratory of Cellular and Comparative Physiology, Gerontology Research Center, National Institute on Aging, National Institutes of Health, PHS, U.S. Department of Health, Education and Welfare, Bethesda, and Baltimore City Hospitals, Baltimore, Maryland.

Thin-sectioning precludes visualization of the entire cell surface without resorting to reconstruction of serial sections (Stackpole *et al.,* 1971), a task that is both difficult and tedious.

Negative staining of isolated membrane fragments and replica techniques permit viewing of larger areas of the membrane surface with TEM. However, results obtained with these procedures can be difficult to interpret because many of the procedures employed are conducive to artifact formation (for a more detailed review, see Zingsheim, 1972).

In contrast to TEM, scanning electron microscopy (SEM) permits three-dimensional analysis of events occurring at the cell surface, allows rapid scanning of thousands of intact cells, and requires a minimum of preparative procedures. With regard to the latter point, excellent results have been obtained by a simple glutaraldehyde fixation of the specimen followed by a 3- to 5-min dehydration in a graded series of six ethanol solutions and critical point drying (Kay, 1974; Anderson, 1951). Glutaraldehyde appears to be the best membrane fixative presently available because it alone preserves a membrane width of 16.5 nm (McMillan and Luftig, 1973), which is in close agreement with the membrane measurements obtained with X-ray diffraction (Zingsheim, 1972); in the same study, osmium produced a membrane width of 9.5 nm and large quantities of protein were detected in the solution. Although the preceding data were obtained with erythrocytes, similar results have been observed when the effect of different fixatives on lymphocytes was investigated (Kay, 1975f).

At present, the three areas in which SEM is being utilized rather extensively are: (a) cell-to-cell interactions, (b) the distribution of specific receptors on the surfaces of young and senescent cells, and (c) membrane events following ligand–receptor interaction. Therefore, it seems appropriate to discuss these in this chapter. However, before discussing these subject areas, I wish to briefly describe the basic SEM techniques for dispersed cells and monolayers in order to make available to the general reader procedures for high-resolution SEM which have been limited to a few laboratories or published in highly specialized journals, on the assumption that there will be increasing demand for their use.

2. SEM Techniques

Because the quality of the specimen generally limits the resolution of biological specimens, extreme care must be taken in its preparation. Osmolarity, temperature, pH, presence of nonautologous serum, and the use of silver membranes as a substrate can alter the surface appearance of cells (Kay *et al.,* 1974; Kay, 1975a; Alexander and Wetzel, 1975). Air-drying and excess heat during specimen coating can also introduce artifacts such as collapse or cracking of surface structures. Hydrocarbon contamination (e.g., oil vapor in an evaporator or fingerprints on the specimen, stub, or holder) often appears as a "halo" around, or a dark area on, the specimen itself and greatly decreases the resolution.

Since incubation of cell suspensions at 37°C requires a humidified atmosphere of 5% CO_2, a bicarbonate buffered medium is recommended. However, for all cellular manipulations that are performed in air, HEPES (20 mM) or phosphate (0.1 M) buffered medium is recommended in order to maintain the pH at approximately 7.4. This protocol increases cell viability (Kay, unpublished), preserves ultrastructural detail (Kay, unpublished), and enhances the response of cultured cells to mitogenic stimulation (Thorpe and Knight, 1974) when compared to protocols utilizing only bicarbonate buffered media which allow an alkaline pH shift at room atmosphere.

137

HIGH-RESOLUTION
SCANNING
ELECTRON
MICROSCOPY AND
ITS APPLICATION TO
RESEARCH ON
IMMUNITY AND
AGING

Cells are generally fixed first with 1% glutaraldehyde in phosphate buffered saline (PBS pH 7.4) for 30–60 min, then with 3% glutaraldehyde in PBS solution for 4–16 hr, followed by dehydration in a graded series of ethanol–water solutions (Kay *et al.*, 1974), and, finally, by CO_2 critical point drying (Anderson, 1951). It has been found that specimens can be critical point dried directly from 100% ethanol without processing through a transitional fluid, such as amyl acetate, since ethanol is miscible with CO_2 (DeBault, 1973). Presumably, this has the advantage of decreasing solvent extraction of membrane lipids and permitting the use of formvar coated TEM grids which would be dissolved by either amyl acetate or acetone. Three changes of 100% ethanol are recommended to ensure complete removal of water (Kay, unpublished).

After critical point drying, specimens may be coated in either an oil-free vacuum evaporator equipped with a rotating stage and liquid nitrogen trap or a "sputtering" device. Gold–palladium (60:40) is widely used because of its relatively small grain size when "sputtered" and its good secondary electron emission. Platinum-carbon coating, using a modification of the Baalzer's freeze-fracture evaporation technique, has also been utilized successfully by the Electron Microscopy Laboratory of the University of California, Berkeley (Carolyn Schooley, personal communication). Chromium has likewise been used successfully because of its small grain size (Timothy Denton, personal communication). In order to maximize surface detail, it is desirable to minimize the coating thickness. Further, metal coating increases the apparent size of structures. For example, tobacco mosaic virus is 15 nm in diameter in negatively stained TEM preparations, but appears to be 33–50 nm in diameter in SEM specimens coated with approximately 10 nm of gold–palladium (Lipscomb *et al.*, 1975). I have obtained good results with a 5 nm coating.

Although various methods for coating specimens in solutions of ammoniacal silver nitrate (Goldman and Leif, 1973), osmium utilizing thiocarbohydrazide (Kelly, *et al.*, 1975), etc., have been developed, these have not proved useful for high-resolution SEM of single cells in some laboratories, including mine. The disadvantages encountered include: (a) the appearance of artifacts such as small holes in cell membranes, (b) fine precipitates which appear as a "fuzz" at higher magnifications (20,000–75,000), and (c) obliteration of cell-surface detail by the thickness of the coating deposited on the surface, which ranges from 20 to 50 nm. However, some of these techniques have been employed successfully by others, particularly on tissues such as kidneys and stomach (T. Denton, personal communication).

A filtered, saturated, aqueous solution of uranyl acetate has been used as the diluent in ethanol-water dehydration solutions to prevent solubilization of membrane lipids and to reduce the amount of metal coating required (Kay, unpublished). Moreover, uranyl acetate does not seem to produce visible artifacts (McMillan and Luftig, 1973; Kay, unpublished); however, its efficacy regarding its intended purpose has not been definitely established.

Ruthenium Red (RR) has been utilized as part of the second glutaraldehyde fixation (i.e., 1% RR in 3% glutaraldehyde solution). It seems to reduce the amount of metal coating necessary to prevent specimen "charging" without introducing visible artifacts (Kay, unpublished). It may also fix mucopolysaccharides.

Lightly coated cell preparations tend to absorb water vapor from the air and should, therefore, be stored in a vacuum desiccator to prevent cracking when placed in the evacuated SEM specimen chamber.

Most of the photographs presented in this chapter were obtained with a field-emission (cold-cathode) SEM with 3 nm resolution. A few were obtained with a conventional (heated-cathode) SEM capable of 7 nm resolution. Photographs were recorded either on Polaroid 55/PN film or on Kodak Plus X 4 × 5 in. sheet film.

Silver-conducting paint tends to be the universal adhesive for attaching coverslips or discs to SEM stubs. However, it has the following disadvantages: (a) it "out-gasses" in high vacuum, unless dried and prepumped in an evaporator, (b) it does not allow for easy removal of the specimen from the stub, and (c) coverslips (if recovered unbroken from a stub) are no longer transparent, thus hindering observation of the sample with light or phase microscopy. An ingenious solution to this problem of specimen mounting was discovered by Dr. Paul Lin and M. K. Lamvik at the Microscope User's Laboratory of the Enrico Fermi Institute, University of Chicago. They designed "stubs" which contained indentations in which the disc or coverslip is placed. The "cap," containing holes through which the specimens are observed, clamps on the top of the stub, holding the specimens in place by slightly overlapping their edge. It should be easy to adapt this design to any type of SEM (Lamvik and Lin, 1974). This stub is inexpensive and facilitates easy, rapid mounting and easy removal of specimens. Only a few stubs are needed, and these can remain with the SEM for use by each successive operator.

3. Cell–Cell Interactions

A representative type of study in this area concerns tumor-cell–antitumor-cell interaction. The interaction between cytolytic T cells and autochthonous cancer cells was examined using lymph node cells. Cells were dissociated from involved lymph nodes of patients with untreated Hodgkin's disease, and incubated on coverslips in RPMI 1640 medium *without* serum at 37°C. Samples were fixed and processed for SEM at 5, 10, 20, and 30 min. Each coverslip was viewed with a phase microscope and the location of cancerous Reed–Sternberg (RS) cells was noted for viewing with SEM. Cells having all the following features were considered RS cells (Kay, 1975b,c): (a) two or more nuclei, (b) thick nuclear membranes, (c) abundant, "foamy" cytoplasm, and (d) large, round or oval nucleoli (Figure 1). Such cells were generally larger than the cells about them and were, therefore, easily located with SEM (Kay, 1975b).

Lymphocytes attacking RS cells were considered to be T cells because (a) they fluoresced when treated with fluorescent labeled anti-T cell sera, (b) they did not fluoresce when treated with fluorescent labeled anti-B cell sera, (c) they formed nonimmune sheep erythrocyte (E) rosettes, and (d) they met the SEM criteria for T cells. The RS cells appear to be macrophage-histiocyte cells because they (a) did not fluoresce when treated with the anti-T cell reagent, (b) did not form nonimmune E rosettes, (c) met the SEM criteria for macrophages, and (d) phagocytized lymphocytes (Kadin *et al.,* 1974; Kay and Kadin, 1975; Kay, 1975b).

139

HIGH-RESOLUTION
SCANNING
ELECTRON
MICROSCOPY AND
ITS APPLICATION TO
RESEARCH ON
IMMUNITY AND
AGING

SEM examination of RS-T cell interactions (Figures 2–6) indicates that "killer" T cells lyse autologous target cells in the following sequential manner: Stage 1, T cells affix the tips of their microvilli onto target cells. Stage 2, T cells subject target cell membranes to tearing and shearing forces which produce gaps progressing to holes between membrane subunits. The formation of gaps and holes may allow leakage of ions and results in an increase in intracellular osmotic pressure which can lead to an influx of extracellular fluid. This, in turn, can induce osmotic swelling causing the cells to assume a spherical shape (Seeman, 1974) and resulting in the loss of surface structures, such as lamellae. Stage 3, target cells lyse as a result of further stretching of the membrane, caused by increasing internal osmotic pressure, and T cells move away. Consistent with the interpretation that lysis is caused by increasing osmotic pressure is the observation that the size of RS cells increased from an average of 9 μm in diameter after 5 min of culture to an average of 15 μm in diameter after 20 min in culture.

Occasionally, "normal" macrophages (i.e., those that did not meet the criteria of RS cells) and monocytes were attacked by lymphocytes (Kay, 1975c). This is unusual, as I have observed over 3000 macrophages from normal individuals with SEM during the past five years and have not observed lymphocytes pulling on their membranes. Further, I have not observed the membrane particles (Figure 1) on macrophages of normal individuals when prepared by the same techniques. These

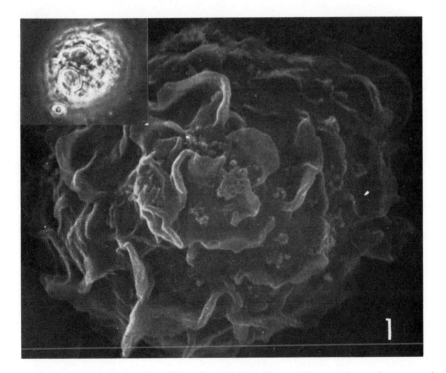

Figure 1. Reed–Sternberg (RS) cells with lamellae and virus-like particles not observed on macrophages of normal individuals prepared by the same techniques ($\times$ 8000). Phase microscopy (inset) demonstrates the identifying features of RS cells in SEM preparations: (a) two nuclei, (b) thick nuclear membranes, (c) abundant, "foamy" cytoplasm, and (d) large, oval nucleoli ($\times$ 896). From Kay, 1975b.

MARGUERITE M. B.
KAY

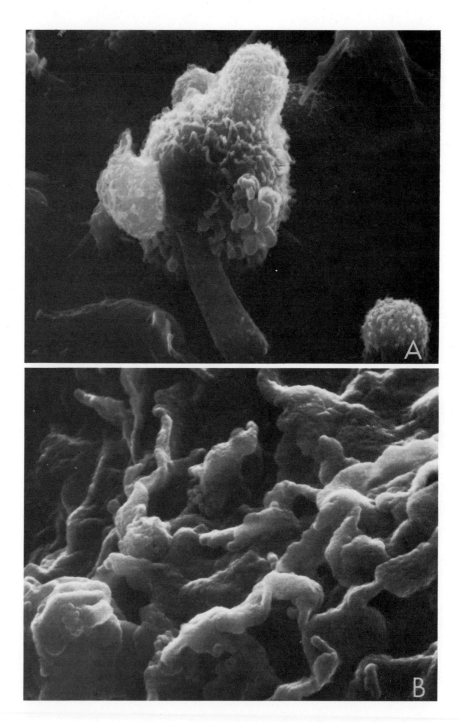

Figure 2(A).   RS cell with lamellae after 5 min of culture ($\times$ 4000).   (B).   A higher magnification of RS cell showing that there are no discontinuities in the membrane ($\times$ 20,000).

HIGH-RESOLUTION
SCANNING
ELECTRON
MICROSCOPY AND
ITS APPLICATION TO
RESEARCH ON
IMMUNITY AND
AGING

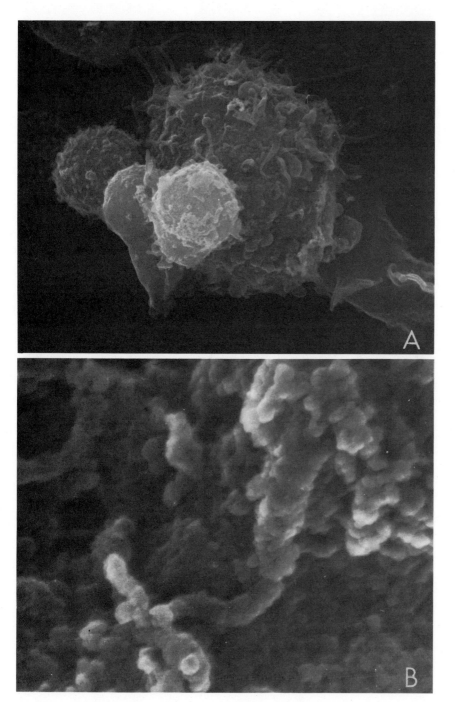

Figure 3 (A). RS cells after 10 min of culture ($\times$ 5540). Most of the RS cell's lamellae have collapsed. Filopodia and microvilli are still visible. (B). A high magnification of the surface of RS cell showing gaps between membrane subunits and membrane subunits ($\times$ 50,000).

MARGUERITE M. B.
KAY

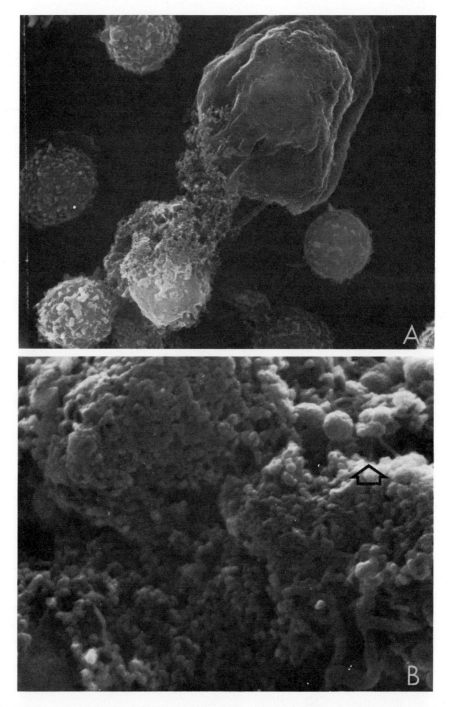

Figure 4 (A).   RS cell devoid of lamellae and filopodia after 15 min of culture (× 4000).   (B).   A higher magnification of RS cell surface showing holes between membrane subunits and larger holes with missing membrane units (× 20,000).

143

HIGH-RESOLUTION
SCANNING
ELECTRON
MICROSCOPY AND
ITS APPLICATION TO
RESEARCH ON
IMMUNITY AND
AGING

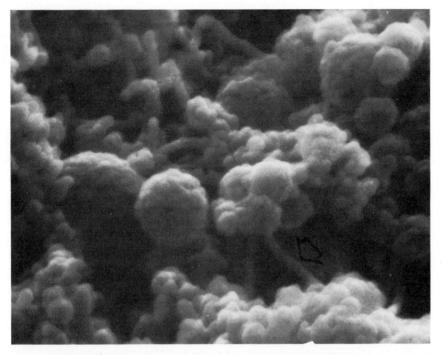

Figure 5. A higher magnification of a hole indicated by an arrow in Figure 4B. Note that cytoplasmic vesicles and inclusions are visible; the arrow indicates microtubules ($\times$ 50,000).

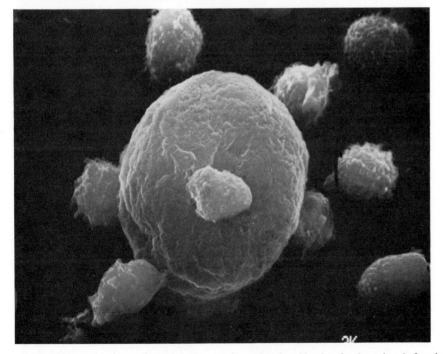

Figure 6. Spherical RS cell devoid of lamellae and filopodia after 20 min of culture just before lysis ($\times$ 3000).

are generally observed on RS cells. This suggests that certain normal macrophages in Hodgkin's disease may be expressing altered surface antigens. If so, the possibility exists that the macrophages of patients with Hodgkin's disease may have been infected with an intracellular parasite, such as a virus, because they could not digest it after engulfment. Suffice it to say, certain viruses can proliferate preferentially inside macrophages (Bang and Warwick, 1960; DeThé and Notkins, 1965; Jones, 1974; Silverstein, 1970).

It has been suggested that this defect in the ability of macrophages to digest certain viruses may be genetically determined and that it may be age dependent. The latter possibility might help to explain the bimodal curve of age-related incidence found with lymphocyte predominant Hodgkin's disease—a peak at approximately puberty, flattening of the curve between 35 to 40 years, and a second rise after 40 years. It is tempting to speculate that the first peak includes individuals with subtle immunodeficiencies, and the second with an age-related decline in T cell competence (Makinodan and Adler, 1975), permitting the ingress of viruses (Kay, 1975d).

4. Distribution of Specific Receptors on the Surfaces of Young and Senescent Cells

A multiple labeling technique developed in this laboratory employs SV 40 virus, keyhole limpet hemocyanin (KLH), T2 bacteriophage, f 2 phage, and ferritin as SEM visible markers (Kay, 1975a). Briefly, a marker is conjugated to an antibody or a lectin with 0.1% glutaraldehyde, and aggregates, unconjugated marker, and unconjugated protein are removed by column chromatography on Sepharose 6B. This technique has proved useful for (a) the detection of small numbers of molecules on cell surfaces (<100), (b) quantitation and mapping of different receptors on individual cells, (c) unambiguous identification of subpopulations of cells, and (d) kinetic studies of changes in membrane fluidity initiated by binding of ligands with their receptors.

This technique was utilized recently to demonstrate visually how macrophages selectively remove senescent RBC (Kay, 1975e). It was shown that attachment of IgG autoantibody to the surface of senescent human RBC initiates their removal by macrophages. The experimental evidence implicating IgG as the initiator of phagocytosis is as follows:

1. When RBC aged *in vitro* for two weeks at 4°C in serum-free medium 199 were incubated with autologous macrophages, the percent phagocytosis of RBC incubated in autologous IgG was essentially the same as that of RBC incubated in autologous serum or an autologous Ig fraction (Table 1). On the other hand, the percent phagocytosis of RBC incubated in IgA or IgM was only slightly higher than that of RBC incubated in medium alone. This indicated that (a) Ig are required for a phagocytosis of aged RBC, (b) normal circulating Ig attach to aged RBC, and (c) that the Ig are of the IgG class.

2. When freshly drawn RBC were separated into young (Y-RBC) and old (O-RBC) populations according to the difference in their densities (Murphy, 1973), washed, and incubated with autologous macrophages, less than 5% of the Y-RBC were phagocytized whereas greater than 30% of the O-RBC were phagocytized, regardless of whether the final incubations were performed in medium without

serum (Y-RBC, 5 ± 2%; O-RBC, 33 ± 1.5%) or autologous Ig depleted serum (Y-RBC, 2 ± 2.5%; O-RBC, 51 ± 17%) or whole serum (Y-RBC, 0%; O-RBC, 43 ± 5%). This indicates that the Ig are attached *in situ* to the aged RBC and that phagocytic recognition is not inhibited by other serum components.

145

HIGH-RESOLUTION
SCANNING
ELECTRON
MICROSCOPY AND
ITS APPLICATION TO
RESEARCH ON
IMMUNITY AND
AGING

3. SEM labeling studies were performed on aliquots drawn from the Y-RBC and O-RBC fractions. The cells were washed with serum-free culture medium and then incubated with SV 40 conjugated to goat antihuman (GAH) IgG, KLH-GAH IgM, and T2-GAH IgA. SEM of the two populations revealed that the Y-RBC were essentially unlabeled, whereas the O-RBC were labeled with SV 40-GAH IgG. On the basis of these findings, it was concluded that IgG attaches *in situ* to senescent RBC making them vulnerable to phagocytosis by macrophages.

4. When Y-RBC are incubated in *Vibrio cholerae* neuraminidase (VCN), washed, and incubated in Medium 199, autologous IgG or Ig, those incubated in IgG and Ig are phagocytized as though they were O-RBC (IgG, 47 ± 4%; Ig, 46% ± 1%); whereas those incubated in medium alone are not (0%). SEM, using ferritin as a marker, demonstrated the presence of IgG on the surface of VCN treated RBC incubated in IgG and Ig (Figure 7). This suggests that IgG binds to antigenic groups exposed by removal of sialic acid, presumably carbohydrate determinants.

Based on these findings with VCN-treated RBC, it is tempting to speculate that molecules intrinsic to an organism which, so long as they remain intact, are not themselves immunogenic, may be rendered immunogenic by the action of microbial enzymes that can cleave groups or fragments of such molecules, thus changing their "identity." This hypothesis, which can be referred to as the microbial–enzyme theory of autoantibody formation, is consistent with the evidence accumulating in the literature that implicates microbes as precipitating agents in autoimmune disease (Kay, 1975d). Further, it would explain the age-dependent onset of certain autoimmune diseases, and the appearance of autoimmune hemolytic anemia and thrombocytopenia in patients who are immunologically hyporesponsive (i.e., those with Hodgkin's disease, lymphocytic lymphoma, or chronic lymphocytic leukemia). A deficiency in cellular immunity is common to all these conditions (Kay, 1975d).

TABLE 1.   Phagocytosis of RBC Aged *in Vitro*,
Preincubated in Various Media, Washed, and Incubated for
3 hr with Autologous Macrophages in Serum-Free Medium
199[a]

Preincubation media	% Phagocytosis (± SEM)
Medium 199	0
Medium 199 + PNH IgM	6.5 ± 0.5
Medium 199 + PNH IgA	7.0 ± 1.5
Autol Ig depleted serum	0
Autol whole serum	44 ± 5
Medium 199 + Autol Ig	42.5 ± 5
Medium 199 + Autol IgG	49 ± 1
Medium 199 + PNH IgG	25.5 ± 3.5

[a]Briefly, the experimental protocol is as follows: macrophages (5 × 10⁵), isolated from human peripheral blood by glass adhesion were incubated with 4–6 × 10⁶ RBC for 3 hr at 37°C. The remaining RBC were counted at the end of the incubation and the percent phagocytosis determined (Kay, 1975e).

MARGUERITE M. B. KAY

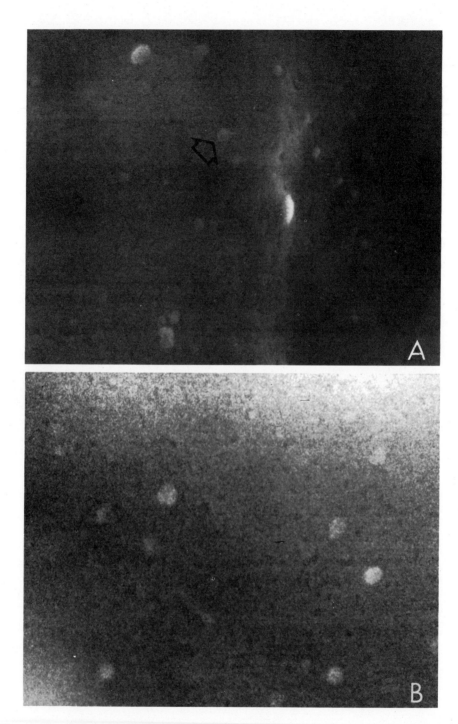

Figure 7 (A).   Surface of young RBC treated with VCN, incubated in IgG, washed, and incubated with ferritin-conjugated antihuman IgG. Arrows indicate ferritin molecules ($\times$ 50,000).   (B).   A higher magnification of ferritin-labeled RBC ($\times$ 75,000).

Decreased T cell responsiveness could permit the entry and prolong the residence of microbes such as bacteria and viruses whose enzymes could alter host molecules so that they are no longer recognized by the immune system as "self" components (Kay, 1975e).

The *in situ* aging experiments with RBC suggest that autoantibodies that are normally present in the blood are essential for the removal of cells that have reached the end of their useful life span. On the basis of these experiments, it appears necessary to revise the popular concept of autoantibody wherein it is considered "bad" by differentiating those autoantibodies with *"physiological"* functions from autoantibodies with *"pathological"* functions. One would predict that the former would be present at birth or appear shortly afterward, while the latter would be age dependent.

147

HIGH-RESOLUTION
SCANNING
ELECTRON
MICROSCOPY AND
ITS APPLICATION TO
RESEARCH ON
IMMUNITY AND
AGING

5. Membrane Events Following Ligand–Receptor Interaction

"Capping" is a membrane event following ligand–receptor interactions observed most commonly with the use of T and B cells under fluorescent microscopy and TEM. In spite of its obvious advantages, SEM has not been utilized extensively to study this phenomenon. Therefore it seems appropriate to discuss it briefly at this time. Using the multiple labeling technique discussed earlier, the following membrane events were observed accompanying the binding of antibody to the Ig molecules on B cell surfaces (Kay, 1975a).

1. Within 2 min of incubation of B cells at 37°C with antibody-marker conjugates, the microvilli on labeled cells migrated to one pole of the cell forming a "cap," while elongated macrovilli and lamellae formed on the other. An average of ten markers were visible on each labeled cell.
2. By 15 min, elongated macrovilli and lamellae covered the surfaces of 70% of the B cells, and an average of 300 markers were visible on each labeled cell.
3. Within 30 min, the surfaces of 50% of the labeled cells were extensively covered with lamellae, and the marker had again "capped."

Throughout this process of "capping," it appeared that globular membrane subunits were extruded from the cell membrane and "capped" at a pole on the surface of the cells, where they are either released into the medium or engulfed by the cell's lamellae (Figure 8). This has not been discussed by those viewing the "capping" process with fluorescent light microscopy; it is, however, consistent with the concept of a "fluid, mosaic membrane." Thus SEM analysis of this event may provide a better understanding of cell membrane components and activities by virtue of its capability for resolving three-dimensional events.

This kinetic approach is currently being utilized to study the membrane fluidity and the fate of receptors on young and old T cells. For example, Hung *et al., 1975* have shown that there is no difference in the binding of PHA between young and old cells, yet the response of cells from old individuals is 10% that of cells from young individuals. Kinetic studies are now in progress to determine whether the difference in responsiveness is reflective of membrane dynamics. Consistent with this view are our preliminary findings showing that human T cells are osmotically more fragile than B cells, and that both the B and T cells of older individuals (>60 years old) are more fragile than those from young adults (20–25 years); unpublished.

MARGUERITE M. B.
KAY

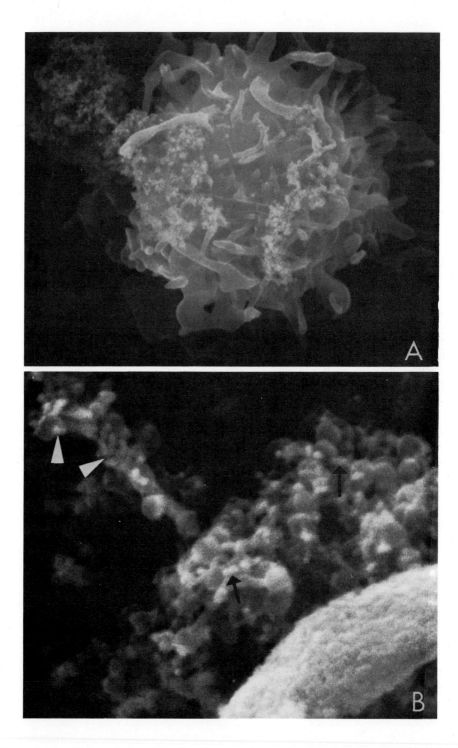

Figure 8 (A). T2-bacteriophage-labeled antihuman IgM, on the surface of a human B cell at low magnification ($\times$ 20,000). Note the "fuzzy" appearance of the label. (B). A higher magnification of the area in upper left of Figure 8B which shows that membrane units (arrows) are attached to the T2-bacteriophage label ($\times$ 75,000).

6. Concluding Remarks

In this chapter, an attempt has been made to introduce the capabilities and potentials of high-resolution SEM as a technique for studying, at membrane level, the decline in certain functional activities of cells of the immune system and to provide technical information that is not readily available. High-resolution SEM has now been developed to the degree that it is probably the best and most convenient technique for studying membrane dynamics and receptors. Thus, e.g., it has been shown that high-resolution SEM can be utilized to study cell-to-cell interactions, distribution of membrane receptors of young and senescent immune cells, and membrane events following ligand–receptor interaction. These are just a few examples. It is apparent that the possibilities for use of SEM to study age effects on immunity at the cellular and molecular levels have barely been "tapped."

References

Alexander, E. L., and Wetzel, B., 1975, Human lymphocytes: similarity of B and T cell surface morphology, *Science* **188**:732–734.

Anderson, T. F., 1951, Techniques for the preservation of three-dimensional structure in preparing specimens for the electron microscope, *Trans. N.Y. Acad. Sci.* **13**:130–133.

Bang, F. B., and Warwick, A., 1960, Mouse macrophages as host cells for the mouse hepatitis virus and the genetic basis of their susceptibility, *Proc. Natl. Acad. Sci.* **46**:1065.

DeBault, L. E., 1973, A critical point drying technique for scanning electron microscopy of tissue culture cells grown on plastic substratum, in: *Scanning Electron Microscopy* (O. Johari and I. Corvin, eds.), pp. 317–324, ITT Research Institute, Chicago.

DeThé, G., and Notkins, A. L., 1965, Ultrastructure of lactic dehydrogenase virus (LDV) and cell-virus relationship, *Virology* **26**:512.

Goldman, M., and Leif, R., 1973, A wet chemical method for rendering samples conductive and observations on the surface morphology of human erythrocytes and Ehrlich ascites cells, *Proc. Nat. Acad. Sci. USA* **70**:3599–3603.

Jones, T. C., 1974, Macrophages and intracellular parasitism, *J. Reticuloendothel. Soc.* **15**:439–450.

Hung, C.-Y., Perkins, E., and Yang, W.-K., 1975, Age related refractoriness of PHA-induced lymphocyte transformation. II: ^{125}I-PHA binding to spleen cells from young and old mice, *Mech. Age. Devel.* **4**:103–112.

Kadin, M., Newcom, S., Gold, S., and Stites, D., 1974, Origin of Hodgkin's cell, *Lancet* **1**:167–168.

Kay, M. M. B., 1975a, Multiple labeling technique used for studies of activated human B lymphocytes, *Nature* **254**:424–426.

Kay, M. M. B., 1975b, Surface characteristics of Hodgkin's cells, Lancet **11**:459–460.

Kay, M. M. B., 1975c, Hodgkin's disease: a war between T lymphocytes and transformed macrophages?, *Congress of the European Organization for Research on Treatment of Cancer,* in press.

Kay, M. M. B., 1975d, Autoimmune disease: the consequence of deficient T cell function?, *J. Am. Soc. Geriat.,* in press.

Kay, M. M. B., 1975e, Mechanism of removal of senescent cells by human macrophages *in situ, Proc. Natl. Acad. Sci. U.S.,* **72**:3521–3525.

Kay, M. M. B., 1975f, High resolution scanning electron microscopy and its application to age-related changes of T and B cells, *Proc. of the 10th International Congress of Gerontology,* Vol 1, Plenary Sessions, Symposia. The Congress, Jerusalem, pp. 84–86.

Kay, M. M. B., and Kadin, M., 1975, Classification of Hodgkin's cells according to surface characteristics, *Lancet* 1, No. 7909:748–749.

Kay, M. M., Belohradsky, B., Yee, K., Vogel, J., Butcher, D., Wybran, J., and Fudenberg, H., 1974, Cellular interactions: scanning electron microscopy of human thymus-derived rosette-forming lymphocytes, *J. Clin. Immunol. Immunopath.* **2**:301–309.

Kelly, R. O., Dekker, R. A. F., and Bluemink, J. G., 1975, Thiocarbohydrazide mediated osmium binding: a technique for protecting soft tissues in the scanning electron microscope, in: *Principles and*

Techniques of Scanning Electron Microscopy (M. A. Hayat, ed.), Vol 4, pp. 34–43, Van Nostrand Reinhold Co., New York.

Lamvik, M. K., and Lin, S. D., 1974, A new specimen mounting system for scanning electron microscopy, *J. Microscopy* **101**:329–331.

Lipscomb, M. F., Holmes, K. V., Vitetta, E. S., Hammerling, U., and Uhr, J. W., 1975, Cell surface immunoglobulin XII. Localization of immunoglobulin on murine lymphocytes by scanning immuno-electron microscopy, *Eur. J. Immunol.* **5**:255–259.

Makinodan, T., and Adler, W., 1975, The effects of aging on the differentiation and proliferation potentials of cells of the immune system, *Fed. Proc.* **34**:153–158.

McMillan, P. N., and Luftig, R. B., 1973, Preservation of erythrocyte ghost ultrastructure achieved by various fixatives, *Proc. Natl. Acad. Sci. U.S.* **70**:3060–3064.

Murphy, J., 1973, Influence of temperature and method of centrifugation on the separation of erythrocytes, *J. Lab. Clin. Med.* **82**:334–341.

Seeman, P., 1974, Ultrastructure of membrane lesions in immune lysis, osmotic lysis, and drug-induced lysis, *Fed. Proc.* **33**:2116–2124.

Silverstein, S. C., 1970, Macrophages and viral immunity, *Semin. Hematol.* **7**:185–214.

Stackpole, C. W., Aoki, T., Boyse, E. A., Old, L. J., Lumley-Frank, J., and deHarven, E., 1971, Cell surface antigens: serial sectioning of single cells as an approach to topographical analysis, *Science* **172**:472–474.

Thorpe, P. E., and Knight, S. C., 1974, Microplate culture of mouse lymph node cells I. Quantitation of responses to allogeneic lymphocytes, endotoxin and phytomitogens, *J. Immunol. Methods* **5**:387–404.

Zingsheim, H. P., 1972, Membrane structure and electron microscopy: the significance of physical problems and techniques (freeze etching), *Biochim. Biophys. Acta* **265**:339–366.

11

Immunological Responsiveness and Aging Phenomena in Germfree Mice

ROBERT E. ANDERSON, WILLIAM E. DOUGHTY, and GARY M. TROUP

1. Introduction

1.1. General

Germfree animals constitute a unique resource for the evaluation of aging phenomena, especially as the latter relates to immune dysfunction. In particular, it is possible to eliminate one important variable, i.e., infection, in studies designed to define the relationship between the immune response and aging. Such infection may be overt or occult. Of perhaps greater importance, in the context of this discussion, is the fact that germfree animals may be utilized to perform experiments that are not possible with their conventional counterparts. For example, neonatal thymectomy in many strains of mice results in an acute, fatal runting phenomenon; this syndrome is not noted in neonatally thymectomized germfree animals of the same strains.

Most of the data referred to herein were obtained with germfree mice. Although more information is available with germfree mice than for other species, numerous important studies have been performed with germfree rats, hamsters, dogs, birds, guinea pigs, and probably other experimental animals.

Germfree, in the context of this report, indicates that the mice did not harbor

ROBERT E. ANDERSON, WILLIAM E. DOUGHTY, and GARY M. TROUP • Department of Pathology, University of New Mexico School of Medicine, Albuquerque, New Mexico, and the Albuquerque Veterans Administration Hospital.

ROBERT E.
ANDERSON,
WILLIAM E.
DOUGHTY, AND
GARY M. TROUP

viable bacteria and fungi and did not react serologically with the following murine viruses: pneumonia virus of mice; Sendai; GD-VII; rat, H-l; simian virus 5; mouse adeno virus; mouse hepatitis; lymphocytic choriomeningitis; polyoma; Theiler's; and K virus.

The question often arises as to what constitutes a comparable study population in experiments with germfree animals. Such a study population may be considered as the "control" or the "experimental" population, depending upon one's frame of reference. In the majority of the aging studies referred to in this report, the conventional and germfree mice were maintained in identical fashion in flexible plastic isolators as described in detail elsewhere (Anderson *et al.*, 1972a). Both groups were fed autoclaved food and sterile water. Monthly surveillance for contamination in the germfree component revealed only antibodies to reovirus 3 at a serum dilution of 1:20. The conventional mice continued to harbor the usual murine viruses and bacteria and did not demonstrate the simplification of their flora often associated with such housing and diet. Conventional mice housed and fed in this fashion will subsequently be referred to as "barrier-maintained." On the other hand, a few of the experiments described herein utilized conventional mice maintained in a standard vivarium. These mice will be referred to as "conventional."

1.2. Characteristics of Germfree Mice

Many of the early experiments with germfree animals were complicated by borderline malnutrition and vitamin deficiencies due to the loss of heat-sensitive nutrients during the sterilization procedure. The nutritional status of the host is known to influence longevity and many aspects of the immune response. The use of hyperfortified food has apparently resolved this problem, as shown in Figure 1. In this figure, body weight is shown as a function of age; no significant difference is apparent between the germfree and conventional groups.

Despite normal growth and development, however, the transit time of food in the gastrointestinal tract is shorter in germfree than in conventional mice. As a reflection of this phenomenon, the feces are generally more liquid. Perhaps related to these phenomena is the observation that the cecum of germfree mice is character-

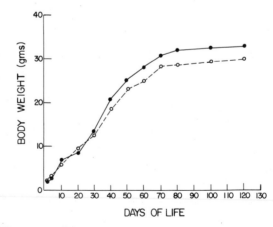

Figure 1. Growth curves of conventional (open circles) and germfree (closed circles) C3H mice (Anderson, unpublished data). Combined data for equal numbers of males and females, 32 mice per group.

istically dilated and thin-walled. As a result, cecal volvulus and infarction is not an infrequent cause of death.

153

IMMUNOLOGICAL
RESPONSIVENESS
AND AGING
PHENOMENA IN
GERMFREE MICE

With respect to comparisons involving other organs, no significant differences have been noted with respect to heart, lungs, kidneys, bone marrow, and endocrine and reproductive organs. Some authors (Thorbecke and Benacerraf, 1959) have reported that the liver is smaller in germfree than conventional mice. Others (Henderson and Titus, 1968) have not observed such a difference, which therefore may be strain-dependent.

In contrast with the above, marked differences are known to exist between the various lymphoid tissues of germfree and conventional mice. Since these discrepancies are of particular relevance to this volume, they will be discussed in detail.

With the possible exception of the thymus, the lymphoid tissues of germfree mice are smaller and less well developed than those of their conventional counterparts. More specifically, the weight of the spleen, lymph nodes, and Peyer's patches is significantly less in germfree than conventional mice (Dukor *et al.*, 1968; Gordon, 1959; Olson and Wostmann, 1966). Some of these differences become less pronounced when the conventional mice are barrier-maintained (Bauer *et al.*, 1964), although most of the histologic differences persisted.

The relationship between thymus weight and the microbial status of the host apparently demonstrates some strain variability. Thus Dukor *et al.* (1968) found no difference in the weight of the thymus of germfree versus conventional C3H/Gif mice, while several other reports have documented a smaller, less cellular organ (Luckey, 1963; Anderson *et al.*, 1972a; Wilson *et al.*, 1965). Perhaps more relevant in this regard are the studies of Bealmer and Wilson (1966) in which there were differences in mitotic activity between the germfree thymus (5–6 mitotic figures per X 197 microscopic field) and conventional thymus (7–8 mitotic figures per X 197 microscopic field) and the related observation of Burns *et al.* (1964) that DNA synthesis, as measured by [^{3}H]thymidine uptake, is considerably slower in the thymus of germfree as opposed to conventional mice. As will be discussed subsequently, these discrepancies in cell turnover are reflected in differences in the size of the recirculation pool of thymic-derived small lymphocytes.

Histologically, the lymphoid tissues of germfree mice are known to lack normally developed germinal centers and to contain few, if any, pyroninophilic blasts and plasma cells (Dukor *et al.*, 1968; Olson and Wostmann, 1966). Histologic comparisons of spleen, lymph nodes, and Peyer's patches obtained from germfree and conventional mice are shown in Table 1. In the spleen of germfree mice, the white pulp is strikingly reduced in cellularity and the numbers of lymphocytes that occupy the periarteriolar sheath are equivocally reduced. Lymph nodes from germfree mice lack germinal centers, while large pyroninophilic cells and plasma cells are absent or sparse. Population of the paracortical areas and medullary cords with lymphocytes is patchy and often limited to only one portion of the node. The appearance of Peyer's patches in germfree mice is similar to that of lymph nodes—an absence of normally developed germinal centers and few, if any, pyroninophilic blasts or plasma cells.

Despite the marked hypoplasia noted in many, if not all, of the lymphoid tissues from germfree mice, alterations in the numbers of formed elements found in the peripheral blood are surprisingly modest. Table 2 summarizes data pertinent to this point for outbred female mice of the Charles River colony sacrificed at 42, 202, 362, and 522 days of life. Of particular interest is the age-related decline in absolute

ROBERT E.
ANDERSON,
WILLIAM E.
DOUGHTY, AND
GARY M. TROUP

TABLE 1. Histologic Observations in Spleen, Lymph Nodes, and Peyer's Patches from Germfree and Conventional Mice[a]

Tissue	Microbial status	Large pyroninophilic cells in periarteriolar sheath		Germinal centers per scored section		Plasma cells		
		Absent or sparse	Numerous	Absent	Present	Absent	Sparse	Numerous
Spleen	Conventional	0	100	0	100	—	—	—
	Germfree	100	0	70	30[b]	—	—	—
Lymph node	Conventional	75	25	25	75	0	100	0
	Germfree	100	0	100	0	57	43	0
Peyer's patch	Conventional	0	100	0	100	0	0	100
	Germfree	100	0	100	0	100	0	0

[a]After Dukor et al., 1968. Results expressed as percentage of mice in group with indicated observation.
[b]Germinal centers of very small size.

TABLE 2. Hematology Values as a Function of Age in Germfree and Barrier-Maintained Mice[a]

Experimental group	Determination	Hematology values in mice sacrificed at various ages			
		42 days	202 days	362 days	522 days
Barrier-maintained	Hematocrit	50	48	53	49
	Reticulocyte count	3.9	3.3	4.5	2.7
	Total leukocyte count	4325	3725	4300	3300
	Absolute lymphocyte count	3794	3166	2850	759
Germfree	Hematocrit	49	49	50	53
	Reticulocyte count	—	—	4.6	5.2
	Total leukocyte count	2262	2260	7850	9100
	Absolute lymphocyte count	1945	1945	5900	4228

[a]After Anderson et al., 1972a. Hematocrit and reticulocyte count expressed as percent; total leukocyte and absolute lymphocyte counts as number of cells per cubic millimeter; each value represents mean determination from four mice.

TABLE 3. Comparison of Thoracic Duct Lymphocyte Production from Conventional and Germfree CBA Mice[a]

Experimental group	Number of mice	Characteristics of thoracic duct output			
		Volume	Number of small lymphocytes $\times 10^{-6}$	Percent of T cells[b]	Percent of B cells[c]
Conventional	22	20.3 ± 3.6	60.4 ± 3.2	78	20
Germfree	14	17.2 ± 7.4	9.7 ± 4.1	85	15

[a]Results expressed as mean for initial 22 hr of cannulation ± S.E.
[b]Cytotoxic assay with anti-θ serum in 1:4 dilution.
[c]Based upon autoradiographic examination of number of cells binding radioiodinated immune complexes.

155

IMMUNOLOGICAL
RESPONSIVENESS
AND AGING
PHENOMENA IN
GERMFREE MICE

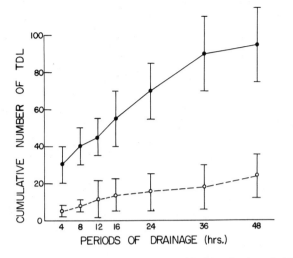

Figure 2. Cumulative total numbers of lymphocytes mobilizable via thoracic duct cannulation in conventional (closed circles) and germfree (open circles) eight- to ten-week-old C3H mice (Anderson, unpublished data).

lymphocyte count in the barrier-maintained group, while the number of lymphocytes found in the peripheral blood of the germfree mice appears to increase with age. Of greater functional importance than these differences among the formed elements of the peripheral blood are the numbers of recirculating small lymphocytes obtainable by thoracic duct cannulation. As shown in Figure 2, there is a marked reduction in the number of thoracic duct lymphocytes (TDL) mobilizable in the germfree group in comparison with their conventional counterparts. Table 3 shows the division of these cells into thymic-derived (T) and bone-marrow-derived (B)

TABLE 4. Mean Serum Proteins as a Function of Age in Germfree and Barrier-Maintained Mice[a]

Experimental group	Determination	\multicolumn{4}{c}{Amounts of protein in mice sacrificed at various ages}
		42 days	202 days	362 days	522 days
Barrier-maintained	Total protein	5.3	5.4	6.1	5.3
	Albumin	2.91	2.94	3.41	3.28
	α_1 globulin	1.20	1.24	1.03	0.91
	α_2 globulin	0.45	0.43	0.49	0.35
	β globulin	0.48	0.63	0.67	0.57
	γ globulin	0.26	0.19	0.52	0.20
Germfree	Total protein	5.3	5.6	4.7	4.9
	Albumin	3.69	3.47	2.28	2.30
	α_1 globulin	0.45	1.28	1.27	1.37
	α_2 globulin	0.40	0.33	0.29	0.55
	β globulin	0.62	0.51	0.69	0.59
	γ globulin	0.16	0.03	0.15	0.09

[a]After Anderson et al., 1972a. Results expressed in grams percent.

ROBERT E.
ANDERSON,
WILLIAM E.
DOUGHTY, AND
GARY M. TROUP

lymphocytes for the initial few hours of cannulation. On the basis of Figure 2 and Table 3, it is clear that the numbers of recirculating T and B cells are reduced by roughly the same proportion in germfree mice in comparison with their conventional counterparts.

Related to the above are the serum protein levels in germfree and conventional mice. Data for individual components are summarized in Table 4. Although the total proteins for the two groups are comparable, most of the globulin fractions are lower in the germfree mice than in the corresponding barrier-maintained groups.

2. Immune Response in Germfree Mice

2.1. General

The preceding discussion has dealt primarily with the morphologic differences between germfree and conventional mice. Now, attention will be focused upon the functional correlates of these differences.

A simplified schematic representation of the events following exposure to a standard antigen, such as sheep erythrocytes, is shown in Figure 3. The subsequent discussion of the immune response in germfree mice will be based upon this schematic representation and therefore will be subdivided, somewhat artificially, into the following components: (a) antigen processing, (b) cell collaboration, (c) antibody formation, (d) delayed-type hypersensitivity responses, and (e) tolerance.

2.2. Antigen Processing

Germfree mice clear carbon particles injected intravenously at approximately the same rate as do conventional animals (Thorbecke and Benacerraf, 1959). Thorbecke and Benacerraf (1959) also investigated the clearance of a nonviable ^{32}P-labeled *Staphylococcus aureus* and *Escherichia coli*. The results are shown in Figure 4. The clearance of *E. coli* by the germfree mice is slower than that found in the conventional group. The clearance of *S. aureus* is much faster than *E. coli* for both groups and there is no significant difference between germfree and conventional mice. Table 5 summarizes the distribution of the cleared organisms among the involved organs; the distribution is approximately the same for the two groups of mice.

Additional important observations that relate to the processing of antigen include the following:

1. Germfree mice appear to demonstrate normal follicular localization of ^{125}I-labeled HGG during the initial ten days after injection (Hanna *et al.*, 1969). In this connection, it is important to note that germfree rats show impaired follicular localization of flagellar antigen (Miller *et al.*, 1968).

2. Germfree mice often show delayed intracellular degradation of antigen (Horowitz *et al.*, 1964; Bauer *et al.*, 1964).

3. Germfree mice, in common with other species, probably exhibit normal, or at most slightly reduced, serum titers of complement and properdin in comparison with their conventional counterparts.

4. The chemotaxis of neutrophils in germfree and conventional mice is comparable (R. E. Anderson, unpublished observations).

5. Opsonins are presumed to be reduced in germfree mice.

157

IMMUNOLOGICAL
RESPONSIVENESS
AND AGING
PHENOMENA IN
GERMFREE MICE

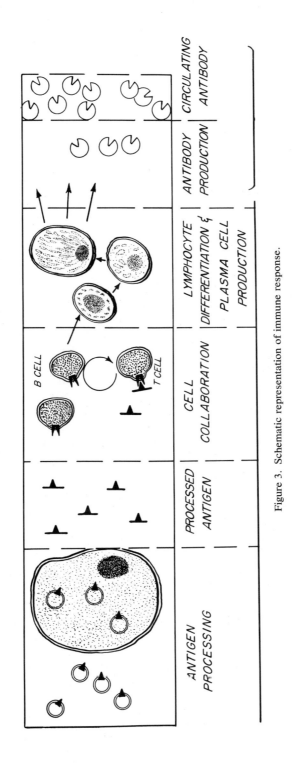

Figure 3. Schematic representation of immune response.

ROBERT E.
ANDERSON,
WILLIAM E.
DOUGHTY, AND
GARY M. TROUP

TABLE 5. Distribution of Radioactivity among Various Organs and Blood after Clearance of ^{32}P-labeled *E. coli* and *S. aureus*[a]

Organ	E. coli		S. aureus	
	Germfree	Conventional	Germfree	Conventional
Liver	21.4	25.0	63.5	74.0
Spleen	14.8	15.4	7.5	5.5
Lungs	7.0	4.9	4.5	1.0
Kidneys	2.5	1.6	0.7	0.3
Blood	30.2	23.8	6.2	4.5
Total recovered	75.9	70.7	82.4	85.3

[a]After Thorbecke and Benacerraf, 1959. Results expressed as percent of total radioactivity injected as found in indicated organs.

2.3. Cell Collaboration

1. *T–B cell collaboration*—The immunologic response to most antigens requires the cooperation of T and B cells. The response of germfree mice to such antigens appears to depend upon the test antigen and the experimental approach. Utilizing intact animals, several investigators have shown that germfree mice are able to mount an equal but delayed antibody response to most antigens thus far evaluated (Bauer *et al.*, 1966). However, the imaginative studies of Bosma *et al.* (1967) suggest that the sluggish character of this response is related to clearance and/or macrophage processing of antigen rather than impaired T–B cell cooperation. These authors were able to negate the former influences by transferring equal numbers of dispersed spleen cells from conventional and germfree mice together with an optimal amount of antigen into lethally irradiated (and therefore immunologically unresponsive) recipients which were subsequently assayed for their antibody response to the test antigen (sheep erythrocytes). The results show that germfree and conventional mice are immunologically comparable in terms of: (a) the number of immunologically competent progenitor cells in the spleens of 3- and 13-week old mice; (b) the kinetics of the hemolysin and hemagglutinin response by dispersed spleen cells from 3-, 9-, and 13-week-old mice; (c) the rate and magnitude of the postnatal maturation of immune competence.

2. *Other forms of cell collaboration*—Recently, considerable attention has been devoted to subpopulations of T and B cells and their role in the modulation of

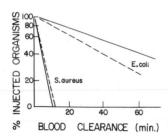

Figure 4. Clearance from the blood of heat-killed ^{32}P-labeled *E. coli* and *S. aureus* for germfree (solid lines) and conventional (dotted lines) Swiss Webster mice (after Thorbecke and Benacerraf, 1959).

159

IMMUNOLOGICAL
RESPONSIVENESS
AND AGING
PHENOMENA IN
GERMFREE MICE

the immune response. Particular attention has been paid to suppressor T cells. At the present time, an attempt to evaluate the ontogeny of suppressor T cells in germfree and conventional mice utilizing a congenic cell transfer system (Warner and Anderson, 1975) is in progress in our laboratories. By inference, we suspect that germfree mice may lose their suppressor population at a faster rate than their conventional counterparts (see below).

2.4. Antibody Formation

As noted above, germfree mice exhibit a slightly delayed primary response to most antigens thus far tested. There is reason to suspect that this delay is related to sluggish processing of antigen by macrophages. In this regard, it is interesting to note that the antibody response is often greater in magnitude and sustained for a longer period of time in germfree, as opposed to conventional, mice. This observation has been attributed to the relatively prolonged period required for antigen processing in germfree mice, associated with a presumably slower release of processed antigen (Bauer et al., 1966).

2.5. Bone-Marrow-Dependent Immune Responses

A few antigens are able to elicit an immune response in the absence of T cells. In fact, the presence of T cells often inhibits the response to these B cell antigens. Insofar as is known, experiments have not as yet been reported that evaluate the response of germfree mice to B cell specific antigens. On the basis of the available information, summarized previously (see T–B cell cooperation), it would be expected that exposure to such antigens would result in a slightly delayed response in the intact germfree mouse but that with a cell transfer system, no difference would be apparent between germfree and conventional animals.

2.6. Thymus-Dependent Immune Responses

1. *Transplantation*—Several early investigators reported delayed rejection of organ and tumor grafts in germfree recipients. Most of these studies were performed in guinea pigs. A more recent study (Miller et al., 1967) with C3H/Gif recipients grafted with CBA skin is shown in Table 6. There is no significant difference between the two groups with respect to either the duration of the survival of the

TABLE 6. Rejection of CBA Skin Grafts by Germfree and Conventional C3H/Gif Mice[a]

Group	Number of mice	Average graft survival[b]	Average time required for rejection[b]
Germfree	12	14	2
Conventional	9	12	2

[a] After Miller et al., 1967.
[b] Results expressed in days.

ROBERT E.
ANDERSON,
WILLIAM E.
DOUGHTY, AND
GARY M. TROUP

homograft or the time required for rejection (i.e., the period between the first sign of rejection and the appearance of a scar).

2. *Neonatal thymectomy*—In many strains of mice, neonatal thymectomy is associated with a wasting disease (Parrott, 1962; Miller, 1962). Even prior to the clinical onset of the wasting phenomenon, however, such mice demonstrate an impairment in the capacity to react to many antigens and to reject skin homografts (Miller, 1962; Parrott, 1962; Miller, 1963; Humphrey *et al.*, 1964; Miller *et al.*, 1965; Sinclair, 1967). On the other hand, germfree mice thymectomized at birth do not develop signs of wasting disease (McIntire *et al.*, 1964; Wilson *et al.*, 1964). These mice exhibit a depressed response to sheep erythrocytes comparable to that noted in conventional mice thymectomized neonatally and an impaired ability to reject skin grafts, although the magnitude of the impairment of graft rejection is generally not as extreme as that noted in thymectomized conventional mice.

As noted above, the number of TDL in germfree mice is much reduced in comparison with their conventional counterparts. As shown in Figure 5, the number of recirculating lymphocytes mobilizable via thoracic duct cannulation is further reduced in germfree mice by neonatal thymectomy. However, the latter effect is much less pronounced than that associated with neonatal thymectomy in conventional mice.

3. *Adult thymectomy*—Conventional mice thymectomized as adults also exhibit an impaired immune response, although expression of this deficit is postponed until several months after surgery. This interval can be shortened by irradiation. Mice operated upon in similar fashion but lethally irradiated and restored with syngeneic bone marrow also demonstrate an impaired responsiveness to homo-

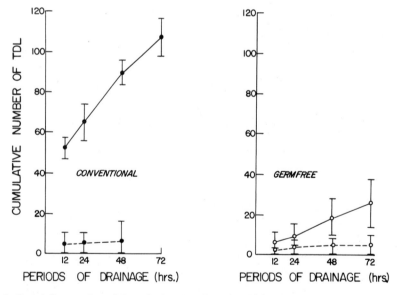

Figure 5. Cumulative number of thoracic duct lymphocytes (TDL) as a function of time in neonatally thymectomized (dotted lines) and sham thymectomized (solid lines) germfree and conventional C3H female mice (Anderson, unpublished data). Note all conventional neonatally thymectomized mice dead at 72 hr.

161

IMMUNOLOGICAL
RESPONSIVENESS
AND AGING
PHENOMENA IN
GERMFREE MICE

grafts and complete loss of the plaque-forming response to sheep erythrocytes (Miller *et al.*, 1963). In this manner, the immune responsiveness of the adult thymec-tomized–irradiated mice closely mimic that associated with neonatal thymectomy.

Adult thymectomy in germfree mice, with or without subsequent irradiation, has seldom been employed experimentally. As a tool to investigate the role of the immune response in aging, such an approach has obvious promise as will be discussed subsequently in more detail.

On the basis of the above experiments, it is assumed that the primary conse-quence of neonatal or adult thymectomy is some degree of immunologic impair-ment. The latter is demonstrable in both germfree and conventional mice. However, in the conventional state, other environmental factors, such as bacterial contamina-tion, endotoxins, cross-reacting antigens, etc., act to commit, and thereby reduce even further, the already compromised numbers of uncommitted thymic-dependent cells available to response to various immunologic insults.

2.7. Tolerance

Very few experiments have been reported that attempt to address experimen-tally the induction of tolerance in germfree animals. There is reason to suspect that such animals may be more susceptible to spontaneous tolerance via cross-reacting antigens (Nossal and Ada, 1971). In this context it is important to note that cross-reactions among antigens are common. A reasonable argument can be advanced that many allegedly primary immune responses involve cells that are, in fact, memory cells. In their cloistered environment, germfree mice would be expected to have a more limited complement of memory cells than their conventional counterparts.

3. Aging in Germfree Mice

An extension of the once popular "toxic" theory of aging suggests that the life span of mammals should be extended by the absence of microorganisms (Koren-chevsky, 1961), especially those microorganisms associated with disease. In this connection, Comfort (1964) has compared the survival curves from several human populations with widely divergent standards of medical care and has concluded that the elimination of infectious disease would be expected to favorably influence mean survival but not appreciably alter the maximum longevity.

To date, at least three studies have been addressed to a definition of the relationship between life span and the microbial status of the host (Gordon *et al.*, 1966; Walburg and Cosgrove, 1967; Anderson *et al.*, 1972a). Some of the data from these experiments are summarized in Table 7. As shown in this table, two of the studies demonstrate that in the mouse absence of the conventional microbial flora is associated with an extension of the mean life span, while the third study documents a reduced longevity in the germfree group in comparison with barrier-maintained mice. Because of these unexpected discrepancies, it may be of value to examine each of the studies in more detail.

ROBERT E.
ANDERSON,
WILLIAM E.
DOUGHTY, AND
GARY M. TROUP

TABLE 7. Influence of Microbial Environment on Mean Age at Death in Three Experiments

Experiment	Number of mice	Sex	Mean age at death (days)			Reference
			Germfree	Barrier-maintained	Conventional	
I	269	Male	708	—	491	Gordon *et al.*,
	355	Female	631	—	526	1966
II	76	Male	535	520	547	Walburg and
	68	Female	556	476	536	Cosgrove, 1967
III	172	Female	564	692	—	Anderson *et al.*, 1972a

1. The earliest experiment was that of Gordon *et al.*, (1966). Animals were added to the experimental groups over a period of five years. Mice which received two different diets are combined in the data of Table 7 even though there were slight differences in longevity between the two groups. In addition, and in contradistinction to the other two studies, the experiment was initiated with 12-month-old mice. This was done to eliminate the effects of early losses and because of the limited availability of germfree animals in the early stages of the study. Also, the "control" animals were kept under open laboratory conditions and were presumably vulnerable to subclinical infections. With these points in mind, reference to Table 7 shows that the mean life-span for both male and female germfree mice is longer than that noted with respect to their conventional counterparts.

2. The experiments of Walburg and Cosgrove (1967) utilized noninbred ICR mice. As shown in Table 8, these authors observed no significant difference in the mortality of conventional, barrier-maintained, and germfree mice. Individual mortality curves for males and females are shown in Figures 6 and 7. From these data, it

TABLE 8. Influence of Microbial Environment upon Mean Age at Death in ICR Mice[a]

Sex	Omitted	Mean age at death (days)		
		Germfree	Barrier-maintained	Conventional
Female	—	535 ± 46(19)	520 ± 38(29)	547 ± 45(20)
Male	—	556 ± 43(22)	476 ± 37(30)	536 ± 41(24)
Female and male (pooled)	—	546 ± 32(41)	498 ± 27(59)	541 ± 31(44)
Female and male (pooled)	Cecal volvulus	586 ± 34(31)	497 ± 25(58)	541 ± 31(44)
Male	Lymphatic leukemia, cecal volvulus, no diagnosis	724 ± 28(11)	—	657 ± 53(16)

[a]After Walburg and Cosgrove, 1967. Results expressed in days ± S.E.; number of mice in parenthesis.

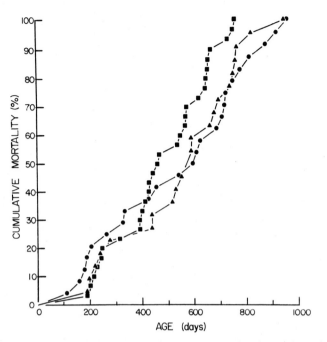

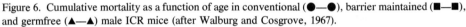

Figure 6. Cumulative mortality as a function of age in conventional (●—●), barrier maintained (■—■), and germfree (▲—▲) male ICR mice (after Walburg and Cosgrove, 1967).

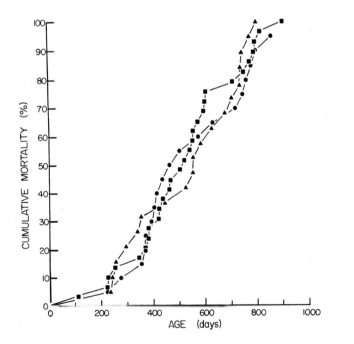

Figure 7. Cumulative mortality as a function of age in conventional (●—●), barrier maintained (■—■), and germfree (▲—▲) female ICR mice (after Walburg and Cosgrove, 1967).

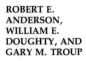

ROBERT E.
ANDERSON,
WILLIAM E.
DOUGHTY, AND
GARY M. TROUP

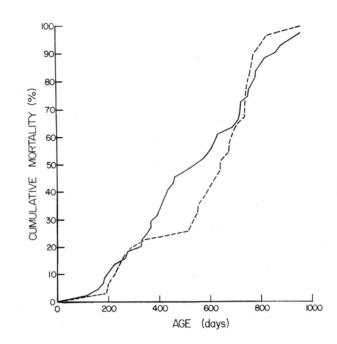

Figure 8. Cumulative mortality as a function of age in conventional (solid line) and germfree (dotted line) ICR mice (after Walburg and Cosgrove, 1967). Combined data for male and female mice; animals with cecal volvulus omitted.

is evident that males reared under barrier conditions showed a slightly accelerated mortality between 400 and 600 days of life. In Figure 8, mice which died with cecal volvulus are omitted and the resultant differences in the character of the mortality curves are apparent. These differences in the shape of the curves are not reflected in significant differences in mean survival, however.

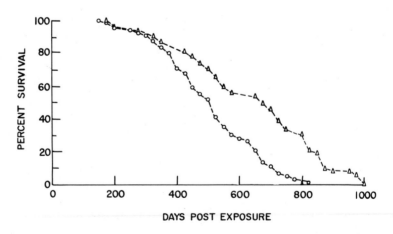

Figure 9. Age-specific cumulative mortality for germfree (open circles) and barrier-maintained (open triangles) female CD-1 mice (after Anderson *et al.*, 1972a).

165

IMMUNOLOGICAL
RESPONSIVENESS
AND AGING
PHENOMENA IN
GERMFREE MICE

3. The experiments of Anderson *et al.* (1972a) utilized noninbred virgin female mice of the Charles Rivers CD-l line. The age-specific cumulative mortality of these animals is shown in Figure 9. Of particular interest is the observation that the barrier-maintained mice have a significantly longer life span than their germfree contemporaries. This discrepancy in death rate appears to influence all age groups in comparable fashion, since the shapes of the mortality curves are almost identical. As will be discussed in more detail subsequently, the germfree mice also developed fewer benign and malignant tumors than their barrier-maintained counterparts, but a similar comparison with respect to the age-specific mortality of animals with neoplasms suggests an accelerated appearance in the germfree group. This observation would be expected to influence the mortality curves of Figure 9. Therefore the cumulative mortality was recalculated with deaths due to neoplasia and cecal volvulus excluded; the latter entity is only encountered in germfree mice. The recalculated mortality data are shown in Figure 10. Again, significant differences between the two experimental groups are apparent.

With a few notable exceptions, the prevalence of benign and malignant tumors increases as a function of age among a variety of mammals. For this reason, the prevalence and age-specific death rate of animals with tumors is of interest in aging studies. Such information for germfree and barrier-maintained mice is shown in Table 9 and Figure 11. Although the barrier mice develop more tumors than their germfree contemporaries, susceptible members of the latter groups are prone to an earlier expression of these entities. This acceleration cannot be attributed to any single neoplasm (Anderson *et al.*, 1972b).

Spontaneous amyloidosis also appears to be age-related and may relate to immune dysfunction. Table 10 shows the incidence of amyloid in germfree and barrier-maintained mice. The former demonstrates a much higher rate of occurrence than the latter. This difference becomes even greater when germfree mice, which succumbed from torsion of the characteristically dilated cecum, often at a young age, are excluded from the calculations. The prevalence of amyloidosis in both groups is age-related (Anderson, 1971).

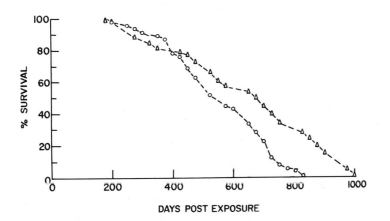

Figure 10. Age specific cumulative mortality for germfree (open circles) and barrier maintained (open triangles) female CD-1 mice, excluding animals with benign and malignant neoplasms and cecal volvulus (after Anderson *et al.*, 1972a).

166

ROBERT E.
ANDERSON,
WILLIAM E.
DOUGHTY, AND
GARY M. TROUP

TABLE 9. Prevalence of Benign and Malignant Tumors as a Function of an Experimental Group[a]

Tumor	Experimental group	
	Barrier-maintained	Germfree
Malignant		
Thymic lymphoma	5.6(4)	8.3(6)
Nonthymic lymphoma	12.8(9)	4.1(3)
Leukemia	4.2(3)	6.9(5)
Hemangioendothelioma (spleen, liver)	4.2(3)	4.1(3)
Adenocarcinoma of breast	2.8(2)	
Alveolar adenocarcinoma of lung	10.0(7)	2.5(2)
Tumors of soft tissue origin (fibrosarcoma, leiomyosarcoma, osteogenic sarcoma)	7.1(5)	
Other	2.8(2)	2.5(2)
Benign		
Granulosa cell tumor of ovary	1.4(1)	
Tubular adenoma of ovary		
Cavernous hemangioma of liver		
Other		1.3(1)
Total	51.4(36)	31.4(22)

[a]After Anderson et al., 1972b. Results expressed as percent of mice in group with indicated tumor; actual number of tumors are in parentheses. Animals with multiple tumors are included more than once. Two animals in the barrier-maintained group each had two primary tumors.

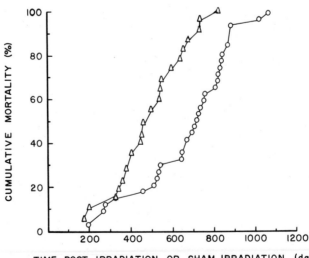

Figure 11. Age-specific cumulative mortality of germfree (open triangles) and barrier-maintained (open circles) female CD-1 mice with benign and malignant neoplasms (after Anderson et al., 1972b).

167

IMMUNOLOGICAL
RESPONSIVENESS
AND AGING
PHENOMENA IN
GERMFREE MICE

TABLE 10. Prevalence of Amyloid in Germfree and
Barrier-Maintained Female CD-1 Mice[a]

Microbial status	Number of mice at risk	Significant amyloid
Germfree	86	55.5
Barrier-maintained	88	8.6

[a]After Anderson, 1971. Results expressed as percent of mice in group with more than trace or equivocal amount of amyloid.

4. Aging in Immune Deficient Germfree Mice

4.1. Effects of Irradiation

Whole-body exposure to significant amounts of ionizing radiation results in a reduced life span. The mechanism(s) involved in this "accelerated" aging is not known but, in general, the irradiated animals die from the same diseases that afflict their nonirradiated counterparts. Irradiation is also known to result in permanent impairment of the immune response and especially the numbers of recirculating T and B cells. The putative relationship of these two radiation-induced abnormalities (shortened life span, decreased numbers of recirculating lymphocytes) is not known. It has been shown, however, that:

1. Whole-body exposure of CD-l female mice at 6 weeks of age significantly shortens life span in both germfree and barrier-maintained mice (Anderson *et al.,* 1972a);
2. This life-shortening effect is slightly more pronounced in the barrier-maintained group, apparently due to infections occasioned by endogenous organisms (Anderson *et al.,* 1972a);
3. Despite the above, the mean life span of irradiated barrier-maintained mice is longer than that of irradiated germfree mice (442 vs. 399 days);
4. In the consideration of the latter observation, it is important to note that the acute (30 day) response after a whole-body irradiation is greatly modified in the germfree state with different survival rates, favoring germfree over barrier-maintained and conventional mice (Anderson *et al.,* 1968). In the longevity experiment referred to above, 18% of the irradiated barrier-maintained group died within 30 days post-exposure as compared with nil percent of the irradiated germfree group. Therefore members of the latter group that would have died in a conventional environment were carried forward and might be presumed to be unusually susceptible to the late effects of such exposure.

4.2. Effects of Thymectomy

One of the first individuals to relate aging to immune dysfunction was Burnet (1959). As an extension of his clonal selection theory, Burnet suggested that aging may relate to a breakdown in immunologic homeostasis. The latter could be due to

ROBERT E.
ANDERSON,
WILLIAM E.
DOUGHTY, AND
GARY M. TROUP

selective loss of tolerance that allows an aberrant clone of immunologically competent lymphoid cells to react against host antigens, which is a pathologic situation that would represent a modified graft-vs.-host response. An accumulation of such autoimmune reactions would be expected to be detrimental to the host and to reduce life span (Walford, 1962). More recently, Burnet has implicated thymic involution as a possible mechanism that could trigger this set of events (Burnet, 1965).

Neonatal thymectomy of conventional mice results in a reduced life span even among those strains that are not susceptible to the runting phenomenon. Adult thymectomy of conventional mice also significantly decreases life span (Jeejeebhoy, 1971). However, the interpretation of these observations is complicated by the known susceptibility of thymectomized mice to overt and occult infection. As observed by Burnet, a large-scale evaluation of the relationship among neonatal thymectomy, life span, and the prevalence of specific diseases, and especially those of an autoimmune or neoplastic character, utilizing germfree mice would have far reaching implications with respect to the role of thymic-dependent immune phenomena in aging. Such a study has yet to be reported.

Neonatal thymectomy appears to increase the prevalence and accelerate the appearance of a variety of viral and chemically induced tumors (Miller, 1969) among those strains of mice that are not susceptible to the runting syndrome. On the basis of a small pilot study, it also appears that the incidence of some spontaneous tumors is increased in neonatally thymectomized germfree mice (Anderson and Doughty, unpublished results). The latter observation raises the possibility of aborting this increment by periodic transfusions of T cells. In this connection, it is important to attempt to achieve an optimal balance between suppressor and enhancer T cells among the infused lymphocytes. Such experiments are currently in progress in our laboratories.

5. Summary and Conclusions

Germfree mice provide a unique resource in the dissection of the role of immune phenomena in aging. Particularly with respect to the thymic-dependent component of the immune response, it is possible to perform experiments on immunologically incompetent mice in the absence of the complicating factors which confuse the interpretation of similar experiments utilizing conventional animals. In addition, the observation that at least one colony of germfree mice, with a marked reduction in the numbers of recirculating lymphocytes, exhibits a shorter life span than their barrier-maintained counterparts may provide an important key to future investigative efforts in this regard. As noted by Burnet (1970), "No life tables have, however, been published comparing the life spans of germ-free, sham operated and thymectomized mice. This is an experiment whose results could be most illuminating."

Burnet then proceeds to ask the following questions:

(1) "What is the longevity and the causes of natural death in neonatally thymectomized mice maintained germ-free? (2) "If such thymectomized mice have a shortened survival time and/or increased tumour incidence, can this be reversed by syngeneic young thymus graft at 12 or 18 months of age?"

Finally, Burnet states,

169

IMMUNOLOGICAL
RESPONSIVENESS
AND AGING
PHENOMENA IN
GERMFREE MICE

"These answers may make it possible to see whether the thymus has a demonstrable influence on ageing and the spontaneous development of malignancy in mice. Until such information is available the approach will have to be almost wholly indirect and will have to analyse carefully the various ways by which immunological processes, notably autoimmune disease and immunological surveillance, *could* influence ageing processes and to what extent the thymus would be involved." In conclusion, he notes the considerable expense of such a project (circa 400,000 Australian dollars of 1970 vintage or approximately 600,000 1975 United States dollars) but concludes "It is a question which in 1969 falls within the art of the soluble."

ACKNOWLEDGMENTS

This investigation was supported by Research Grant Number CA14270 awarded by the National Cancer Institute, DHEW, and the John and Mary R. Markle Foundation.

References

Anderson, R. E., 1971, Disseminated amyloidosis in germ-free mice, *Amer. J. Path.* **65**:43–49.

Anderson, R. E., Howarth, J. L., and Stone, R. S., 1968, Acute response of germfree and conventional mice to ionizing radiation, *Arch. Path* **122**:676–680.

Anderson, R. E., Scaletti, J. V., and Howarth, J. L., 1972a, Radiation-induced life shortening in germfree mice, *Exp. Geront.* **7**:289–301.

Anderson, R. E., Doughty, W. E., Stone, R. S., and Howarth, J. L., 1972b, Spontaneous and radiation-related neoplasms in germfree mice, *Arch. Path.* **94**:250–254.

Bauer, H., Horowitz, R. E., Watkins, K. C., and Popper, H., 1964, Immunologic competence and phagocytosis in germ-free animals with and without stress, *J.A.M.A.* **187**:715–718.

Bauer, H., Paronetto, F., Burns, W. A., and Einheber, A., 1966, The enhancing effect of the microbial flora on macrophage functions and the immune response. A study in germ-free mice, *J. Exp. Med.* **123**:1013–1024.

Bealmer, M., and Wilson, R., 1966, Histological comparison of the thymus of germ-free (axenic) and conventional CFW mice, *Anat. Rec.* **154**:261–273.

Bosma, M. J., Makinodan, T., and Walburg, H. E., Jr., 1967, Development of immunologic competence in germ-free and conventional mice, *J. Immunol.* **99**:420–430.

Burnet, M., 1959, *The Clonal Selection Theory of Acquired Immunity,* Cambridge University Press, London.

Burnet, M., 1965, Somatic mutation and chronic disease, *Brit. J. Med.* **5431**:338–342.

Burnet, M., 1970, *Immunological Surveillance,* p. 217, Pergamon Press, New York.

Burns, W., Bauer, H., and Einheber, A., 1964, Quantitative morphology in the thymus in normal and irradiated germ-free mice, *Fed. Proc., Fed. Amer. Soc. Exp. Biol.* **23**:547.

Comfort, A., 1964, *Aging: The Biology of Senescence,* p. 31, Holt-Rinehart and Winston, New York.

Dukor, P., Miller, J. F. A. P., and Sacquet, E., 1968, The immunological responsiveness of germ-free mice thymectomized at birth. II. Lymphoid tissue and histopathology, *Clin. Exp. Immunol.* **3**:191–212.

Gordon, H. A., 1959, Morphological and physiological characterization of germ-free life, *Ann. N. Y. Acad. Sci.* **78**:208–220.

Gordon, H. A., Bruckner-Kardoss, E., and Wostmann, B. S., 1966, Aging in germ-free mice: Life tables and lesions observed at natural death, *J. Gerontol.* **21**:380–387.

Hanna, M. G., Jr., Nettesheim, P., and Walburg, H. F., Jr., 1969, Advances in experimental medicine and biology, in: *Germfree Biology,* Vol. 3 (E. A. Mirand and N. Black, eds.), Plenum Press, New York.

Henderson, J. D., Jr., and Titus, J. L., 1968, Growth rates and morphology of germfree and conventional mice, *Mayo Clin. Proc.* **43**:517–529.

ROBERT E.
ANDERSON,
WILLIAM E.
DOUGHTY, AND
GARY M. TROUP

Horowitz, R. E., Bauer, H., Paronetto, F., Abrams, G. D., Watkins, K. C., and Popper, H., 1964, The response of the lymphatic tissue to bacterial antigen. Studies in germ-free mice, *Amer. J. Path.* **44**:747–761.

Humphrey, J. M., Parrott, D. M. V., and East, J., 1964, Studies on globulin and antibody production in mice thymectomized at birth, *Immunology* **7**:419–439.

Jeejeebhoy, H. F., 1971, Decreased longevity of mice following thymectomy in adult life, *Transplantation* **12**:525–526.

Korenchevsky, V., 1961, *Physiological and Pathological Aging,* pp. 5–6, Karger, Basel.

Luckey, T. D., 1963, *Germfree Life and Gnotobiology,* pp. 362–366, Academic Press, New York.

McIntire, K. R., Sell, S., and Miller, J. F. A. P., 1964, Pathogenesis of the post-neonatal thymectomy wasting syndrome, *Nature* **204**:151–155.

Miller, J. F. A. P., 1962, Effect of neonatal thymectomy on the immunological responsiveness of the mouse, *Proc. Roy. Soc. (London)* **156**:415–428.

Miller, J. F. A. P., 1963, Tolerance in the thymectomized animal, *Tolérance Acquisé et Tolérance Naturelle á l'égard de Substances Antigéniques Définines,* p. 47, Centre National de la Recherche Scientifique, Paris.

Miller, J. F. A. P., 1969, Thymus and immunocompetence, *Aust. J. Sci.* **32**:87–94.

Miller, J. F. A. P., Doak, S. M. A., and Cross, A. M., 1963, Role of the thymus in recovery of the immune mechanism in the irradiated adult mouse, *Proc. Soc. Exp. Biol. Med.* **112**:785–792.

Miller, J. F. A. P., de Burgh, P. M., and Grant, G. A., 1965, Thymus and the production of antibody-plaque-forming cells, *Nature* **208**:1332–1334.

Miller, J. F. A. P., Dukor, P., Grant, G., Sinclair, N. R. St. C., and Sacquet, E., 1967, The immunological responsiveness of germ-free mice thymectomized at birth. I. Antibody production and skin homograft rejection, *Clin. Exp. Immunol.* **2**:531–542.

Miller, J. J., III, Johnson, D. O., and Ada, G. L., 1968, Differences in localization of Salmonella Flagella in lymph node follicles of germ-free and conventional rats, *Nature* **217**:1059–1061.

Nossal, G. J. V., and Ada, G. L., 1971, *Antigens, Lymphoid Cells and the Immune Response,* p. 257, Academic Press, New York.

Olson, G. B., and Wostmann, B. S., 1966, Lymphocytopoiesis, plasmacytopoiesis and cellular proliferation in non-antigenically stimulated germfree mice, *J. Immunol.* **97**:267–274.

Parrott, D. M. V., 1962, Strain variation in mortality and runt-disease in mice thymectomized at birth, *Transplant. Bull.* **29**:102–104.

Sinclair, N. R. St. C., 1967, Effects of neonatal thymectomy on the haemolysin response to sheep erythrocytes in Swiss albino mice. A time-course study of total 19S and 7S antibody, *Immunology* **12**:549–557.

Thorbecke, G. J., and Benacerraf, B., 1959, Some histological and functional aspects of lymphoid tissue in germ-free animals. II. Studies on phagocytosis *in vivo, Ann. N. Y. Acad. Sci.* **78**:247–253.

Walburg, H. E., Jr., and Cosgrove, G. E., 1967, Aging in irradiated and unirradiated germ-free ICR mice, *Exp. Geront.* **2**:143–158.

Walford, R. L., 1962, Auto-immunity and aging, *J. Gerontol.* **17**:281–285.

Warner, N. L., and Anderson, R. E., 1975, Helper effect of normal and irradiated thymus cells on transferred immunoglobulin production, *Nature* **254**:604–606.

Wilson, R., Sjodin, K., and Bealmear, M., 1964, The absence of wasting in thymectomized germ-free (axenic) mice, *Proc. Soc. Exp. Biol. Med.* **117**:237–239.

Wilson, R., Bealmear, M., and Sobonya, R., 1965, Growth and regression of the germfree (axenic) thymus, *Proc. Soc. Exp. Biol. Med.* **118**:97–99.

12

Congenitally Athymic (Nude) Mice and Their Application to the Study of Immunity and Aging

JOHN W. JUTILA

1. Introduction

Numerous studies in several mammalian species, including man, mice, rats, and hamsters have established a strong relationship between the aging process and a decline in the functional capacity of the immune system (Walford, 1969). The so-called immunologic theory of aging predicts that genetic and induced defects in the immune apparatus may seriously compromise the general health of man or animals by failing to thwart infections and neoplasia on the one hand, and, on the other, by responding to self-antigens to produce destructive autoimmune disorders.

There is compelling evidence to support the concept that a major factor contributing to an age-related decline in immune function involves the thymus, whose functional decline corresponds with the onset of many signs and diseases of aging (Walford, 1974; Yunis *et al.*, 1975). In all mammalian species, the thymus undergoes a progressive decrease in size and function with age, posing the possibility that programmed events paced by the "thymic clock" (Burnet, 1970) are set into motion early in life and diminish with time. Experimental evidence in support of this concept is provided by the observation that neonatal thymectomy contributes to a severe impairment of the development of the immune response (Miller, 1961), while adult thymectomy is considerably less effective in this regard. As a consequence of neonatal thymectomy, a wasting syndrome develops and mimics, in appearance and pathology, the aging process (Parrott, 1962). The loss or absence of thymus-dependent immunity and immunoregulation appears to be associated with an

JOHN W. JUTILA • Department of Microbiology, Montana State University, Bozeman, Montana.

increased incidence of autoimmune disorders, infections, and malignancies (Yunis *et al.,* 1971).

Further opportunities to critically examine the role of thymus (T) cell-mediated immunity in the aging process have been offered by the discovery of the congenitally athymic (nude) mouse (Flanagan, 1966). Several excellent reviews describing the biology of the nude mouse have recently been published (Rygaard, 1973; Wortis, 1974) and serve to illustrate the remarkable versatility of this animal in studies of diverse biological phenomena. Because of its genetic constitution, profound immunoincompetent state, and rapid onset of signs of accelerated aging, this unique "experiment of nature" presents the investigator with an opportunity to examine the nature of primary and secondary events contributing to aging as implied in the immunologic theory.

2. Nature of the Primary Defect

Nude is a mutant allele of the *nu* locus of the VII linkage group. The original mutation was detected in noninbred stock and, in the intervening years since its discovery, a recessive gene transfer scheme (Rygaard, 1973) has been employed to produce congenic lines of C3H, Balb/c, C57B1/6, and AKR mice.

The athymic condition of the nude mouse was first reported by Pantelouris (1968), who later (Pantelouris and Hair, 1970) described two primitive structures in the thymic region, totally devoid of lymphoid tissue. Colonization of these primitive structures fails to occur when normal bone marrow cells are injected into nude mice (Wortis, 1971). Wortis (1971) also demonstrated that nudes possess functional stem cells capable of differentiating into T cells, which further suggests that a defect associated with the development of the thymic epithelium (Cordier and Heremans, 1975) contributes to the athymic condition. Nudes appear to lack a thymic hormone (Bach *et al.,* 1973), are markedly deficient in cells sensitive to cytotoxic anti-θ serum (Raff and Wortis, 1970), and possess large numbers of B (bone-marrow-derived) cells (Bankhurst and Warner, 1972).

3. Natural History of the Nude Mouse

Nude mice are readily identified at birth by the absence of, or poorly developed, vibrissae. Some animals display a sparse hair growth while an infrequent few show abundant hair growth about the eyes and along the spine. The body weight of nudes and normal-appearing littermates is similar at birth but within 10 days a disparity in weight gain becomes apparent. By 60 days of age, nudes usually have body weights about 60 to 70% of those of normal-appearing littermates.

Nude females rarely produce offspring and, if matings are successful, the females generally fail to suckle their young for more than 3 or 4 days. In our laboratory, only one litter has been successfully reared to weaning age by a nude female maintained under specific pathogen-free (SPF) conditions. On the other hand, at least 25% of the nude males are fertile. The fertility of nude males and females dramatically improves when they are grafted with thymic tissue (Wortis, 1974).

Nude mice have a life span of 2 to 4 months when reared under conventional animal-room conditions and most are dead within 25 weeks. Nudes reared under

SPF conditions survive for up to 6 to 10 months (Rygaard, 1973) while those reared as germfree animals live for 20 months or more (Outzen, 1975). Antibiotic treatment also serves to maintain nudes in good health for periods up to nine months.

All nudes reared under conventional or SPF conditions eventually suffer and die from a wasting syndrome similar to that described in neonatally thymectomized mice. Nudes show a rapid loss of body weight, thinning of skin, loss of subcutaneous fat, rapid dehydration with hypothermy and hypotony, diarrhea and cachexia. Although bacteria have been isolated from organs of older nudes (unpublished observations), there are no specific organ changes associated with infections. Animal parasite infections, involving chiefly pinworm and intestinal flagellates, are commonly encountered and may contribute to early death of nudes. Death from spontaneous malignant disease has been rarely observed in nude mice (Rygaard, 1973; Wortis, 1974).

173

CONGENITALLY
ATHYMIC (NUDE)
MICE AND THEIR
APPLICATION TO THE
STUDY OF IMMUNITY
AND AGING

4. Immunology of the Nude Mouse

4.1. Phagocytosis

The phagocytic mechanism of the nude mouse has not been extensively studied, but preliminary studies in our laboratory have revealed that nudes appear to phagocytize sheep erythrocytes (SRMC), *Candida albicans,* and pneumococci in a normal fashion. Experimentally induced inflammatory reactions, whether produced subcutaneously or in the peritoneal cavity, are characterized by normal cellular infiltrates and production of and reaction to chemotactic factors (J. Cutler, Montana State University, unpublished observations). That the phagocytic mechanism is important for the survival of the nude is suggested by the observation that nude mice whose B cell population and immunoglobulin levels have been profoundly depleted by treatment with antiheavy chain serum (Manning and Jutila, 1974) experience no increased mortality when compared to nudes treated with normal serum.

4.2. The Humoral Response

The serum levels of immunoglobulins (Ig) in nude mice have been extensively studied by numerous investigators (Crewther and Warner, 1972; Manning and Jutila, 1972; Bloemmen and Eyssen, 1973; Pritchard *et al.,* 1973). The facts derived from these studies can be summarized briefly. IgM levels of nudes are comparable to those of littermates, whereas IgA and IgG_1 levels are markedly decreased to values varying from 5 to 65% of normal. IgG_{2a} and IgG_{2b} are only slightly depressed. These results essentially support the conclusion that IgM synthesis and secretion is thymus-independent, whereas IgG_1 and IgA are both highly thymus-dependent.

A large number of antigens from the so-called thymus-dependent and independent class have been carefully studied in nudes and cell-culture systems containing nude lymphoid cells. Following immunization with SRBCs, the spleens of nude mice produce many fewer direct plaque-forming cells (PFC) than do normal littermates (Wortis, 1971; Pantelouris, 1971; Reed and Jutila, 1972). Nudes do not produce a secondary response to SRBC; instead they produce a meager second primary (Kindred, 1971a). Additional evidence generated from *in vitro* studies confirm the findings in intact animals; i.e., nude spleen cells produce a weak direct PFC response to SRBC (Aden and Reed, 1972). As measured by indirect plaque-forming cell assays, there is a marked depression of IgG antibody produced in response to SRBC (Kindred, 1971a; Reed and Jutila, 1972). Reed and Jutila (1972) have also reported that rosette-forming cells (RFC) in nude mice fail to increase following immunization.

The results of studies in nudes with other thymus-dependent antigens, including rat and cat erythrocytes, chicken gamma-globulin (Jutila *et al.*, 1975), bacteriophage T4 (Kindred, 1971a), and *Brucella abortus* (Crewther and Warner, 1972) have confirmed the thymus-dependent status of these antigens.

Studies employing thymus-independent antigens have shown that nude mice produce a normal, predominantly IgM response to these antigens. Thus Manning *et al.* (1972) have shown that nudes respond to *Escherichia coli* lipopolysaccharide (LPS) as effectively as do normal littermates. Similar results have been obtained with polyvinylpyrrolidone (Lake and Reed, 1975) and Vi antigen (Reed *et al.*, 1974). In general, the results of *in vivo* work have been confirmed in tissue culture systems but, in the case of *in vitro* responsiveness to LPS, a cellular LPS was found to be necessary to provoke a response in nude spleen cultures; i.e., there was no response to soluble, phenol-water extracted LPS (Aden and Reed, 1973).

Antibody-mediated hypersensitivity phenomena have been investigated in nude mice by Reed and his colleagues in our laboratory. These studies (1976) have shown that nudes fail to produce reaginic IgE in response to hen egg albumin or crude ascaris extracts mixed with alum, saline extracts of *Bordetella pertussis*, or complete Freunds adjuvant. Antigen-specific IgE was quantitated in normal CFW mice by the passive cutaneous anaphylaxis (PCA) reaction. Passive sensitization of nudes with normal littermate IgE-positive serum produced typical responses, suggesting that nudes possess the necessary mechanism to elicit normal PCA reactions. These results clearly indicate that the IgE response is thymus-dependent and are in accord with those of Michael and Bernstein (1973).

4.3. Cellular Immunity

Following Rygaard's report (1969) that rat skin will survive for long periods in nude mice, many investigators sought to extend these findings to include a wide variety of tissue from many animal species. As a rule, skin allografts are retained for the life of the nude (Kindred, 1971b; Pantelouris, 1971; Manning *et al.*, 1973). Surprisingly, nudes also fail to reject xenografts from many species, including cat, human, chicken, lizard, and tree frog, provided that care is taken to prevent damage to the graft by scratching or biting (Manning *et al.*, 1973). Rygaard and Poulsen (1969) first showed that human tumors grow in nude mice, and many investigators now employ nudes as means of cultivating human tumor lines for chemotherapeutic and immunologic studies.

Studies in nudes have demonstrated that immunity to parasitic infections requires the participation of thymus-derived cells. Thus Jacobsen and Reed (1974) have demonstrated that nude mice maintain, for their lifetime, infections with *Nippostrongylus brasiliensis,* while normal littermates expel the nematode by day 10–12 of postlarval inoculation. The worm expulsion mechanism is produced in nude mice given thymus transplants 30 days prior to larval inoculation.

Other cell-mediated immune responses, including contact sensitivity to oxazalone (Pritchard and Micklem, 1972), graft-vs.-host reactivity (Lowenberg *et al.*, 1972 and unpublished observations), or killer cells with specificity for alloantigens (Wagner, 1972) have not been demonstrated in nude mice or their cell cultures.

175

CONGENITALLY
ATHYMIC (NUDE)
MICE AND THEIR
APPLICATION TO THE
STUDY OF IMMUNITY
AND AGING

4.4. Restoration of Immunity

After thymus transplantation with either intact glands or by infusion of cell suspensions, nude mice enjoy a restoration of most cell-mediated immune functions (Pantelouris, 1971; Pritchard and Micklem, 1972; Jutila *et al.*, 1975). In many studies, total restoration with thymic transplants has not been accomplished because of the genetic disparity between the thymus donor and nude recipients. Thymus cell transplantation enables nudes to respond to SRBC in a near normal fashion (Kindred, 1971b; Jutila *et al.*, 1975) and leads to the development of normal levels of IgA, IgG_1, and IgG_2 (Pritchard *et al.*, 1973; Rampy and Jutila, unpublished). Normal immunoglobulin levels are reached by 30 days after transplantation with syngeneic thymus glands, whereas restoration of immunoglobulin levels is delayed an additional month when allogeneic thymic transplants are used (Rampy and Jutila, 1975, unpublished). A singular observation made in these studies was that allogeneic thymic grafts restore immunoglobulin levels but fail to significantly restore helper cell function in nudes.

Other studies (Jutila *et al.*, 1975) have shown that immunologic responsiveness in nudes is not restored with thymus glands contained in cell-impermeable diffusion chambers. In a similar "diffusion chamber of nature" experiment, female nudes, mated previously to Balb/c males to yield litters bearing normal mice, demonstrated no restoration of responsiveness to SRBC or skin allografts. Thus it appears that nude mice are not reconstituted by the *in utero* passage of a thymic humoral factor or passage of such factors through cell impermeable membranes. Further support for these findings is provided by the observation that the immune response of nudes is not restored with large doses of thymosin (Wortis, 1974).

After transplantation, the improved health of nude mice, when compared to nongrafted nudes, is readily apparent. The mice begin to gain weight more rapidly, the skin develops a rubbery, wrinkled appearance, and their general vigor and overall health, especially as they grow older, is in marked distinction to nongrafted nudes. Nudes receiving two intact semisyngeneic or allogeneic thymi have remained healthy for over 550 days in our laboratory. Infections in restored nudes are rare. Nudes transplanted with allogeneic thymi often display symptoms of graft-vs.-host reaction two to three weeks following transplantation and experience a mortality of about 20%.

The fertility of nude males and females improves markedly and their gonads appear to be histologically normal (Wortis, 1975). In marked contrast to nongrafted nudes, thymus-bearing nudes begin to develop spontaneous tumors at an early age (Wortis, 1974) and develop tumors following cutaneous application of dimethyl-benzanthracene (Johnson, Reed, and Jutila, unpublished).

5. Diseases Associated with Aging

Numerous diseases and pathological changes in tissues and organs have been associated with aging in man and animals, including an increased incidence of malignancies, infections, and autoimmune disorders. Because it has been established that thymic deficiencies predispose to an increased incidence of age-related diseases, the nude mouse would be expected to develop many, if not all, such diseases.

5.1. Autoimmunity

It has been suggested that lack of responsiveness to autoantigens is the result of regulation exerted by a subpopulation of T cells (suppressor cells). A functional decrease in suppressor cells is speculated to increase reactivity to self and other antigens (Allison *et al.*, 1971). Nude mice should be free of T-cell-regulatory influences and should experience higher incidence of autoimmune diseases than their normal littermates. In this regard, Rygaard (1973) detected autoantibodies against thyroid and liver autoantigens in only 3 of 30 nude mice. He concluded that there is no greater incidence of autoimmune disorders in nudes than in littermate controls.

Morse *et al.* (1974) have shown, however, that nude mice develop serum factors capable of binding with double-stranded DNA, which apparently increase in titer as they grow older. Significantly, nudes showing signs of wasting disease demonstrate a greater serum DNA-binding capacity than nudes experiencing good health. The introduction of an immunoregulatory mechanism by thymus grafting yielded a serum DNA-binding capacity in nudes comparable to normal littermates. Immunofluorescent staining of kidneys revealed the presence of significant amounts of IgM, IgG_1, IgG_2, and IgA in the glomeruli of nudes but not littermate mice. The authors conclude that nudes lack a "regulatory" T cell population which allows nudes to develop anti-DNA antibodies. These results are consistent with those obtained using neonatally thymectomized mice and New Zealand mice, both of which suffer from a high incidence of autoimmune disorders and other symptoms of aging (Yunis *et al.*, 1971).

5.2. Infections and Endotoxin Sensitivity

The major pathological changes found in the nudes are, in all probability, the consequence of infection. In limited studies in our laboratory, at least 50% of nudes, 2 to 4 months of age, reared under conventional animal-room conditions, suffer from infections. Harderian gland infections are frequently encountered and, in severe cases, exophthalmos becomes apparent. Acute inflammatory reactions leading to necrosis of ducts is commonly observed (Rygaard, 1973). Rygaard (1973) has also reported infections of the parotid gland accompanied by massive granulocyte infiltration and marked tissue degeneration.

The infectious agents involved in infections in nude mice have not been precisely defined, but Jutila (1973) has provided evidence that the intestinal tract may serve as a source of opportunistic organisms that are not usually pathogenic. In this regard, he reported a massive coliform colonization of the bowel of nudes in association with reduced fecal IgA levels. Coliform organisms and fecal streptococci, presumed to be derived from the gut, have been isolated from the spleen and liver of wasting nudes, but never in overwhelming numbers. The nonpathogenic organism *Staphylococcus albus* has also been isolated from Harderian gland infections of the nude (unpublished). Flanagan (1966) and Rygaard (1973) have both reported that nudes may suffer from *Toxoplasma gondii* infections of the liver but attempts to isolate the organism have been unsuccessful. Other etiological agents from other environmental sources may be involved in infection of the nudes but little evidence has been published to support this supposition.

177

CONGENITALLY
ATHYMIC (NUDE)
MICE AND THEIR
APPLICATION TO THE
STUDY OF IMMUNITY
AND AGING

Few studies have been conducted on the susceptibility of nudes to bacterial, viral, and fungal pathogens. Our studies (unpublished) indicate that nudes are no more susceptible to challenge with type 19 *Streptococcus pneumoniae* than are normal littermates. Resistance to this agent may be associated with protective factors generated in the serum which enhance phagocytosis. Similarly, nudes appear to be slightly more resistant to challenge with *C. albicans* than normal littermates (J. Cutler, personal communication). It appears that nudes possess some form of antibacterial and antifungal immune mechanism, most likely in the form of a phagocytic response. Phagocytosis may be enhanced by a humoral (IgM) response directed against thymus-independent antigens such as pneumococcal capsular polysaccharide (Manning *et al.,* 1972).

Jutila *et al.* (1975) have reported that nude mice exhibit a profound age-related sensitivity to endotoxin, which is similar to that reported in neonatally thymectomized mice (Salvin *et al.,* 1965). It has been proposed that the marked increase in susceptibility to endotoxin in nudes as they grow older may be the factor contributing to wasting of these mice. Because nudes may develop intestinal overgrowth phenomena due to impaired cellular and secretory immune functions, they may experience frequent "bursts" of organisms or their endotoxins from the gut into the vascular system, which leads to an increased state of "hypersensitivity" to these agents as they age. It is speculated that these microorganisms establish themselves as microcolonies in liver, spleen, lung, etc., which in turn attract inflammatory cells. Shwartzman-like reactions (Kelly *et al.,* 1957) may develop as a consequence of sensitization by colonization or direct stimulation with endotoxin and ultimately give rise to a systemic reaction recognizable as signs of wasting.

The observation that nudes maintained under germfree conditions fail to waste and that antibiotic treatment delays the onset of wasting strongly supports an infectious etiology for wasting. It is tempting to speculate that infections and endotoxin sensitivity, manifest as signs of wasting in immunodeficient animals, may also contribute to signs and diseases of immunodeficiency and aging in man.

5.3. Spontaneous and Induced Tumors in Nudes

The vast majority of neoplasms are thought to be eliminated by a T-cell-influenced immunological surveillance mechanism (Burnet, 1970), which, as it declines in function with aging, allows nascent spontaneous tumor cells to "sneak through" and develop into rapidly growing tumors. Since nudes are profoundly T-cell-deficient and are presumed to lack an immunological surveillance system, it was expected that they would suffer from a high incidence of spontaneous tumors of all types. In contradistinction to the surveillance hypothesis, numerous investigators (Rygaard, 1973; Wortis, 1974; Reed and Jutila, unpublished) have reported few, if any, spontaneous tumors following observations on several thousand nudes reared under SPF and conventional conditions. The shortened life span of the nudes has been considered to be the most likely explanation for these observations (Outzen *et al.,* 1975). Outzen *et al.* (1975) have reported an increased incidence of spontaneous lymphoreticular neoplasms in germfree nudes when there is a virtual absence of similar tumors in their normal germfree littermates. The latency of the tumors ranged from a minimum of 95 days to a maximum of 483 days. Only 2% of 261 male and female nudes had developed tumors by 35 weeks of age. The authors suggest that the low incidence of this tumor type in germfree mice up to nine months of age accounts for the failure to detect such tumors in nudes maintained in the conventional or SPF environment. These observations may be correlated with those made on human patients suffering from naturally acquired or therapeutically induced immunologic defects (Penn *et al.*, 1971). The increased incidence of lymphoreticular tumors in nudes, as in humans, may reflect compensatory hyperplasia in damaged tissue that eventually undergoes malignant change.

Outzen *et al.* (1975) and Stutman (1974) have also presented another challenge to the concept of T-cell-mediated immunosurveillance by demonstrating that nudes are no more prone to develop tumors in response to methylcholanthrene than are normal littermates. In these studies, nude mice and normal littermates showed no differences in either latent period or incidence of local or systemic tumors. Jutila and Reed (unpublished) have shown that nudes painted with dimethylbenzanthracene (DMBA) fail to develop tumors unless previously thymus grafted, suggesting that skin oncogenesis may involve the participation of T cells or an intact immune response. The hairless condition of nudes apparently did not contribute to these results since genetically hairless *(hr/hr)* mice bearing normal thymi develop tumors in response to DMBA painting. The possibility that immunostimulation (Prehn, 1972) may help the growth of tumor cells has been proposed to explain these results.

The finding that there is an increased incidence of tumors in young nudes injected with polyoma virus (Allison *et al.,* 1974; Stutman, 1975) suggests a role for T-cell-mediated immunosurveillance of some virus-induced tumors. It has been shown, however, that as nudes age they become partially resistant to polyoma virus; only 25% develop tumors when infected at 120 days of age. The partial resistance can be transferred with spleen cells to newborn mice and appears to be associated with spleen cells bearing immunoglobulin receptors (Stutman, 1975). Perhaps related to this observation is the finding that nudes can be made more susceptible to polyoma virus by prior treatment with antilymphocyte serum (Allison *et al.,* 1974). These results strongly suggest that a weak secondary immune surveillance system involving B cells may operate to prevent the development of certain virus-induced tumors as well as the development of small foci of nascent spontaneous tumor cells in nude mice.

Because nudes possess the necessary complement of B and S (stem) cells for infection, it was anticipated that murine leukemia viruses, having a B cell requirement, such as Friend and Rauscher virus, would produce a typical leukemic process in these animals. In this regard, a puzzling observation has been made by Kouttab and Jutila (1974), in which nudes, given 2 LD_{50} of Friend leukemia virus (FLV), fail to develop a typical disease but die within a 60-day observation period. Littermates developed typical signs of the disease, including lymphocytosis and splenomegaly in 100% of the cases, as did nudes receiving thymus grafts one month earlier. This would suggest that FLV induced leukemias may have a T cell requirement for proper manifestations of the disease. Stutman and, separately, Kouttab (personal communication) have found, however, that FLV does produce typical leukemia in nudes. Resolution of these conflicting findings may reside in determining the target cell requirements of different strains of FLV (N-tropic vs. B-tropic) and the relative concentrations of defective and helper virus components in each virus preparation which may influence viral replication and malignant transformation.

179

CONGENITALLY
ATHYMIC (NUDE)
MICE AND THEIR
APPLICATION TO THE
STUDY OF IMMUNITY
AND AGING

5.4. Other Pathological Changes

The possible role of the athymic condition on endocrine functions and morphology in nudes has been investigated by Pierpaoli and Sorkin (1972) and Wortis (1975). Pierpaoli and Sorkin (1972) have reported that nudes possess lower concentrations of thyroxine in the blood when compared to normal littermates. Although the thyroid gland was observed to be histologically normal in healthy nudes, hypofunction and atrophy of the thyroid was detected in nudes suffering from wasting disease. The athymic condition also appeared to contribute to alteration of the adrenal cortex, which was prevented by thymus grafting. The authors suggest that the thymus in fetal or early postnatal life secretes a hormonal factor that influences the structure of the adrenal cortex and the function of the thyroid gland.

Wortis (1975) showed that nudes suffer from abnormal development of gonads and salivary glands but experience no abnormalities of the thyroid, parathyroid, or adrenals. Their reproductive defects were shown to be overcome by grafting with intact thymus glands.

6. Application of the Knowledge of the Nude Mouse to the Aging Problem

The nude mouse represents an interesting animal model for aging studies because of its unique genetic constitution, i.e., a rare mutant gene deprives the animal of a normal thymus gland. The ultimate effect of the athymic condition is a profound immunodeficiency state that contributes to a rapid onset of pathological changes and early death reminiscent of an accelerated aging process. Numerous studies over the past seven years have revealed the following salient features of the genetically thymusless condition of the nude.

1. Nudes lack functional T cells but possess normal numbers of functional S (stem) and B (bone-marrow-derived) cells.
2. The lack of cellular immunity prevents nudes from rejecting skin and tumor allografts or xenografts, expelling parasites, developing graft-vs.-host reactions, forming killer cells, and resisting infections.
3. The humoral response of nudes to thymus-dependent antigens is weak or nonexistent, whereas the response to thymus-independent antigens is essentially normal.
4. The athymic condition increases the incidence and accelerates the development of many age-related diseases and pathological changes, including autoimmune diseases, certain types of malignancies, and infections.
5. Restoration of immunity can be readily accomplished with thymus transplants and reduces the rapid onset of age-related diseases.

The availability of the "nude" gene in many inbred backgrounds presents the investigator of the aging problem with a tool to critically explore a number of events associated with primary and secondary aging. Parenthetically, studies in the germfree nude would be desirable in order to accommodate long-term studies and to avoid the secondary complications of infection. The incorporation of the gene into the genome of long-lived as well as short-lived strains of mice would help dissociate the role of T cells in the aging process from other intrinsic primary aging events.

Other applications of nude mouse technology to the problems of aging would serve to (a) identify the nature of the secondary immune surveillance mechanism operative against tumors in the nudes and which may be enhanced in aging man or animals, (b) determine the effect of age-related changes in B cell populations with and without the regulatory effects of the thymus gland, (c) further explore the role of thymus immunoregulation by suppressor cells in autoimmune disorders and tumor immunity, (d) better define the role of the immune response in tumor development, and (e) define *in vivo* cellular and molecular events associated with malignant change in the absence of tumor immune responses.

References

Aden, D. P., Reed, N. D., and Jutila, J. W., 1972, Reconstitution of the *in vitro* immune response of congenitally thymusless (nude) mice, *Proc. Soc. Exp. Biol. Med.* **140**:548–552.

Aden, D. P., and Reed, N. D., 1973, In vitro immune response to lipopolysaccharide: Thymus-derived cells not required, *Immunol. Comm.* **2**:335–340.

Allison, A. C., Denman, A. M., and Barnes, R. D., 1971, Cooperating and controlling of thymus derived lymphocytes in relation to autoimmunity, *Lancet* **ii**:135–137.

Allison, A. C., Monga, J. N., and Hammond, V., 1974, Increased susceptibility to virus oncogenesis of congenitally thymus deprived nude mice, *Nature* **252**:746.

Bach, J. F., Dardenne, M., and Bach, M. A., 1973, Detection of a circulating thymic hormone using T-rosette forming cells, in: *Proceedings of the Seventh Leucocyte Culture Conference* (F. Daguillard, ed.), pp. 271–287, Academic Press, New York.

Bankhurst, A. D., and Warner, N. L., 1972, Surface immunoglobulins on the thoracic duct lymphocytes of the congenitally athymic (nude) mouse, *Aust. J. Exp. Biol. Med. Sci.* **50**:661.

Bloemmen, J., and Eyssen, H., 1973, Immunoglobulin levels of sera of genetiacally thymusless (nude) mice, *Eur. J. Immunol.* **3**:117–118.

Burnet, F. M., 1970, *Immunological Surveillance,* Pergamon, Oxford.

Cordier, A. C., and Heremans, J. F., 1975, Nude mouse embryo: Ectodermal nature of the primordial thymic defect, *Scand. J. Immunol.* **4**:193–196.

Crewther, P., and Warner, N. L., 1972, Serum immunoglobulins and antibodies in congenitally athymic (nude) mice. *Aust. J. Exp. Biol. Med. Sci.* **50**:625–635.

Flanagan, S. P., 1966, "Nude," a new hairless gene with pleiotropic effects in the mouse, *Genet. Res. (Camb.)* **8**:295–301.

Jacobsen, R. H., and Reed, N. D., 1974, The immune response of congenitally athymic (nude) mice to the intestinal nematode *Nippostrongylus braciliensis, Proc. Soc. Exp. Biol. Med.* **147**:667–670.

Jutila, J. W., 1973, Etiology of the wasting diseases, in: *Bacterial Lipopolysaccharides* (E. Kass and S. Wolff, eds.), pp. 91–95, University of Chicago Press.

Jutila, J. W., Reed, N. D., and Isaac, D., 1975, Studies on the immune response of congenitally athymic (nude) mice, in: *Immunodeficiency in Man and Animals,* Birth defects: original article series, Vol XI, pp. 522–527, Sinauer Assoc. Inc., Sunderland, Mass.

Kelly, M. G., Smith, N. H., Wodinsky, I., and Rall, D. P., 1957, Strain differences in local hemorrhagic response (Shwartzman-like reaction) of mice to a single intradermal injection of bacterial polysaccharides, *J. Exp. Med.* **105**:653–663.

Kindred, B., 1971a, Immunological unresponsiveness of genetically thymusless (nude) mice, *Eur. J. Immunol.* **1**:59–62.

Kindred, B., 1971b, Antibody response in genetically thymusless nude mice injected with normal thymus cells, *J. Immunol.* **107**:1291–1295.

Kouttab, N., and Jutila, J. W., 1973, The role of the thymus in the leukemic process, *Mont. Acad. Sci.* **33**:56–66.

Lake, J., and Reed, N. D., 1975, Immunological responsiveness of congenitally athymic mice to polyvinylpyrrolidone, *Bact. Proc.* (abstract).

Lowenberg, B., Nieuwerkerk, H. T. M., and Kekkum, D. W., 1972, Effect of thymus extracts on *in vitro* graft-versus-host activity of nude mouse spleen cells, TNO-REP 72, p. 105.

Manning, J. K., Reed, N. D., and Jutila, J. W., 1972, Antibody response to *Escherichia coli* lipopolysaccharide and Type III pneumococcal polysaccharide by congenitally thymusless (nude) mice, *J. Immunol.* **108**:1470–1473.

Manning, D. D., and Jutila, J. W., 1972, Immunosuppression of mice injected with heterologous anti-immunoglobulin heavy chain antisera, *J. Exp. Med.* **135**:1316–1333.

Manning, D. D., Reed, N. D., and Schafffer, C., 1973, Maintenance of skin xenografts of widely divergent phylogenetic origin on congenitally athymic (nude) mice, *J. Exp. Med.* **138**:488–494.

Manning, D. D., and Jutila, J. W., 1974, Immunosuppression of congenitally athymic (nude) mice with heterologous anti-immunoglobulin heavy-chain antisera, *Cell. Immunol.* **14**:453–459.

Michael, J. G., and Bernstein, T. L., 1973, Thymus dependence of reaginic antibody formation in mice, *J. Immunol.* **111**:1600–1601.

Miller, J. F. A. P., 1961, Immunological function of the thymus, *Lancet* **2**:748:749.

Morse, H. C., Steinberg, A. D., Schur, P. H., and Reed, N. D., 1974, Spontaneous "autoimmune disease" in nude mice, *J. Immunol.* **113**:688–697.

Outzen, H. C., Custer, R. P., Eaton, G. J., and Prehn, R. T., 1975, Spontaneous and induced Tumor incidence in germfree "nude" mice, *J. Reticulo Soc.* **17**:1–9.

Pantelouris, E. M., 1968, Absence of thymus in a mouse mutant, *Nature* **217**:370–371.

Pantelouris, E. M., and Hair, J., 1970, Thymus dysgenesis in nude *(nu/nu)* mice, *J. Embryol. Exp. Morph.* **24**:615–621.

Pantelouris, E. M., 1971, Observation on the immunobiology of "nude" mice *Immunology* **20**:247–252.

Parrott, D. M. V., 1962, Strain variation in mortality and runt disease in mice thymectomized at birth, *Transpl. Bull.* **29**:102–104.

Penn, I., Halgrimson, C. G., and Starzl, T. E., 1971, *De novo* malignant tumors in organ transplant recipients, *Transplant Proc.* **3**:773.

Pierpaoli, W., and Sorkin, E., 1972, Alterations of adrenal cortex and thyroid in mice with congenital absence of the thymus, *Nature New Biol.* **238**:282–285.

Prehn, R. T., 1972, The immune reaction as a stimulator of tumor growth. *Science* **176**:170–171.

Pritchard, H., and Micklem, H. S., 1972, Immune responses in congenitally thymusless mice I. Absence of response to oxazolone, *Clin. Exp. Immunol.* **10**:151.

Pritchard, H., Riddaway, J., and Micklem, H. S., 1973, Immune responses in congenitally thymusless mice II-Quantitative studies of serum immunoglobulins, the antibody response to sheep erythrocytes and the effect of thymus allografting, *Clin. Exp. Immunol.* **13**:125–138.

Raff, M. C., and Wortis, H., 1970, Thymus dependence of O-bearing cells in the peripheral lymphoid tissues of mice, *Immunology* **18**:931–942.

Reed, N. D., and Jutila, J. W., 1972, Immune response of congenitally thymusless mice to heterologous erythrocytes, *Proc. Soc. Exp. Biol. Med.* **139**:1234–1237.

Reed, N. D., Manning, J. K., Baker, P. J., and Ulrich, J. T., 1974, Analysis of thymus-independent immune responses using nude mice, in: *Proc. First International Workshop on Nude Mice* (J. Rygaard and C. Poulsen, eds.), Stuttgart.

Rygaard, J., 1969, Immunobiology of the mouse mutant "nude." Preliminary investigations, *Acta Pathol. Microbiol. Scand.* **77**:761–762.

Rygaard, J., 1973, *Thymus and Self*, F.A.D.L., Copenhagen.

Rygaard, J., and Poulsen, C. O., 1969, Heterotransplantation of a human malignant tumor to "nude" mice, *Acta Pathol. Microbiol. Scand.* **77**:758–759.

Salvin, S., Peterson, R. B., and Good, R. A., 1965, The role of the thymus in resistance to infection and endotoxin toxicity, *J. Lab. Clin. Med.* **65**:1004–1022.

Stutman, O., 1974, Tumor development after 3-methylcholanthrene in immunologically deficient athymic-nude mice, *Science* **183**:534–536.

Stutman, O., 1975, Tumor development after polyoma infection in athymic nude mice, *J. Immunol.* **114**:1213–1217.

Wagner, H., 1972, The correlation between the proliferative and the cytotoxic responses of mouse lymphocytes to allogeneic cells in vitro, *J. Immunol.* **109**:630–637.

Walford, R. L., 1969, *The Immunologic Theory of Aging*, Munksgaard, Copenhagen.

Walford, R. L., 1974, Immunologic theory of aging: Current status, *Fed. Proc.* **33**:2020–2027.

CONGENITALLY
ATHYMIC (NUDE)
MICE AND THEIR
APPLICATION TO THE
STUDY OF IMMUNITY
AND AGING

Wortis, H., 1971, Immunological responses of "nude" mice, *Clin. Exp. Immunol.* **8**:305–317.

Wortis, H., 1974, Immunological studies of nude mice, *Contemporary Topics in Immunobiology,* Vol. 3, pp. 243–263, Plenum, New York.

Wortis, H. H., 1975, Pleiotropic effects of the nude mutation, in: *Immunodeficiency in Man and Animals,* Birth defect: original article series, Vol. XI, pp. 528–530, Sinauer Assoc., Inc., Sunderland, Mass.

Yunis, E. J., Fernandes, G., Teague, P. E., and Good, R. A., 1971, in: *Tolerance, Immunity, and Molecular Aging* (S. Sigel and R. Good, eds.), Charles Thomas, Springfield.

Yunis, E. J., Fernandes, G., and Greenberg, L. J., 1975, Immune deficiency, autoimmunity and aging, in: *Immunodeficiency in Man and Animals,* Birth defects: original article series, Vol. XI, pp. 185–192, Sinauer Assoc., Inc., Sunderland, Mass.

13

Immunoengineering: Prospects for Correction of Age-Related Immunodeficiency States

ROY L. WALFORD, PATRICIA J. MEREDITH, and KAY E. CHENEY

1. Introduction

The term *immunoengineering* in the context used here refers to procedures that may serve to ameliorate the immunologic abnormalities associated with aging. Such amelioration would be important for both theoretical and practical reasons. From the standpoint of theory, it has been repeatedly emphasized that the only valid test of an aging hypothesis requires significant extension of the life span of long-lived strains of animals, including extension of the longest-lived or tenth decile survivorship (Walford, 1969, 1974). Considered in these terms, life span cannot be extended merely by eliminating specific diseases (Strehler, 1975). A major extension of longest-lived survivorship by measures that can only be interpreted immunologically would constitute formal proof of the immunologic theory of aging, at least in terms of pathogenesis (Walford, 1974).

Even if age-related immune abnormalities are not involved in basic aging, but are secondary or epiphenomenal, their amelioration should still favorably influence most so-called diseases of aging, including amyloidosis, cancer, maturity-onset diabetes, vascular disease (chiefly atherosclerosis and hypertension), and senile dementia. This prospect constitutes the practical aspect of immunoengineering procedures. The developing use of bone marrow transplantation in therapy of leukemias, aplasias, and certain pediatric immunodeficiency states in humans

ROY L. WALFORD, PATRICIA J. MEREDITH, and KAY E. CHENEY • Department of Pathology, UCLA School of Medicine, Los Angeles, California.

ROY L. WALFORD,
PATRICIA J.
MEREDITH, AND KAY
E. CHENEY

(Good and Bach, 1974; Thomas *et al.*, 1975) attests to the potential immediacy of such an application for geriatrics.

Two broad classes of immune dysfunction are associated with aging (Figure 1). These consist of (1) a developing severe deficiency in humoral and cellular immune response capacities, and (2) an increasing incidence of autoimmune manifestations in older animals. Which of these is primary or whether both are coequal is difficult to say. For example, normal aging and the chronic graft-vs.-host reaction, which we have taken as a model for autoimmunity and aging (Walford, 1962; Cheney and Walford, 1974), show the following features in common: lymphoid depletion and hypoplasia; thymic atrophy; small reticuloendothelial aggregates in the liver; an increase in plasma cells in lymphoid organs; hyaline changes in renal glomeruli; renal atrophy; deposition of amorphous hyaline material in lymphoid organs; generalized weight loss and a "shriveling up" of the body; characteristic changes in skin and hair; amyloidosis; hypergammaglobulinemia; a decreased response to alloantigens, particularly those requiring T and B cell cooperation; positive tests for autoantibodies; and a tendency toward activation of latent tumor viruses.

In NZB and related strains of mice, autoimmunity may precede the onset of immunodeficiencies (Morton and Siegel, 1968). On the other hand, certain primary immunodeficiencies in humans and mice are associated with autoimmune manifestations (Good and Yunis, 1974). We do note that most of these, specifically excepting common variable immunodeficiency (Park and Good, 1974), lack one feature characteristic of accelerated aging, namely, an increase in incidence of a wide variety of tumors and not merely, e.g., lymphomas. Be that as it may, and whatever the precise sequence and relationships, immunoengineering has two

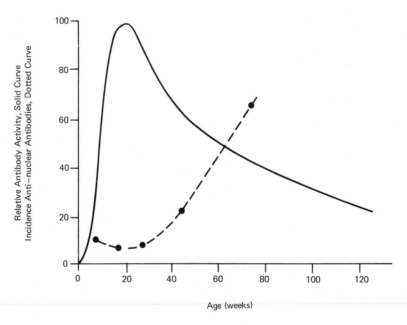

Figure 1. Solid curve shows relative primary antibody response, dotted curve the incidence of antinuclear antibodies in relation to age in long-lived mouse strains (Walford, 1974).

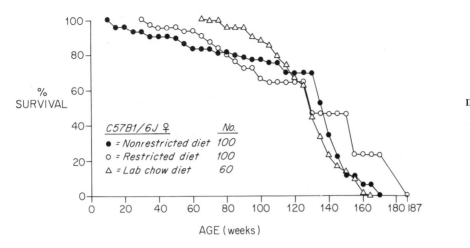

185

IMMUNO-
ENGINEERING:
PROSPECTS FOR
CORRECTION OF
AGE-RELATED
IMMUNODEFICIENCY
STATES

Figure 2. Survival curves of C57B1/6J female mice on restricted, nonrestricted, and *ad lib* lab chow diets (updated from Gerbase-DeLima *et al.*, 1975).

points of attack: restoration of the immune response capacity of the immunodeficient animal and/or prevention of the autoimmune aspects of aging.

The procedures discussed here may concern either or both points. Some can be interpreted as exerting their life-span-prolonging, age-decelerated effects via immunologic mechanisms, but other interpretations may be equally plausible. Certain other procedures, which can probably be interpreted only in strict immunologic terms, have not yet been evaluated vis-a-vis life span. Success in prolonging life by these latter methods would constitute a more fundamental experiment.

2.   Nutritional Manipulation, Life Span, and Immune Function

McCay and associates (1935) discovered that a calorically restricted but nutritionally supplemented diet (i.e., undernutrition without malnutrition) markedly prolongs the life span of rats. Later work, largely of a biochemical nature and also limited to rats, confirmed that controlled dietary restriction decelerates aging (Ross, 1969). Previous restriction studies in mice, on the other hand, have been almost meaningless gerontologically because only short-lived, high-tumor-incidence strains, such as AKR, were employed.

In the past few years we have studied the effects of controlled dietary restriction in long-lived C57BL/6 and (C57BL/10 × C3H)F$_1$ hybrid mice with regard to longevity, disease pattern, and age-specific immune response capacity. Nutritional requirements are much less well known for mice than for rats. Nevertheless, some prolongation of longest-lived survivorship has already been obtained (Figure 2). Dietary restriction in this experiment was not, in fact, severe, judging by body weights at 108–118 weeks of age (average of 20.7 g for restricted, 24.5 g for control mice). Studies on more severely restricted animals, in which a 60% difference in body weights between test and controls has been maintained, appear to be showing an even more enhanced survival.

Compared to controls, the lymphoid cells from mice on both moderately and

ROY L. WALFORD,
PATRICIA J.
MEREDITH, AND KAY
E. CHENEY

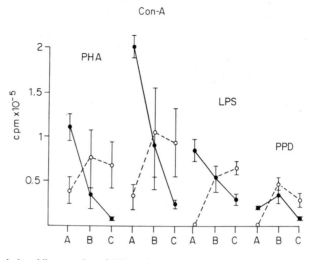

Figure 3. Tritiated thymidine uptake of PHA, Con-A, LPS, and PPD stimulated spleen cells from restricted (○---○) and nonrestricted (●—●) mice of three different ages (A = 31–34 weeks, B = 56–61 weeks, C = 75–85 weeks) (adapted from Gerbase-DeLima *et al.*, 1975).

severely restricted diets demonstrate the same kind of response to T and B cell mitogens (Figure 3). At a young age, they show a diminished immune response; however, by one year of age and continuing through a later period they respond better than cells from control mice. A similar relationship obtains with the response to injected sheep red blood cells (Walford *et al.*, 1974). Skin allograft survival is greatly prolonged in dietarily restricted mice and does not reach normal values until over 1 year of age. These studies add up to a "reversal effect," as illustrated schematically in Figure 4. The restricted diet delays the early maturation of immune response capacity but retards the age-related decline in that capacity. Our studies do not prove that dietarily induced immune alterations cause a deceleration of the rate of aging; however, failure to find consistent changes in the immune system under a regime that prolongs life span in long-lived mice would be strong evidence against an immunologic interpretation of aging.

Since it has been suggested that the thymus is fundamentally involved in the aging process (Walford, 1969; Burnet, 1970), we may reemphasize its extreme susceptibility to dietary manipulation (Walford, 1969; McFarlane and Hamid, 1973) and the fact that it may contain a higher population of potentially "self"-reactive cells than other lymphoid organs (Micklem and Asfi, 1971).

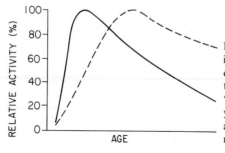

Figure 4. The reversal effect. Solid line represents immune response of control mice, dotted line of dietarily restricted mice. If restriction delays maturation of immune response capacity and maintains a "younger" immune system into a later age, then young restricted mice would show a decreased reactivity and older restricted mice an increased reactivity compared to controls.

Deficiencies of essential amino acids may influence the immune system in different ways (Jose and Good, 1973). For example, a deficit in valine alters humoral more than cellular immunity, whereas a deficit in lysine decreases both responses. The apparent deceleration of aging obtained with a tryptophan-deficient diet (Segall and Timiras, 1975) might reflect immune functional alterations equally as well as alterations of brain monoamines (Timiras, 1975). Factors such as temperature and nutritional status, which affect the rate of aging, might do so by mediation of the hypothalmic-pituitary-peripheral endocrine system (Everitt, 1975). There may be an important relationship between neuroendocrine and immune systems, the one being the "clock" and the other the "pacemaker" for aging.

187

IMMUNO-
ENGINEERING:
PROSPECTS FOR
CORRECTION OF
AGE-RELATED
IMMUNODEFICIENCY
STATES

3. Internal Body Temperature, Aging, and Immune Function

Early observations by naturalists, e.g., that fence lizards enjoy a longer life span in New England than in Florida, stimulated us to undertake controlled laboratory investigations of the effect of body temperature on life span in poikilothermic vertebrates. We were aware from work by Hildemann (1957) that the immune system may be extremely sensitive to body temperature variables. We have studied several species of annual fish of the genus *Cynolebias* (Walford and Liu, 1965) obtained originally from a field expedition to South America. Populations maintained at about 20°C live 60% longer than those at 15°C and show deceleration of the rate of aging as judged by collagen solubility. The life-span prolongation at reduced temperature cannot be attributed merely to general metabolic slowdown (Liu and Walford, 1972). Recent observations suggest that the effect of lowered temperature is exerted most prominently during the last half of life (Liu and Walford, 1975).

The temperature phenomenon is paradoxical in terms of the relation between immunology and aging. Lowering body temperature greatly suppresses both humoral and cellular immunity (Trump and Hildemann, 1970; Cone and Marchalonis, 1972). This would seem likely to accentuate the immunodeficiency of aging; nevertheless, life span is greatly prolonged. The fact that reduced body temperature especially prolongs the last half of life may indicate that suppression of age-related autoimmunity overrides any disadvantages accruing from adding, by such a regime, to the general immunodeficiency of aging. Lending mild support to this view is the observation that long-term, late-life administration of immunosuppressive drugs may, despite toxic side effects, favorably influence the 50% survival point in mouse populations (Walford, 1967).

With normal aging in rodents, a mild decrease in average temperature and in circadian amplitudes has been observed (Yunis *et al.*, 1974). Attempts to achieve prolonged low-grade hypothermia in homeothermic animals by drug administration have been disappointing (Liu and Walford, 1972; Liu, 1974). On the other hand, certain yogic practices may indeed lower internal body temperature (Walford *et al.*, 1975), and these practices might significantly extend life span according to calculations by Rosenberg *et al.* (1973). Under discussion in our laboratory is the possibility of achieving long-term mild hypothermia in laboratory animals by biofeedback techniques. We believe this might be approached by negative feedback reinforcement of the peak amplitudes of circadian temperature rhythms in mice.

It seems reasonable to emphasize at this point that the life-span-prolonging effects of caloric undernutrition and of lowering body temperature are maximally effective at the opposite extremes of life span: nutritional manipulation during the first half and temperature lowering during the last half. One of these regimes delays the immunodeficiency of normal aging, the other probably ameliorates the autoimmunity that develops with age. The situation may reflect the operation of dual, age-related, immune dysfunctional processes (Figure 1). A combination of underfeeding and mild lowering of body temperature should lead to very striking increases in life span without interfering with normal activity.

4. Reconstitution Experiments with Injected or Grafted Lymphoid Cells

Several investigators have injected young mice with lymphoid and/or bone marrow cells from old animals, and old mice with cells from young animals. Bone marrow but not thymus, lymph node, or thoracic duct lymph contains stem cells capable of repopulating the lymphoid system (Miller and Phillips, 1975), but long-term survival and regeneration of functional capacity seems quite complex.

We will first briefly review old → young injection experiments. Yunis *et al.* (1972) reported that marrow cells from young or old NZB or CBA mice were both capable of repopulating the hematopoietic tissues of lethally irradiated young recipients. Assessment of comparative effects on immune and gerontologic parameters must be tempered by the finding, at least in some strains, of a striking difference in cellular constituency of aged vs. young mouse marrows: an increase in the frequency of differentiated lymphoid cells may occur with age (Farrar *et al.*, 1974), giving a speciously better performance for cell suspensions from old marrows. This might explain why Micklem *et al.* (1973) observed no great difference in capacity to generate functional B cells from marrow cells of 3- or 22-month-old mice, whereas, correcting for the constituency differences, Farrar *et al.* (1974) noted a difference between young and old marrow B cell responses. We do note, however, that different mouse strains were used, and that the CBA mouse employed by Micklem *et al.* (1973) may show less age-related immune decline than most other strains. Injecting irradiated mice with bone marrow cells, thymocytes, and sheep red blood cells, and examining their antibody forming capacity 4 and 8 days later, Farrar *et al.* (1974) found that even in the presence of optimal sources of T helper cells, the B cells of aged BC3F1 mice showed a two- or threefold decreased capacity. On the other hand, performing similar experiments but examining the injected, irradiated young recipients 3–10 months after marrow transplantation, Harrison and Doubleday (1975) reported that bone marrow cells from old CBA donors functioned as well as cells from young donors unless the recipients had been thymectomized before irradiation. After allowing for the strain difference, these results might still suggest that bone marrow lymphoid precursor cells from old animals may show a delayed ability to reach functional capacity under thymic influence, rather than an absolute decrease in capacity.

Teague and Friou (1969) and Teague (1974) found that injecting thymocytes from old into moderately young strain A mice led to the appearance of antideoxyribonucleoprotein (anti-DNP) antibodies in the latter, although very young mice were resistant to this adoptive transfer. According to Albright *et al.* (1969), injection of spleen cells from 112- to 137-week-old donors into lethally irradiated 76-week-old recipients caused a greatly decreased survival compared to irradiated but noninjected mice, or to mice injected with 14-week-old cells.

Young → old injection experiments have also been performed. Teague and Friou (1965, 1969) reported that injection of spleen cells from young into old A/J mice prevented the development of antibodies to DNP, or led to disappearance of the spontaneously occurring anti-DNP present in the old mice. Formation of anti-DNP in susceptible mouse strains can be reversed or delayed by treatment with thymus as well as spleen cells (Yunis et al., 1971). Grafting of thymectomized young B/W mice with young (2 week) but not older (10 week) syngeneic thymus cells caused a reduction of serum anti-DNA titers (Steinberg et al., 1970). Yunis et al. (1973) treated the autoimmune hemolytic disease of adult NZB mice with cyclophosphamide plus administration of 2-month-old spleen cells. The erythrocyte antiglobulin test (Coomb's test) was converted from positive to negative for as long as three months. Into old irradiated mice, Perkins et al. (1972) transplanted spleen cells from young mice immunized with a vaccine to S. typhimurium, then challenged the old mice with multiples of LD_{50} doses of the bacterium. Normally very susceptible to S. typhimurium, the old mice were substantially protected for as long as 10–12 weeks. Gelfand and Steinberg (1973) found that skin allograft rejection in old intact B/W mice could be reverted to a youthful rate by intravenous administration of young spleen cells, or more effectively by lymph node cells. The restored function could be abrogated by cortisone and antithymus serum.

Although Yunis and Greenberg (1974) reported a slight increase in survival of old NZB mice following treatment with young T cells, significant extension of life span by lymphoid cell reconstitution has been achieved only in very short-lived abnormal mice. Fabris et al. (1972) obtained a threefold prolongation of life span of hypopituitary dwarf mice (whose lymphoid system is atrophic) by injection of 150 million lymph node cells, but no prolongation with either thymus or bone marrow cells. The lymph node is a particularly rich source of so-called T_2 or T_y cells. Our own work has suggested that a major immunological defect in long-lived aged mice resides in depressed T_2 cell function (Meredith et al., 1975a,b). Figure 5 depicts results of our pilot study involving monthly injections of lymph node cells from young into old mice. No extension of longest-lived survivorship was obtained with lymph node cells alone. Addition of a single irradiation of the old recipients with 200R at 150 weeks of age may have allowed a slight extension, possible by providing space for the injected cells to home in to. Albright et al. (1969) were unable to extend the life span of 78-week-old (C57BL/6 × C3H/Anf)F_1-hybrid mice by injecting young spleen or bone marrow cells.

Whereas bone marrow grafts (Nordin and Loughman, 1972) or thymus grafts (Metcalf et al., 1966) seem individually incapable of extending the life span of aged mice, recent investigations suggest that a suitable combination of the two merit trial. Hirokawa (1975) and Hirokawa and Makinodan (1975) grafted thymuses from donor mice of different ages into young, T cell deprived syngeneic, thymectomized and lethally irradiated BC3F$_1$ mouse recipients reconstituted with young syngeneic bone marrow cells. The reemergence of T cell function was assessed by several parameters including histology, recolonization of T-cell-dependent areas of lymph nodes, total number of T cells responsive to antitheta serum, response to injected sheep erythrocytes, and mitogenic response to PHA, Con-A and allogeneic cells. Full recovery of T cell function as judged by all criteria was achieved only with neonatal thymus grafts. Teague and coworkers (Mercer et al., 1976; Pachciarz and Teague, 1976b) obtained somewhat different results in reconstituting young adult, thymectomized irradiated A/J and DBA/1J mice with combinations of young (four to six

189

IMMUNO-
ENGINEERING:
PROSPECTS FOR
CORRECTION OF
AGE-RELATED
IMMUNODEFICIENCY
STATES

ROY L. WALFORD,
PATRICIA J.
MEREDITH, AND KAY
E. CHENEY

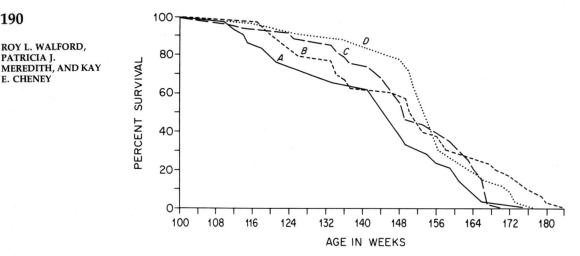

Figure 5. Survival of C57BL/6J male mice injected intraperitoneally at monthly intervals with 45–50 x 10⁶ lymph node (LN) cells from 35–50-day-old C57BL/6J male donors. Injections started in populations A and B at 112 weeks of age. — A (29 mice) = LN cell injections. --- B (30 mice) = LN cell injections, plus 200R total body irradiation at 150 weeks of age. — — C (34 mice) = 200R irradiation only. · · · · D (33 mice) = untreated control population.

weeks) and aged (18–20 months) thymus and bone marrow. In these experiments the thymus grafts were irradiated *in vitro* prior to grafting, to eliminate thymocytes, leaving intact the epithelial component. Whereas best results in terms of cellular immune function were obtained when both thymus and bone marrow were replaced, the age of the injected bone marrow seemed more important than age of the thymus. On the other hand, when old mice were reconstituted with young thymus or bone marrow or both, the thymus graft seemed the most critical (Pachciarz, J. A., and Teague, P. O., personal communication).

The possible role of hormones in maturation and performance of a reconstituted lymphoid system deserves consideration because old recipients of young transplants might be deficient in these ancillary factors. Growth hormone may influence maturation of the thymus-dependent system, and thyroxin and insulin play a role in maintaining the efficiency of the immune system in adult life (Fabris and Piantanelli, 1975).

A potential complicating factor to immune reconstitution was mentioned by Yunis *et al.* (1973). Strains of mice such as NZB which display vertical transmission of virus infection might be resistant to reconstitution if it were done too late in life. Genetic alterations resulting from virus interaction with thymus-dependent lymphocytes might not be susceptible to replacement therapy because the donor populations would suffer the same fate. Indeed slow viruses, which are probably of considerable importance in aging (Gajdusek, 1972), may be activated by age-related autoimmune or graft-vs.-host-like reactions. Hence old animals could be more resistant to life-span prolongation following lymphoid reconstitution than middle-aged animals in whom viruses had not yet been activated. An observation of Stutman *et al.* (1969) may be quite pertinent. They found that neonatally thymectomized animals could be restored with thymus cells only if therapy was not delayed too long. Analogously, beyond a certain age the thymic replacement might be too late.

191

IMMUNO-
ENGINEERING:
PROSPECTS FOR
CORRECTION OF
AGE-RELATED
IMMUNODEFICIENCY
STATES

5. Thymic Humoral Factors

In a consideration of autoimmunity in the absence of somatic cell variation one of us suggested some years ago that the thymus might be fundamentally involved in aging because of its possible relationship to tolerance, immunological homeostasis, and self-recognition (Walford, 1969). Later investigations do support the view that autoimmunity can result from defects in homeostatic control mechanisms as well as from genesis of new, mutant antiself clones (Orgad and Cohen, 1974; Kolata, 1974; Roberts *et al.,* 1973). Certain evidence indicates an aberration in suppressor cells affecting cellular immunity with age in mice (Gerbase-DeLima *et al.,* 1974; Gerbase-DeLima and Walford, 1975). These might operate via interference with T cell activation (Roder *et al.,* 1975). It has been proposed that disturbances in suppressor mechanisms play a role in aging of the immune system (Walford, 1974), as well as in autoimmunity (Teague and Friou, 1969).

One category of suppressor T cells might normally prevent autoantibody formation (Allison, 1974). A decline in suppressor T cells has, in fact, been reported with age in B/W mice (Talal and Steinberg, 1974). The idea of a specific T-cell-mediated feedback control of autoantibody formation by B cells has been entertained (Allison *et al.,* 1971). The subject is quite open but clearly corresponds to a homeostasis/tolerance control mechanism. This approach represents a somewhat different orientation than that later proposed by Burnet (1970) who, tying thymus involution to a Hayflick clock limit, envisaged a decline in immune surveillance with age as allowing mutant clones to proliferate and lead to autoimmune manifestations. It is no longer necessary to postulate an actual mutation, although such is not ruled out.

The role of the thymus in vertebrate aging including man (Mackay, 1972) could be quite complex, and further studies of its various functional components should be rewarding. Investigation of thymic hormonal factors represents one such approach. In past years thymic extracts have been found to influence various physiological processes such as calcium and phosphate metabolism, and to contain a myositis-inducing factor, and a myasthenic neuromuscular blocking factor (Galante *et al.,* 1968; Goldstein and Manganaro, 1971; Goldstein, 1974; and Kalden *et al.,* 1973). Most notably, however, cell-free thymic extracts affect cellular immunity. One protein preparation isolated from bovine thymus and termed "lymphocyte stimulating hormone" (LSHr, molecular weight 80,000) augmented the antibody response of newborn mice injected with sheep red blood cells (Robey *et al.,* 1972; Robey, 1975). A second polypeptide (THF, mol. wt. 1000), obtained from calf and mouse thymus, restored the capacity to produce *in vivo* and *in vitro* graft-vs.-host responses of spleen cells from neonatally thymectomized mice (Trainin and Small, 1970; Kook and Trainin, 1975); increased the reactivity of responding cells in the mixed lymphocyte reaction; conferred resistance upon thymocytes to hydrocortisone; prevented wasting disease in neonatally thymectomized mice; and increased the cytotoxic reactivity of mouse spleen cells sensitized *in vitro* against syngeneic tumor cells (Umiel and Trainin, 1975; Trainin *et al.,* 1974; Trainin *et al.,* 1966;

ROY L. WALFORD,
PATRICIA J.
MEREDITH, AND KAY
E. CHENEY

Carnaud *et al.,* 1973). Thymopoietin (thymin, mol. wt. 7000), another thymic humoral factor, induces surface antigenic markers characteristic of T cells on lymphoid stem cell precursors when used in subnanogram concentrations (Basch and Goldstein, 1974; G. Goldstein, 1975; Basch and Goldstein, 1975). A fourth extract, thymosin (molecular weight approximately 12,200) (Hooper *et al.,* 1975; A. L. Goldstein *et al.,* 1972), has been shown to restore cell-mediated immunity in neonatally thymectomized mice; to accelerate first- and second-set allograft rejection in adult mice; to enhance resistance to Moloney sarcoma virus-induced tumor growth in neonatal mice; and to induce both immunocompetence and T-cell-surface markers in lymphoid precursors in normal and nude mice (Law *et al.,* 1968; Goldstein *et al.,* 1970; Hardy *et al.,* 1968; Zizblatt *et al.,* 1970; Hardy *et al.,* 1971; Bach *et al.,* 1971; Scheid *et al.,* 1973; Komuro and Boyse, 1973).

It is clear from the above that much evidence supports the existence of a thymic hormone or hormones influential in inducing maturation of thymus-derived lymphocytes (Mandi and Glant, 1973; Bach *et al.,* 1975; Dardenne *et al.,* 1974). During gestation and in the neonate this factor may stimulate development of peripheral lymphoid tissues toward full competence (Bach *et al.,* 1975). In the adult it perhaps maintains T cell populations involved in cellular immunity. During aging the thymus atrophies, serum thymic hormone levels fall dramatically, and the functional capacity of the immune system declines (Bach *et al.,* 1972, 1973; Walford, 1969; A. L. Goldstein *et al.,* 1974). There is also clearly an increased decline of cellular immunity in presenile adult thymectomized mice (Pachciarz and Teague, 1975). The question arises, whether the age-related decline of cell-mediated immunity, and perhaps the incidence of the diseases of aging can be influenced by supplying thymic hormonal factors.

Direct evidence pertaining thereto is scant. Using an *in vitro* graft-vs.-host assay, Friedman *et al.* (1974) found that cells derived from spleens of 33-month-old (C3H × C57BL)F$_1$-hybrid mice were less capable of eliciting a GVH reaction than those from 3-month-old animals. The addition of THF to the culture increased the ability of old spleen cells to mount a GVH reaction, but no such effect was observed with cells from young mice. They postulated that the decline in GVH response of spleen cells from old mice was not due to decreased numbers of progenitor cells but to failing maturation from inadequate thymic activity. Strausser *et al.* (1971) reported that the normal age-related decline in response to sheep red blood cells in 18-month-old mice could be modified by treatment with either calf thymosin or similarly prepared calf spleen fractions.

The effects of thymic hormones on various immunologic "models" of accelerated aging, such as NZB mice (Teague *et al.,* 1972), may also be cited. Using a rosette assay, Bach *et al.* (1972, 1973, 1975) found an age-related decline of thymic factor (TF) levels in serums of normal humans and mice. In CBA, C57BL/6, Balb/c, and A strain mice the level declined progressively after 6 months of age and was no longer detectable beyond 15 months. In NZB and B/W mice the decline was more rapid, paralleling the early fall in T lymphocyte reactivity in these strains (Bach *et al.,* 1973). NZB mice showed deficient circulating TF by two months of age, probably correlating with the early abnormality of NZB thymic medullary epithelial cells (De Vries and Hijmans, 1967).

Antigen-induced depression of spleen DNA synthesis, as a measure of suppressor T cell activity, decreases during aging in NZB mice, but could be restored to normal with thymosin (Dauphinee and Talal, 1975). Furthermore, abnormal DNA proliferation patterns of thymocytes from 8-week-old NZB mice transplanted into lethally irradiated C57BL/6J recipients could be corrected with thymosin (Dauphinee *et al.*, 1974). Dauphinee and coworkers suggested that thymosin might suppress autoimmunity by inducing the appearance of new T cells with suppressor activity, or by causing aberrant T cells to revert to normal function. Thymosin has also been reported to stimulate mitogenic responsiveness, mixed lymphocyte reactivity, graft rejection, and the direct splenic plaque-forming cell response of aging NZB and nude mice after prolonged treatment (Gershwin *et al.*, 1974; Thurman and Goldstein, 1975).

193

IMMUNO-
ENGINEERING:
PROSPECTS FOR
CORRECTION OF
AGE-RELATED
IMMUNODEFICIENCY
STATES

In systemic lupus erythematosus, TF levels in patients ranging from 15–60 years of age have been consistently found low compared to age-matched normal subjects, analogous to the situation in NZB mice (Bach *et al.*, 1975).

Human patients with certain immunodeficiency diseases have been considered possible "models" for accelerated aging. Patients with T cell deficiencies demonstrate low serum thymus hormone levels. In six cases of pure agammaglobulinemia Bach *et al.* (1975) found normal TF levels. However, in two cases of DiGeorge syndrome hormone levels were undetectable, analogous to the situation in nude mice (Bach *et al.*, 1975). In several cases of ataxia-telangiectasia and variable combined immunodeficiency, the levels were normal or low. Wara *et al.* (1975b) reported partial restoration of cell-mediated immunity in a patient with thymic hypoplasia after daily injections of thymosin. Numerous other investigators have reported that exposure to thymic factors *in vitro* may profoundly affect the lymphoid cells from patients with primary immunodeficiency diseases including the DiGeorge syndrome, ataxia-telangiectasia, Wiskott-Aldrich syndrome, IgA deficiency, and secondary immunodeficiency disease (viral upper respiratory infection, and nasopharyngeal carcinoma), but not with congenital combined immunodeficiency (Aiuti *et al.*, 1975; Touraine *et al.*, 1975a,b; Wara and Amman, 1975a).

It appears from the above that thymus hormonal factors might favorably influence the immunodeficiency of aging. Evaluation of available data, however, is difficult not only because of the diversity of substances of thymic origin which have been described, but also in view of the enormous range of biological effects claimed.

6. Polynucleotides

Although largely unexplored in the realm of aging, synthetic polynucleotides may have potential for immunologic restoration. The history of their use as enhancers of immunity can be traced back to studies showing that naturally-occurring DNA and RNA could restore the immune response in X-irradiated animals (Simic and Kanazir, 1968). Braun and Nakano (1967) then discovered that commercially available poly AU could enhance the anti-SRBC response in a manner resembling that of oligonucleotides obtained from digestion of calf thymus DNA (Braun and Nakano, 1965), and Braun and Firshein (1967) that various oligo- and polynucleotides could stimulate macromolecular synthesis and cell division in both bacterial and mammalian systems.

Only one report has appeared regarding the effect of polynucleotides on the immune system with age. Braun *et al.* (1970) observed that poly AU and other polynucleotides, given in conjunction with SRBC, caused a five- to tenfold increase

ROY L. WALFORD,
PATRICIA J.
MEREDITH, AND KAY
E. CHENEY

in the number of plaque-forming cells (PFC) in 11–14-month-old C57BL mice. The response equaled or exceeded that found in 6- to 10-week-old mice challenged with SRBC only and approximated their response resulting from the addition of polyAU. Since 11–14 months of age is only young- or midadulthood for C57BL mice, the significance of the observations for aging and senescence is not clear.

Evidence from the literature suggests that polyAU may stimulate both B and T cells. Campbell and Kind (1971) noted an earlier appearance and increased numbers of PFC to SRBC after polyAU administration. However, when lethally irradiated mice reconstituted with normal spleen cells were challenged with SRBC + polyAU, no increase was found in hemolytic focus-forming cell units (FFU) in the spleen compared with animals challenged with SRBC only. Since the number of FFU are assumed to reflect the number of thymus-derived cells in the reconstituting inoculum, polyAU was considered in these experiments to raise the number of PFC by acting on the B cells, either by increasing their proliferation, or by increasing the number interacting with T cells. In another study (Hanjan and Talwar, 1975) polyAU increased the electrophoretic mobility of avian bursal cells, of a subpopulation (77%) of B cells from normal rat spleen, and a subpopulation (70–83%) of splenic lymphocytes from nude mice. The authors suggested that polyAU may contribute to the net negative surface charge on B cells, thereby allowing them to engage more effectively in electrostatic interaction with antigen (or with T cells?).

In contrast to Campbell and Kind (1971), Jaroslow and Ortiz-Ortiz (1972) concluded that the primary effect of polyAU in the PFC response is on T cells. They could detect no acceleration in the rate of formation of PFC, and suggested that polyAU probably did not increase proliferation of the T cells but rendered more of these cells susceptible to activation by antigen. This would in turn increase the number of B cells that become PFC. In line with these interpretations Chess *et al.* (1972) could detect no polyAU-dependent increase in the rate of [^{3}H]thymidine incorporation in lymphoid cells.

In another series of experiments, suggesting an effect of polyAU on T cells, Cone and Johnson (1971) were able to restore the splenic rosette-forming cells (RFC) to normal or near-normal levels in adult mice that had been neonatally thymectomized or treated with antimouse thymocyte serum (ATS). Skin graft rejection was also restored in neonatally thymectomized adult mice. PolyAU was thought to cause restoration by amplification of a small number of residual T cells that may have been thymus-influenced *in utero* before thymectomy, or that had survived treatment with ATS. Restoration of the RFC response was less in mice treated with ATS in addition to neonatal thymectomy.

In additional experiments it was shown that lethally irradiated mice reconstituted with excess bone marrow cells and as few as 4×10^4 thymocytes were able to produce RFC when challenged with SRBC and polyAU, whereas without polyAU the minimal threshold for response was 10^7 thymocytes (Cone and Johnson, 1971). By contrast, where thymocytes were in excess and bone marrow cells limiting, polyAU did not exert an adjuvant effect. Furthermore, when either thymocytes or bone marrow cells were incubated *in vivo* or *in vitro* with polyAU prior to transfer to an irradiated syngeneic host, a tenfold enhancement of the RFC assay was noted only in animals receiving thymocytes preincubated with polyAU (Cone and Johnson, 1972). In an *in vitro* system Cone and Marchalonis (1972) found

195

IMMUNO-
ENGINEERING:
PROSPECTS FOR
CORRECTION OF
AGE-RELATED
IMMUNODEFICIENCY
STATES

that polyAU enabled 10^4 thymocytes to cooperate with spleen cells from nude mice to produce an RFC response. At least 10^5 thymocytes were required to give a response in the absence of polyAU.

Synthetic polynucleotides may exert their immunological effect by raising the intracellular levels of cAMP. Spleen cells exposed *in vitro* to polyAU, and other oligonucleotides show a rise in adenyl cyclase activity (Winchurch *et al.*, 1971). In this respect the action of polynucleotides may be similar to that of other agents which raise intracellular cAMP levels, such as catecholamines (Braun, 1973; Scheid *et al.*, 1973, 1975) and thymic humoral factors (Scheid *et al.*, 1973, 1975). Also the stimulatory effect of polyAU on antibody responses can be magnified by simultaneous administration of theophylline (Ishizuka *et al.*, 1970), which is a phosphodiesterase inhibitor and stabilizer of cAMP levels.

Cone and Wilson (1972) found that 45–55% of RFC in mice were theta-positive 4 days after immunization with SRBC + polyAU, whereas after SRBC alone the theta-positive population was insignificant. Scheid *et al.* (1973, 1975) noted that polyAU, dibutyryl cAMP, endotoxin, and thymic extracts all induced the appearance of THY-1 (theta) and TL antigens on a fraction of spleen cells from normal mice as well as from nude mice, and polyAU, dibutyryl cAMP, endotoxin, and epinephrine induced the appearance of the *C'3* receptor in B cells. Elevation of intracellular cAMP levels may thus be involved in maturation of both T and B cells. Thymopoietin, although capable of inducing the TL antigen on T cells, did not induce the C'3 receptor on B cells (Scheid *et al.*, 1975). Ubiquitin, on the other hand, was able to induce both T and B cell maturation as judged by specific cell markers. The maturation was blocked by propanolol, a β-adrenergic antagonist, whereas TL induction by thymopoietin was unaffected by this agent. In another study, enhancement of anti-SRBC antibodies by polyAU was also unaffected by propranolol (Braun and Rega, 1972).

Thus the possibility exists that polyAU may act via the same membranal adenyl cyclase receptor on T cells as does thymopoietin and probably other thymic extracts. Kook and Trainin (1974) showed that polyAU can induce an *in vitro* GVH response in spleen cells from neonatally thymectomized mice similar to that induced by THF. Synthetic polynucleotides such as polyAU might be able to function as replacements for thymic factors in T cell (and possibly B cell) maturation.

Ishizuka *et al.* (1971) demonstrated that the stimulatory effect of polyAU could be abolished by trypsinization of the cells following exposure to the nucleotide. Apparently the cell membrane is altered by exposure to polyAU. It may be relevant to note here that, in contrast to the great decline with age in the blastogenic response to PHA (Hori *et al.*, 1973; Mathies *et al.*, 1973), no difference could be detected in [^{125}I]PHA binding to spleen cells of young (4-month) compared to old (30-month) BC3F$_1$ mice (Hung *et al.*, 1975), nor in binding of [^{125}I]ricin and [^{125}I]Con A, both of which attach to receptor sites which are biochemically distinct from each other and from that of PHA. These membranal receptors may be resistant to changes with age. The age-related decline in blastogenic response to PHA (and other immune stimuli) could conceivably be due to an insufficient mitogenic signal—possibly an initial rise and subsequent decline in cAMP (Yamamoto and Webb, 1975)—secondary to a decline in circulating thymic humoral factors. Indeed, Heidrick and Makinodan (1972) attributed the age-related func-

196

ROY L. WALFORD,
PATRICIA J.
MEREDITH, AND KAY
E. CHENEY

tional decline in immunity to an inability of both T cells and B cells to proliferate. Inasmuch as synthetic polynucleotides are believed to stimulate proliferation and/or differentiation of B and/or T cells, they may be useful in treating the immunodeficiency of aging, perhaps by replacing the lost thymic functions. Studies in this direction are in progress in our laboratory.

ACKNOWLEDGMENT

This study was supported by NIH grant HD-00534.

References

Aiuti, F., Schirrmacher, V., Ammerati, P., and Fiorilli, M., 1975, Effect of thymus factor in human precursor T lymphocytes, *Clin. Exp. Immunol.* **20**:499–503.

Albright, J. F., Makinodan, T., and Deitchman, J. W., 1969, Presence of life-shortening factors in spleens of aged mice of long lifespan and extension of life expectancy by splenectomy, *Exp. Geront.* **4**:267–276.

Allison, A. C., 1974, Interactions of T and B lymphocytes in self-tolerance and immunity, in: *Immunologic Tolerance* (D. H. Katz and B. Benecerraf, eds.), pp. 25–59, Academic Press, New York.

Allison, A. M., Denman, A. M., and Barnes, R. D., 1971, Cooperating and controlling functions of thymus-derived lymphocytes in relation to autoimmunity, *Lancet* **1**:135–140.

Bach, J. F., Dardenne, M., Pleau, J. M., and Bach, M. A., 1975, Isolation, biochemical characteristics, and biological activity of a circulating thymic hormone in the mouse and in the human, *Ann. N. Y. Acad. Sci.* **249**:186–210.

Bach, J. F., Papiernik, M., Levasseur, P., Dardenne, M., Barsis, A., and Le Brigard, H., 1972, Evidence for a serum-factor secreted by the human thymus, *Lancet* **2**:1056–1058.

Bach, J. F., Dardenne, M., and Saloman, J. C., 1973, Studies on thymus products. IV. Absence of serum thymic activity in adult NZB and (NZB × NZW)F₁ mice, *Clin. Exp. Immunol.* **14**:247–256.

Bach, J. F., Dardenne, M., Pleau, J. M., and Bach, M. A., 1975, Isolation, biochemical characteristics, and biological activity of a circulating thymic hormone in the mouse and in the human, *Ann. N. Y. Acad. Sci.* **249**:186–210.

Basch, R., and Goldstein, G., 1974, Induction of T-cell differentiation *in vitro* by thymin, a purified polypeptide hormone of the thymus, *Proc. Nat. Acad. Sci. U.S.* **71**:1474–1478.

Basch, R., and Goldstein, G., 1975, Antigenic and functional evidence for the *in vitro* inductive activity of thymopoietin (thymin) on thymocyte precursors, *Ann. N. Y. Acad. Sci.* **249**:290–307.

Braun, W., 1973, RNAs as amplifiers of specific signals in immunity, *Ann. N. Y. Acad. Sci.* **207**:17–28.

Braun, W., and Firshein, W., 1967, Biodynamic effects of oligonucleotides, *Bact. Rev.* **31**:83–94.

Braun, W., and Nakano, M., 1965, Influence of oligodeoxyribonucleotides on early events in antibody formation, *Proc. Soc. Exp. Biol. Med.* **119**:701–707.

Braun, W., and Nakano, M., 1967, Antibody formation: stimulation by polyadenylic and polycytidylic acid, *Science* **157**:819–821.

Braun, W., and Rega, M. J., 1972, Adenyl cyclase-stimulating catecholamines as modifiers of antibody formation, *Immunol. Commun.* **1**:523–532.

Braun, W., Yajima, Y., and Ishizuka, M., 1970, Synthetic polynucleotides as restorers of normal antibody forming capacities in aged mice, *J. Reticuloendothel. Soc.* **7**:418–424.

Burnet, F. M., 1970, An immunological approach to aging, *Lancet* **1**:358–360.

Campbell, P. A., and Kind, P., 1971, Bone marrow-derived cells as target cells for polynucleotide adjuvants, *J. Immunol.* **107**:1419–1423.

Carnaud, C., Ilfeld, S., Brook, I., and Trainin, N., 1973, Increased reactivity of mouse spleen cells sensitized *in vitro* against syngeneic tumor cells in the presence of a thymic humoral factor, *J. Exp. Med.* **138**:1521–1532.

Cheney, K., E., and Walford, R. L., 1974, Immune function and dysfunction in relation to aging, *Life Sci.* **14**:2075–2084.

Chess, L., Levy, C., Schmukler, M., Smith, K., and Mardiney, M. R., Jr., 1972, The effect of synthetic polynucleotides on immunologically induced tritiated thymidine incorporation, *Transplantation* **14**:748–755.

197

IMMUNO-
ENGINEERING:
PROSPECTS FOR
CORRECTION OF
AGE-RELATED
IMMUNODEFICIENCY
STATES

Cone, R. E., and Johnson, A. G., 1971, Regulation of the immune system by synthetic polynucleotides. III. Action on antigen-reactive cells of thymic origin, *J. Exp. Med.* **133**:665–671.

Cone, R. E., and Johnson, A. G., 1972, Regulation of the immune system by synthetic polynucleotides. IV. Amplification of proliferation of thymus-influenced lymphocytes, *Cell. Immunol.* **3**:283–293.

Cone, R. E., and Marchalonis, J. J., 1972, Cellular and humoral aspects of the influence of environmental temperature on the immune response of poikilothermic vertebrates, *J. Immunol.* **108**:952–957.

Cone, R. E., and Marchalonis, J. J., 1972, Adjuvant action of poly (A:U) on T-cells during the primary immune response *in vitro, Aust. J. Exp. Biol. Med. Sci.* **50**:69–77.

Cone, R. E., and Wilson, J. D., 1972, Adjuvant action of poly A:U on T and B rosette-forming cells in SRBC-immunized mice, *Int. Arch. Allergy* **43**:123–130.

Dardenne, M., Papiernik, M., Bach, J. F., and Stutman, O., 1974, Studies on thymus products. III. Epithelial origin of the serum thymic factor, *Immunology* **27**:299–304.

Dauphinee, M. J., and Talal, N., 1975, Reversible restoration by thymosin of antigen-induced depression of spleen DNA synthesis in NZB mice, *J. Immunol.* **114**:1713–1716.

Dauphinee, M. J., Talal, N., Goldstein, L., and White, A., 1974, Thymosin corrects the abnormal DNA synthetic response of NZB mouse thymocytes, *Proc. Nat. Acad. Sci. U.S.* **71**:2637–2641.

De Vries, M. J., and Hijmans, W., 1967, Pathologic changes of thymic epithelial cells and autoimmune disease in NZB, NZW, (NZB/NZW)F$_1$ mice, *Immunology* **12**:179–196.

Everitt, A. V., 1975, Hypothalmic-pituitary factors in ageing, 10th Internat. Congr. Gerontol., Jerusalem, Israel (June 22–27), in: *Congress Abstracts* **1**:46–47.

Fabris, N., and Piantanelli, L., 1975, Hormones, lymphocytes, and ageing, 10th Internat. Congr. Gerontol, Jerusalem, Israel (June 22–27), in: *Congress Abstracts* **1**:76–78.

Fabris, N., Pierpaoli, W., and Sorkin, E., 1972, Lymphocytes, hormones and ageing, *Nature* **240**:557–559.

Farrar, J. J., Loughman, B. E., and Nordin, A. A., 1974, Lymphopoietic potential of bone marrow cells from aged mice: comparison of cellular constituents of bone marrow from young and aged mice, *J. Immunol.* **112**:1244–1249.

Friedman, D., Keiser, V., and Globerson, A., 1974, Reactivation of immunocompetence in spleen cells of aged mice, *Nature* **251**:545–546.

Gajdusek, D. C., 1972, Slow virus infection and activation of latent infections in aging, *Advan. Gerontol. Res.* **4**:201–219.

Galante, L., Gudmundsson, T. V., Matthews, E. W., Williams, E. D., Tse, A., Woodhouse, N. J. Y., and MacIntyre, I., 1968, Thymic and parathyroid origin of calcitonin in man, *Lancet* **2**:537–538.

Gelfand, M. E., and Steinberg, A. D., 1973, Mechanisms of allograft rejection in New Zealand mice I. Cell synergy and its age-dependent loss, *J. Immunol.* **110**:1652–1662.

Gerbase-DeLima, M., and Walford, R. L., 1975, Effect of cortisone in delineating thymus cell subsets in advanced age, *Proc. Soc. Exp. Biol. Med.* **149**:562–564.

Gerbase-DeLima, M., Meredith, P., and Walford, R. L., 1974, Age-related changes including synergy and suppression in the mixed lymphocyte reaction in long-lived mice, *Fed. Proc.* **34**:159–161.

Gerbase-DeLima, M., Liu, R. K., Cheney, K. E., Mickey, R., and Walford, R. L., 1975, Immune function and survival in a long-lived mouse strain subjected to undernutrition, *Gerontologia* **21**:184–202.

Gershwin, M. E., Ahmed, A., Steinberg, A. D., Thurman, G. B., and Goldstein, A. L., 1974, Correction of T cell function by thymosin in New Zealand mice, *J. Immunol.* **113**:1068–1071.

Goldstein, A. L., Asanuma, Y., Battisto, J. R., Hardy, M. A., Quint, J., and White, A., 1970, Influence of thymosin on cell-mediated and humoral immune responses in normal and in immunologically deficient mice, *J. Immunol.* **104**:359–366.

Goldstein, A. L., Guha, A., Zatz, M. M., Hardy, M. A., and White, A., 1972, Purification and biological activity of thymosin, a hormone of the thymus gland. *Proc. Nat. Acad. Sci. U.S.* **69**:1800–1803.

Goldstein, A. L., Hooper, J. A., Schulof, R. S., Cohen, G. H., Thurman, G. B., and McDaniel, M. C., 1974, Thymosin and the immunopathology of aging, *Fed. Proc.* **33**:2053–2056.

Goldstein, G., 1974, Isolation of bovine thymin: A polypeptide hormone of the thymus, *Nature* **247**:11–14.

Goldstein, G., 1975, The isolation of thymopoietin (thymin), *Ann. N. Y. Acad. Sci.* **249**:177–185.

Goldstein, G., and Manganaro, A., 1971, Thymin: A thymic polypeptide causing the neuromuscular block of myasthenia gravis, *Ann. N. Y. Acad. Sci.* **183**:230–240.

Good, R. A., and Bach, F. H., 1974, Bone marrow and thymus transplants: cellular engineering to correct primary immunodeficiency, *Clin. Immunobiol.* **2**:63–114.

ROY L. WALFORD,
PATRICIA J.
MEREDITH, AND KAY
E. CHENEY

Good, R. A., and Yunis, E., 1974, Association of autoimmunity, immunodeficiency and aging in man, rabbits, and mice, *Fed. Proc.* **33**:2040–2050.

Hanjan, S. N. S., and Talwar, G. P., 1975, The selective action of poly A:U on the electrophoretic mobility and surface charge of a subpopulation of B cells, *J. Immunol.* **114**:55–58.

Hardy, M. A., Quint, J., Goldstein, A. L., State, D., and White, A., 1968, Effect of thymosin and anti-thymosin serum on allograft survival in mice, *Proc. Nat. Acad. Sci. U.S.* **61**:875–882-

Hardy, M. A., Zizblatt, M., Levine, N., Goldstein, A. L., Lilly, F., and White, A., 1971, Reversal by thymosin of increased susceptibility of immunosuppressed mice to Maloney sarcoma virus, *Transplant. Proc.* **3**:926–928.

Harrison, D. E., and Doubleday, J. W., 1975, Normal function of immunologic stem cells from aged mice, *J. Immunol.* **114**:1314–1317.

Heidrick, M. L., and Makinodan, T., 1972, Nature of cellular deficiencies in age-related decline of the immune system, *Gerontologia* **18**:305–320.

Hildemann, W. H., 1957, Scale homotransplantation in goldfish *(Carassius auratus), Ann. N. Y. Acad. Sci.* **64**:775–780.

Hirokawa, K., 1975, Thymus and aging, 10th Internatl. Congr. Gerontol., Jerusalem, Israel (June 22–27), in: *Congress Abstracts* **1**:79–80.

Hirokawa, K., and Makinodan, T., 1975, Thymic involution: effect of T cell differentiation, *J. Immunol.* **114**:1659–1664.

Hooper, J. A., McDaniel, M. C., Thurman, G. B., Cohen, G. H., Schulof, R. S., and Goldstein, A. L., 1975, The purification and properties of bovine thymosin, *Ann. N. Y. Acad. Sci.* **249**:125–144.

Hori, Y., Perkins, E. H., and Halsall, M. K., 1973, Decline in phyto-hemagglutinin responsiveness of spleen cells from aging mice, *Proc. Soc. Exp. Biol. Med.* **144**:48–53.

Hung, C., Perkins, E. H., Yang, W., 1975, Age-related refractoriness of PHA-induced lymphocyte transformation. II. ^{125}I-PHA binding to spleen cells from young and old mice, *Mech. Ageing Dev.* **4**:103–112.

Ishizuka, M., Gatni, M., and Braun, W., 1970, Cyclic AMP effects on antibody synthesis and their similarities to hormone-mediated events, *Proc. Soc. Exp. Biol. Med.* **134**:963–967.

Ishizuka, M., Braun, W., and Matsumoto, T., 1971, Cyclic AMP and immune responses. I. Influence of poly A:U and cAMP on antibody formation *in vitro, J. Immunol.* **107**:1027–1035.

Jaroslow, B. N., and Ortiz-Ortiz, L., 1972, Influence of poly A-polyU on early events in the immune response *in vitro, Cell. Immunol.* **3**:123–132.

Jose, D. G., and Good, R. A., 1973, Quantitative effects of nutritional essential amino acid deficiency upon immune responses to tumors in mice, *J. Exp. Med.* **137**:1–9.

Kalden, J. R., Williamson, W. C., and Irvine, W. J., 1973, Experimental myasthenia gravis, myositis and myocarditis in guinea pigs immunized with subcellular fractions of calf thymus or calf skeletal muscle in Freund's complete adjuvant, *Clin. Exp. Immunol.* **13**:79–88.

Kolata, G. B., 1974, Autoimmune diseases in animals: useful models for immunology, *Science* **184**:1360.

Komuro, K., and Boyse, E. A., 1973, Induction of T lymphocytes from precursor cells *in vitro* by a product of the thymus, *J. Exp. Med.* **138**:479–482.

Kook, A. I., and Trainin, N., 1974, Hormone-like activity of a thymus humoral factor on the induction of immune competence in lymphoid cells, *J. Exp. Med.* **139**:193–207.

Kook, A. I., and Trainin, N., 1975, Intracellular events involved in the induction of immune competence in lymphoid cells by a thymus humoral factor, *J. Immunol.* **114**:151–157.

Law, L., Goldstein, A. L., and White, A., 1968, Influence of thymosin on immunological competence of lymphoid cells from thymectomized mice, *Nature* **219**:1391–1392.

Liu, R. K., 1974, Hypothermic effects of marihuana, marihuana derivatives and chlorpromazine in laboratory mice, *Res. Comm. in Chemical Path. and Pharmacol.* **9**:215–228.

Liu, R. K., and Walford, R. L., 1972, The effect of lowered body temperature on lifespan and immune and non-immune processes, *Gerontologia* **18**:363–388.

Liu, R. K., and Walford, R. L., 1975, Mid-life temperature-transfer effects on lifespan of annual fish, *J. Gerontol.* **30**:129–131.

MacKay, I. R., 1972, Ageing and immunological function in man, *Gerontologia* **18**:239–245.

McCay, C. M., Crowell, M. F., and Maynard, L. A., 1935, The effect of retarded growth upon the length of life span and upon the ultimate body size, *J. Nutrition* **10**:63–79.

McFarlane, H., and Hamid, J., 1973, Cell mediated immune response in malnutrition, *Clin. Exp. Immunol.* **1**:153–164.

Mandi, B., and Glant, T., 1973, Thymosin-producing cells of the thymus, *Nature New Biol.* **246**:25.

199

IMMUNO-
ENGINEERING:
PROSPECTS FOR
CORRECTION OF
AGE-RELATED
IMMUNODEFICIENCY
STATES

Mathies, M., Lipps, L., Smith, G. S., and Walford, R. L., 1973, Age-related decline in response to phytohemaglutinin and pokeweed mitogen by spleen cells from hamsters and long-lived mouse strains, *J. Gerontol.* **28**:425–430.

Mercer, W. D., Pachciarz, J. A., and Teague, P. O., 1976, Serum IgA levels and autoantibody formation in mice. *Proc. Soc. Exp. Biol. Med.* (in press).

Meredith, P., Tittor, W., Gerbase-DeLima, M., and Walford, R. L., 1975a, Age-related changes in the cellular immune response of lymph node and thymus cells in long-lived mice, *Cellular Immunol.* **18**:324–330.

Meredith, P., Gerbase-DeLima, M., and Walford, R. L., 1975b, Age-related changes in the PHA:Con A stimulatory ratios of cells from spleens of a long-lived mouse strain, *Exp. Gerontol.* **10**:247–250.

Metcalf, D., Moulds, R., and Pike, B., 1966, Influence of the spleen and thymus on immune responses in ageing mice, *Clin. Exp. Immunol.* **2**:109–120.

Micklem, H. S., and Asfi, C., 1971, Cells carrying receptors for "self" constituents: their possible significance in the evolution of the vertebrate immune system, *Arch. Zool. exp. gen.* **112**:105–111.

Micklem, H. S., Ogden, D. A., and Payne, A. C., 1973, Ageing, haemopoietic stem cells and immunity, in: *Haemopoietic Stem Cells* (Ciba Found. Symp.), pp. 285–297, Elsevier/North Holland.

Miller, R. G., and Phillips, R. A., 1975, Development of B lymphocytes, *Fed. Proc.* **34**:145–150.

Morton, J. I., and Siegel, B. V., 1968, Relation between immunodepression and autoimmune disease in NZB mice, *J. Reticuloendothel. Soc.* **5**:567.

Nordin, A. A., and Loughman, B. W., 1972, Cellular deficiencies resulting in reduced immunological responsiveness, *The Gerontologist* **12**:30.

Orgad, S., and Cohen, I. R., 1974, Autoimmune encephalomyelitis: activation of thymus lymphocytes against syngeneic brain antigens *in vitro, Science* **183**:1083–1085.

Pachciarz, J. A., and Teague, P. O., 1976a, Age-associated involution of cellular immune function I. Accelerated decline of mitogen reactivity in spleen cells in adult thymectomized mice, *J. Immunol.* **116**:982–988.

Pachciarz, J. A., and Teague, P. O., 1976b, Age-associated involution of cellular immune function II. Reconstitution of cellular immunity of young adult thymectomized and lethally irradiated mice by young and aged lymphoid tissue (unpublished).

Park, B. H., and Good, R. A., 1974, *Principles of Modern Immunobiology,* Lea and Febiger, Philadelphia.

Perkins, E. H., Makinodan, T., and Seibert, C., 1972, Model approach to immunologic rejuvenation of the aged, *Infection and Immunity* **6**:518–524.

Roberts, I. M., Whittingham, S., and MacKay, I. R., 1973, Tolerance to an autoantigen-thyroglobulin. Antigen-binding lymphocytes in thymus and blood in health and autoimmune disease, *Lancet* **2**:936–940.

Robey, W. G., 1975, Further characterization of an antibody-stimulatory factor isolated from bovine thymus, *Ann. N. Y. Acad. Sci.* **249**:211–219.

Robey, W. G., Campbell, B. J., and Luckey, T. D., 1972, Isolation and characterization of a thymic factor, *Infect. Immunol.* **6**:682–688.

Roder, J. C., Bell, D. A., and Singhal, S. K., 1975, T-cell activation and cellular cooperation in autoimmune NZB/NZW F_1 hybrid mice, *J. Immunol.* **115**:466–472.

Rosenberg, B., Kerney, G., Smith, L. G., Skurnick, I. D., and Barduski, M. J., 1973, The kinetics and thermodynamics of death in multicellular organisms, *Mech. Ageing and Develop.* **2**:275–293.

Ross, M. H., 1969, Aging, nutrition, and hepatic enzyme activity patterns in the rat, *J. Nutrition,* Suppl. 1, part 2, **97**:565–601.

Scheid, M. P., Hoffman, M. K., Komuro, K., Hammerling, U., Abbott, J., Boyse, E. A., Cohen, G. H., Hooper, J. A., Schulof, R. S., and Goldstein, A. L., 1973, Differentiation of T-cells induced by preparations from thymus and by non-thymic agents. The determined state of the precursor cell, *J. Exp. Med.* **138**:1027–1032.

Scheid, M.P., Goldstein, G., Hammerling, U., and Boyse, E. A., 1975, Lymphocyte differentiation from precursor cells *in vitro, Ann. N. Y. Acad. Sci.* **249**:531–540.

Segall, P. E., and Timiras, P. S., 1975, Age-related changes in thermoregulatory capacity of tryptophan-deficient rats, *Fed. Proc.* **38**:83–85.

Simic, M. M ., and Kanazir, D. T., 1968, Restoration of immunologic capacities in irradiated animals by nucleic acids and their derivatives, in: *Nucleic Acids in Immunology* (O. J. Plescia and W. Braun, eds), pp. 386–403, Springer-Verlag, New York.

ROY L. WALFORD,
PATRICIA J.
MEREDITH, AND KAY
E. CHENEY

Steinberg, A. D., Law, L. D., and Talal, N., 1970, The role of NZB/NZW F_1 thymus in experimental tolerance and auto-immunity, *Arthritis Rheum.* **13**:369–377.

Strausser, H. R., Bober, L. A., Bucsi, R. A., Shillock, J. A., and Goldstein, A. L., 1971, Stimulation of the hemagglutinin response of aged mice by cell-free lymphoid tissue fractions and bacterial endotoxin, *Exp. Gerontol.* **6**:373–378.

Strehler, B. L., 1975, Implications of aging research for society, *Fed. Proc.* **34**:5–8.

Stutman, O., Yunis, E. J., and Good, R. A., 1969, Carcinogen-induced tumors of the thymus. IV. Humoral influences of normal thymus and functional thymomas and influence of post thymectomy period on restoration. *J. Exp. Med.* **130**:809–819.

Talal, N., and Steinberg, A. D., 1974, The pathogenesis of autoimmunity in New Zealand black mice, in: *Current Topics in Microbiology and Immunology,* pp. 79–103, Springer-Verlag, New York.

Teague, P. O., 1974, Spontaneous autoimmunity and involution of the lymphoid system, *Fed. Proc.* **33**:2051–2052.

Teague, P. O., and Friou, G. J., 1965, Inhibition of autoimmunity in A/J mice by transfer of isogenic thymic or spleen cells from young animals, *Arthritis Rheum.* **8**:474.

Teague, P. O., and Friou, G. J., 1969, Antinuclear antibodies in mice. II. Transformation with spleen cells; inhibition or prevention with thymus or spleen cells, *Immunology* **17**:665–675.

Teague, P. O., Friou, G. J., Yunis, E. J., and Good, R. A., 1972, Spontaneous autoimmunity in aging mice, in: *Tolerance, Autoimmunity, and Aging,* pp. 33–61, Charles C Thomas Co., Illinois.

Thomas, E. D., Storb, R., Clift, R. A., Fefer, A., Johnson, F. L., Neiman, P. E., Lerner, K. G., Glucksberg, H., and Buckner, C. D., 1975, Bone marrow transplantation, *New Eng. J. Med.* **292**:832–843 and 895–902.

Thurman, G. B., and Goldstein, A. L., 1975, Thymosin induced amplification of T-cell responses in mice, *Fed. Proc.* **34**:4479.

Timiras, P. S., 1975, Neurophysiological factors in aging: recent advances, 10th Internat. Congr. Gerontol., Jerusalem, Israel (June 22–27), Symp. on Manual Regulatory Mechanisms, in *Congress Abstracts* **1**:50–52.

Touraine, J. L., Touraine, F., Dietruge, J., Gilly, J., Colon, S., and Gilly, R., 1975a, Immunodeficiency diseases I. T-lymphocyte differentiation in partial Di George syndrome, *Clin. Exp. Immunol.* **21**:39–46.

Touraine, J. L., Touraine, F., Incify, G. S., and Good, R. A., 1975b, Effect of thymic factors on the differentiation of human marrow cells into T-lymphocytes *in vitro* in normals and patients with immunodeficiencies, *Ann. N. Y. Acad. Sci.* **249**:335–342.

Trainin, N., and Small, M., 1970, Studies on some physicochemical properties of a thymus humoral factor conferring immunocompetence on lymphoid cells, *J. Exp. Med.* **132**:885–897.

Trainin, N., Bejerano, A., Strahilevitch, M., Goldring, D., and Small, M., 1966, A thymic factor preventing wasting and influencing lymphopoiesis in mice, *Israel J. Med. Sci.* **2**:549–559.

Trainin, N., Levo, Y., and Rotter, V., 1974, Resistance to hydrocortisone conferred upon thymocytes by a thymic humoral factor, *Eur. J. Immunol.* **4**:634–637.

Trump, G. N., and Hildemann, W. H., 1970, Antibody responses of goldfish to bovine serum albumin. Primary and secondary responses, *Immunology* **19**:621–626.

Umiel, T., and Trainin, N., 1975, Increased reactivity of responding cells in the mixed lymphocyte reaction by a thymic humoral factor, *Eur. J. Immunol.* **5**:85–88.

Walford, R. L., 1962, Auto-immunity and aging, *J. Gerontol.* **17**:281–285.

Walford, R. L., 1967, The role of autoimmune phenomena in the aging process, in: *Aspects of the Biology of Ageing,* 21st Symp. Soc. Exper. Biol. (H. W. Woodhouse, ed.), pp. 351–372, Cambridge Univ. Press.

Walford, R. L., 1969, *The Immunologic Theory of Aging,* Munksgaard, Copenhagen.

Walford, R. L., 1974, The immunologic theory of aging, current status, *Fed. Proc.* **33**:2020–2027.

Walford, R. L., and Liu, R. K., 1965, Husbandry, life span, and growth rate of the annual fish *Cynolebias Adloffi, Exp. Gerontol.* **1**:161–171.

Walford, R. L., Liu, R. K., Gerbase-DeLima, M., Mathies, M., and Smith, G. S., 1974, Longterm dietary restriction and immune function in mice; response to sheep red blood cells and to mitogenic agents, *Mech. Ageing and Develop.* **2**:447–454.

Walford, R. L., Gerbase-DeLima, M., Liu, R. K., and Smith, G. S., 1975, Immunologic engineering, 10th Internat. Congr. Gerontol., Jerusalem, Israel, (June 22–27), in: *Congress Abstracts* **2**:39 (103).

Winchurch, R., Ishizuka, M., Webb, D., and Braun, W., 1971, Adenyl cyclase activity of spleen cells exposed to immunoenhancing synthetic oligo- and polynucleotides, *J. Immunol.* **106**:1399–1400.

Wara, D. W., and Ammann, A. J., 1975a, Activation of T-cell rosettes in immunodeficiency patients by thymosin, *Ann. N. Y. Acad. Sci.* **249**:308–315.

Wara, D. W., Goldstein, A. L., Doyle, N. E., and Ammann, A. J., 1975b, Thymosin activity in patients with cellular immunodeficiency, *New Eng. J. Med.* **292**:70–74.

Yamamoto, I., and Webb, D. R., 1975, Antigen-stimulated changes in cylcic nucleotide levels in the mouse, *Proc. Nat. Acad. Sci. U.S.* **72**:2320–2324.

Yunis, E. J., and Greenberg, L. J., 1974, Immunopathology of aging, *Fed. Proc.* **33**:2017–2019.

Yunis, E. J., Fernandes, G., and Stutman, O., 1971, Susceptibility to involution of the thymus-dependent lymphoid system and autoimmunity, *Am. J. Clin. Path.* **56**:280–292.

Yunis, E. J. Fernandes, G., Smith, J., Stutman, O., and Good, R. A., 1972, Involution of the thymus-dependent lymphoid system, in: *Microenvironmental Aspects of Immunity,* pp. 301–306, Plenum Press, New York.

Yunis, E. J., Fernandes, G., and Greenberg, W. J., 1973, Immune deficiency, autoimmunity and aging, in: *2nd Internat. Workshop on the Primary Immunodeficiency Diseases in Man* (Feb. 4–8), Nat. Sci. Found.

Yunis, E. J., Fernandes, G., Nelson, W., and Halberg, F., 1974, Circadian temperature rhythms and aging in rodents, Proc. Soc. Internat. Study of Biol. Rhythm, in: *Chronobiology* (L. E. Scheving, F. Halberg, and J. E. Pauley, eds.), pp. 358–363, Igaku Shoin Ltd, Tokyo.

Zizblatt, M., Goldstein, A. L., Lilly, F., and White, A., 1970, Acceleration by thymosin of the development of resistance to murine sarcoma versus induced tumor in mice, *Proc. Nat. Acad. Sci. U.S.* **66**:1170–1174.

201

IMMUNO-
ENGINEERING:
PROSPECTS FOR
CORRECTION OF
AGE-RELATED
IMMUNODEFICIENCY
STATES

Abbreviations

A—Amboceptor (Forssman antibody)
Ab—antibody
Ag—antigen
AFC—antibody-forming cell
AFCP—antibody-forming cell precursor
ATC—activated thymus cells

B cells—bone-marrow-derived cells
BSA—bovine serum albumin

C_{na}, C_{nb}, C_{nc}, C_{nd}—fragments of complement
    components produced by enzymatic
    cleavage mostly during the activation
    process
C—complement
C1 . . . C9—complement components
$\overline{C1}$, etc.—the overbar indicates an activated
    component that has acquired enzymatic or
    other biological activity
Con A—concanavalin A

DMBA—dimethylbenzanthracene
DNCB—dinitrochlorobenzene
DNP—2,4-dinitrophenol
DNP-6L—2,4-dinitrophenyl conjugated with L-
    glutamic acid and L-lysine copolymer
DPFC—direct plaque forming cells
DTH—delayed thymus hypersensitivity

E—erythrocytes (sheep red blood cells)
EA—sensitized erythrocytes
EDTA—ethylenediaminetetraacetate

Fab—fraction ab of the immunoglobulin
    molecule

Fc—fraction c of the immunoglobulin molecule
FLV—Friend leukemia virus

GH—growth hormone
GVH—graft versus host

I—the immune region of the major
    histocompatibility complex
Ia—immune region associated
IBS—immunologic burst size
Ig—immunoglobulin
IgA—immunoglobulin A
IgG—immunoglobulin G
IgM—immunoglobulin M
IgT—immunglobulin on T cells
IO—immunocompetent precursor
IR—immune response

LPS—lipopolysaccharides
Ly—designation of a T cell subset

MCA—methylcholanthrene
MHC—Major histocompatibility complex
MLC—mixed lymphocyte culture

NIP 4—hydroxy-3-iodo-5-nitrophyenylacetic
    acid

OVA—ovalbumin

PHA—phytohemagglutinin
PFC—plaque forming cells
PTU—propylthiouracil

RBC—red blood cells
RFC—rosette-forming cells
RS—Reed–Sternberg cells

S–Con A—succinyl–concanavalin A

SRBC—sheep red blood cells

T cells—thymus-derived cells

TL—thymus lymphocyte antigen

TL−—thymus lymphocyte antigen (negative)

TL+—thymus lymphocyte antigen (positive)

TXB—thymectomized, irradiated, and bone marrow reconstituted

TXB-NT—TXB mouse with new born thymus graft

TXB-3T—TXB mouse with three-month-old thymus graft

TXB-33T—TXB mouse with 33-month-old thymus graft

Index

M